Sexual Chemistry

Sexual Chemistry

A History of the Contraceptive Pill

Lara V. Marks

Yale University Press
New Haven and London

For information about this and other Yale University Press publications, please contact:
U.S. Office: sales.press@yale.edu   www.yale.edu/yup
Europe Office: sales@yaleup.co.uk   www.yaleup.co.uk

Set in FFScala by Northern Phototypesetting Co. Ltd, Bolton, Lancs.
Printed in Great Britain by Biddles Ltd, Guildford and King's Lynn

Library of Congress Cataloging-in-Publication Data

Marks, Lara, 1963–
    Sexual chemistry : a history of the contraceptive pill / Lara V. Marks.
       p. cm.
    Includes bibliographical references and index.
    ISBN 0-300-08943-0 (cloth: alk. paper)
       1. Oral contraceptives—History. 2. Oral contraceptives—Social aspects—History.
RG137.5 M327 2001
    613.9'432—dc21   2001017784

A catalogue record for this book is available from the British Library.

10 9 8 7 6 5 4 3 2 1

Contents

Illustrations, Figures, Tables

Illustrations

Figures

Tables

Acknowledgements

This book is dedicated to my son Daniel, who has a very special place in it. His planned but slightly early conception delayed its completion; his smiles and continual babbling have not only enriched my life and taught me the joys of motherhood, but also widened my understanding of the pill and the importance of contraception.

When I first started my research for this book, my cousin, Ori Winokur, who was about thirteen at the time, was curious to know why on earth I had chosen such a topic. He could not understand why a pill that 'was so small' had any importance at all, or how could it take years of research. I do not know if since that time he has changed his mind about the contraceptive pill, but I do hope that this book goes some way to answering his question. I am greatly indebted to Cathy Crawford who gave me the idea of working on the history of the pill.

Since beginning my research I have found myself having many different kinds of conversations about the pill and have incurred many debts in its completion. First I would like to thank all the archivists and librarians who have helped me in the research, including those who work at the following places: Archives and Manuscripts, Wellcome Library for the History and Understanding of Medicine; Francis Countway Library; Family Planning Association library; International Planned Parenthood Federation library; Library of Congress; Rockefeller Archive; Sophia Smith Collection at Smith College; Ford Foundation Archive; Public Records Office; Royal College of Obstetricians and Gynaecologists; Schlesinger Library; the pharmaceutical company G. D. Searle, based in High Wycombe in England; Worcester Foundation for Experimental Biology; the Smithsonian Collection; and the US Food and Drug Administration.

Special thanks also go to Lesley Hall and Julia Shepard who alerted me to the rich British archival material on the subject held in the Wellcome Library. I am also grateful to Lesley for having read and commented extensively on the book in manuscript form. Much gratitude also goes to Patricia Gossell who was not only generous in hospitality but found financial support to allow me to examine the material at the Smithsonian Institute and inspired me to think about the packaging of the pill; and to Suzanne White Junod at the History Office at the Food and Drug Administration for her warm hospitality and immense help in finding the relevant files on the first oral contraceptives. I am also grateful to Suzanne for reading numerous drafts of chapters and challenging my thinking on the subject, as well as for providing extra finance to support my research in Washington.

I would also like to thank the following people for having shared their personal papers with me and recalling their personal experiences of the pill: Ridgeley C. Bennett, Philip Corfman, William Inman, Stephen Lock, Klim McPherson, Barbara Seaman, Susan Szasz, Margaret Thorogood, Geoffrey Venning, Martin Vessey and Victor Wynn. In addition I would like to thank the clinicians who helped me in the preparation of the book, particularly Michael Gillmer, Valerie Beral and Colin Duncan. Thanks also go to Walli Bounds for helping me to find women who originally participated in clinical trials of the pill in Britain. I am also grateful to the numerous women who responded to my letter in the *Daily Mail*. The book is much richer for the generous time and recollections they gave me. In many ways it could not have been completed without them.

Many thanks also go to the Wellcome Trust for an Award Fellowship which supported much of the research undertaken for the project. I am also indebted to the sponsorship of the Rockefeller Archive, the Smithsonian Institute and the Food and Drug Administration, which aided my research in the United States. Thanks also go to *Social Science and Medicine* which first published much of the material in chapter 6.

During the course of the research I have also greatly benefited from the knowledge and ideas of many colleagues, including those who commented on various papers I presented at seminars and conferences. Special thanks go to the staff at the London School of Hygiene and Tropical Medicine where I began the project, particularly Virginia Berridge and Jenny Stanton. I am also grateful to my former colleagues in the Centre for the History of Science, Technology and Medicine, including Elsbeth Heaman, Robert Iliffe, and Andrew Warwick, and countless colleagues in the Medical School at Imperial College who listened to my ideas about the book. In addition I would like to thank Rima Apple, Jordan Goodman, Irvine Loudon, Hilary Marland, Majorie Melluish, Marilyn Plant, Anne-Marie Rafferty and Anne Summers, all of whom provided much intellectual f̶... ̶...̶...̶ ̶...̶...̶... drafts of the manuscript. Thanks also go ... Vayena, whose interest ... ... ͏ͦm I also owe a great de̶... ... gness to listen to my idea̶ ... ... ͏g the book. I am also ver̶... ... ̶ript from start to finish. S ... and constructive criticis͏n ... University Press during ...

I als̶... ... ͏ndy Neil, Helen Wickha... ... vide me with vital informa̶... ... I could not otherwise ha... ... ̶d Sylvia Frenk for their de...

This ... e generous hospitality o̶ḻ ̶c̶o̶u̶n̶t̶l̶e̶s̶s̶ ̶p̶e̶o̶p̶l̶e̶.̶... ... ̶c̶ially like to thank Ed and Claire Manwell in Northampton, Massachusetts; Annette Schulz in Mexico City; Felicia Shapiro in New York; Richard Shapiro in Boston; and Corky and Ralph Bryant in Washington DC. I am also grateful to Laura Bryant, whose friendship and laughter during my stay in Washington enlivened my research.

Very special thank yous also go to my parents, Shula and Yitz, as well as to my brother, Rafi; their constant support has been invaluable in helping me complete the project.

Lastly, but definitely not least, my thanks go to Emmett. His continual companionship and intellectual challenges opened up new dimensions in my research, while his electronic skills assisted in the drawing of the graphs for the book. His love and continual generosity have been an inspiration throughout.

Introduction:
'A Whole New Bag of Beans'

The contraceptive pill of today is not the same as it was yesterday, neither will it be the same in the future. Today the pill comes in all sorts of colours, including white, yellow, pink, peach, mauve, strawberry-rose, red and blue. Round or pentagonal in shape, these pills are attractively packaged in foil blister packs with arrows and instructions elaborately designed to aid the memory of those taking the contraceptive, and to warn them of its possible hazards. Such pills could not be more of a contrast to the first oral contraceptive marketed in 1960, which came as a little tablet issued in a drab little brown glass bottle with minimal labelling and few directions or warnings.

Such changes in the appearance and the packaging of the pill between 1960 and today represent the shifting nature of the contraceptive over time. Heralded as the catalyst of the sexual revolution, the contraceptive pill is often regarded as one of the most important landmarks in the twentieth century. The pill, just a quarter of an inch in diameter, was once optimistically hailed as a scientific cure for the world's rising population and its consequent social and political ills. As *Sexual Chemistry* shows in chapters 9 and 10, however, the pill did not prove itself to be the social panacea envisaged by its inventors. The Pope has never sanctioned its use, and countries such as India and Japan have, for both political and cultural reasons, largely rejected it. Remaining far too expensive a regime for most women in poor countries, the pill has also proved far from satisfactory in the campaign to control the world's growing population. Even in industrialized countries, where the pill rapidly became incorporated into many women's daily routines by the early 1960s, it fell from popularity in the late 1960s, when its links with cardiovascular disease began to be publicized.

Nonetheless, the pill remains one of several revolutionary new drugs introduced in the 1960s (including Librium and thalidomide) which reshaped pharmacology, altered social perceptions of medication, and changed the regulatory process for new drugs during the second half of the twentieth century. Although not identified as such at the time it was created, the pill can truly be called the first 'designer' or 'lifestyle' drug of the twentieth century. As with many drug 'firsts', there are many lessons to be learned from its development and use.

Challenging previous histories, which have championed the pill as a North American product that fuelled the sexual revolution, this book suggests that its roots and the effects of its adoption were much more diverse and can only be understood within a wider international framework. As chapters 2 and 3 suggest, much of its chemical evolution lies in the rise of the lucrative sex hormone industry in Europe during the early twentieth century, and the migration of refugee scientists to the American continent in the wake of fascism and the Second World War. Born out of the race to find easier and cheaper methods of making sex hormones, and the discovery of the anti-arthritic drug cortisone in 1949, the pill emerged from the research of an ingenious yet fickle chemist called Russell Marker (1902–95) on the *Dioscorea* plant, a wild yam vine which clings to the trees in the mountains of southern Mexico. As chapter 4 shows the initial clinical testing took place in Japan, Israel, Puerto Rico, Haiti, Mexico, Hong Kong and Britain, as well as a number of states in the United States (Massachusetts, New York, Kentucky, Texas and California). Within ten years of its first marketing in the United States in 1960, at least a dozen major inter-national pharmaceutical companies in France, Germany, Hungary, the Netherlands, Switzerland and the United States, with manufacturing facilities around the world, were producing, packaging and distributing different formulations of oral contraceptives. While the raw material for these pills was mostly derived from the yam plant in Mexico, much of the production of the contraceptive took place at the location of the major companies as well as in Italy, Puerto Rico and the Bahamas.[1]

Not only was the development and production of the pill international, so was its distribution. Initially most popular in English-speaking countries – the United States, then Britain, New Zealand, Canada and Australia – by the late 1960s the pill had become even more popular in northern Europe, particularly Belgium, Germany, the Netherlands and Scandinavia. During the 1970s pill consumption spread to the developing world, partly encouraged by international subsidization of family planning after 1968. In Latin America, for instance, oral contraceptives became increasingly popular in Brazil, Venezuela and Argentina from the late 1970s.[2]

From the time of its first clinical trials to the present, nearly 200 million women have swallowed the contraceptive pill. By the end of the twentieth century the contraceptive had become a feature of everyday life, with over 70 million women reaching for their pill packet on a daily basis around the globe.[3] Within six years of its first appearance in the United States, the oral contraceptive had become one of the leading pharmaceutical products sold around the world. In some places the numbers of oral contraceptive pills sold had even begun to exceed any other single pharmaceutical product of an ethical nature, and in some cases was outselling many proprietary items such as aspirin. Many contemporaries felt that the pharmaceutical community had never before seen a product that sold so widely and had such a wide impact.[4]

Although the pill is commonly cited as one of the factors that caused the sexual revolution of the 1960s, surprisingly few scholars have examined in detail its impact on sexual behaviour since its first appearance. Challenging the assumption of the association between the pill and the sexual revolution, I indicate in this book that the drug nonetheless had a profound influence on attitudes towards sex and contraception. The novelty of the pill was the fact that, unlike all previous forms of contraception, it could be taken by mouth and did not require use at the moment of intercourse. Effectively separating contraception from the sexual act, the oral contraceptive was also original in that women could use it discreetly without any knowledge on the part of their male partners. As chapter 8 shows, this had major implications for the ways in which men and women began to view the interaction between contraception and the spontaneity of the sexual act. It also influenced attitudes relating to whether it should be women or men who shouldered the responsibility for contraception. Among the issues considered is also the degree to which the pill freed women from the age-old fear of pregnancy and transformed their ideas about reproduction and health. Promoted as almost 100 per cent effective, the pill altered people's expectations about contraception and what it could achieve. Making older and less effective forms of contraception seem less desirable and less effective, the pill has essentially raised the standards by which all contraceptives are judged today. Even now, with the emergence of the HIV and AIDS epidemic across the world, the pill continues to influence people's perceptions of what forms of contraception are acceptable.

The pill has not only had a major impact on attitudes towards sex and contraception, but, as chapters 5, 6 and 7 suggest, it has been the lynchpin in many heated discussions about the role of the medical profession in contraception and the overall safety and efficacy of drugs. Pharmacologically, the pill is unique. Most drugs are intended for the treatment of organic diseases. By contrast the pill is aimed at preventing pregnancy, a condition not usually considered an illness. The fact that it is a contraceptive designed to be consumed by healthy women of reproductive age for long periods of time has magnified concerns about its potential dangers. As was pointed out by Dr Pasquale DeFelice, who was largely responsible for the final approval of the first oral contraceptive, 'When a new drug application came in for the birth control pills, it was – needless to say – revolutionary for that indication! It was a whole new bag of beans.'[5]

Much of the history of the pill written since the late 1960s has promoted the idea that its early review by the American regulatory authority, the Food and Drug Administration, was so inadequate that a dangerous drug was allowed on to the market. Some critics have gone further, claiming that women were used as guinea pigs in a massive international experiment.[6] Written after the cardiovascular risks of the pill were announced, such histories forget the historical context in which the pill was developed and tested. Most importantly they fail to take into account the fact that it was reviewed and marketed before 1962, when the worldwide epidemic of birth deformities associated with the drug thalidomide prompted stronger laws governing the regulation and marketing of new drugs in Britain, the United States, and most of Europe. In chapter 4, I explore the degree to which the testing of the pill conformed to the standards of pharmaceutical testing at the time. It shows that while some of the procedures used during the pill trials might not stand up to the ethical requirements of today, they more than adequately matched those for many drugs tested at the same time. Moreover, many of the complications later associated with the pill would have been difficult to determine before it was consumed on a large scale.

Lingering suspicions about the pill's safety have made it one of the most heavily scrutinized drugs in the world. As chapters 6 and 7 reveal, the contraceptive has continuously pushed at the limits of drug monitoring and regulatory frameworks. Serious concerns about the implications of long-term use by healthy women, for instance, have led to the implementation of new and innovative medical approaches to tracking patients for long periods of time, and to detecting and reporting serious adverse reactions. Resulting in some of the biggest medical investigations in history, the oral contraceptive required international collaboration on a large scale. Opening up new avenues for epidemiological research and possibilities of funding, this work has not always been harmonious. This can be seen most clearly in the case of the studies into the associations between the pill and cancer, where tensions not only surfaced because of the popularity of the contraceptive and the large number of women's lives that were at stake, but also because of the threat to the status and egos of individual health professionals.

While medical scientists were battling over which were the most appropriate and accurate methods to use, questions about the safety of the drug and how it should be handled were also being shaped by larger political, economic and social issues confronting national governments. Some of the most striking differences in policy can be seen within the context of the United States and Britain in relation to the risk of blood clots. In 1969, in the wake of the news that high doses of oestrogen caused this problem, the British government, at a time when it was facing serious unpopularity, decided to limit the pills prescribed to those with the lowest dose of oestrogen. By contrast, the American government decided to insert warnings inside the pill's packaging to alert women of the drug's side-effects and dangers. Arising partly in response to strong pressure from women's groups and a vigorous debate over the adequacy of drug information provided to patients, such warnings were to become a standard component in nearly all consumer packaging of drugs.

Despite the detection of side-effects and long-term adverse reactions and its fall in popularity as a contraceptive, the medical uses to which the pill has been put have increased over time. From the start the pill was promoted as more than just a contraceptive. When first introduced into Britain and the United States in 1957, for instance, it was marketed not as a contraceptive but as a medication for the treatment of gynaecological and menstrual disorders, as well as infertility. Much of this marketing was part of a carefully orchestrated strategy to test the market for the acceptability of oral contraceptives at a time when the issue of contraception was considered highly sensitive. While it was not advertised directly as a contraceptive, warnings were given to doctors that the drug could prevent ovulation. In some senses this acted as a 'free ad' for people to take it as a contraceptive. By 1959 over 500,000 American women were taking the pill for menstrual disorders, a problem which had never surfaced on such a large scale before.[7]

In later years, once contraception had become an openly discussed feature of everyday life, new opportunities began to be sought for the expansion of the market for the drug. During the 1970s the announcement that the pill could have a protective effect against ovarian and endometrial cancer allowed it to be turned into a major public health tool in the fight against cancer.

With the decline in the popularity of the pill and the increasing saturation of the contraceptive market since the 1960s, the new conditions for which the drug has been advanced have provided an ideal means of expanding its market. Johnson and Johnson, for instance, have witnessed a tripling of sales of their oral contraceptive Ortho Tri-Cyclen since it was officially approved as an effective treatment against acne. Prescriptions for the drug in the United States increased from 330,000 per month in January 1997 to 1.2 million by January 1999. Moreover, once it began to be used for this purpose, it leapt from being the fourth most popular oral contraceptive to being the first. This contrasts with the other three leading brands of oral contraceptives, whose market shares remained the same during this period.[8]

The sales of Ortho Tri-Cyclen have partly been boosted by the way it was widely advertised in leading US women's magazines with photographs of gorgeous models and the caption 'beauty aid for women 15 and over'.[9] Such advertising, permitted in the United States only after 1997, is particularly striking when we consider the fact that when the first oral contraceptive went on the market it could not be advertised directly to the consumer. Like all pharmaceutical drugs in the 1960s, the pill could legally only be advertised through medical journals and direct mailings to physicians.

The pill, however, was unlike any other drug at the time in that patients were aware of its existence long before it had been approved as a contraceptive. Many had been alerted to it by numerous articles on early experiments and its potential to curb the threat of world population growth that began to appear in local and national newspapers as well as women's magazines in Britain, the United States and elsewhere from the mid-1950s. Some of these articles were deliberately planted to test the climate of public opinion towards an oral contraceptive.[10]

As early as 1957, Gregory Pincus (1903–67), a key figure in the early development and testing of the pill, began to receive floods of letters from people desperate to know how to obtain the drug. The excerpts from the following letter show both the effectiveness of such publicity and the eagerness with which its appearance was greeted:

> I am about 30 years old have 6 children, oldest little over 7, youngest a few days. My health dont seem to make it possible to go on this way. We have tried to be careful and tried this and that, but I get pregnant anyway. When I read this article [in *Science Digest* (Sept. 1957)] I couldn't help but cry, for I thought there is my ray of hope.[11]

Another correspondent wrote in 1960, 'Like thousands of others my wife and I bought a recent issue of *Coronet* because of the blurb on the cover concerning birth control pills.'[12] Some went so far as to offer themselves as volunteers for the clinical trials. As one 36-year-old woman wrote to Pincus in 1957:

> I read of your experiments which have resulted in a pill that will induce sterility ... If it is at all possible, I would like to secure some pills, whatever the cost. I would also be more than glad to offer myself as a subject if you are still conducting experiments.[13]

G. D. Searle, the first pharmaceutical company to market the pill, itself recognized that such publicity was the 'main and major source of increased and continued acceptance of the drug'.[14]

The fact that patients began to ask for the pill from their doctors was highly unusual in the early 1960s. Prior to the appearance of oral contraceptives most patients were dependent on the doctor for diagnosis of their problem and the drug that they were to use. Now women were beginning to determine not only what their medical problem was (avoidance of pregnancy) but also the kind of medication they should be prescribed. Moreover, it radically altered the ways in which many women began to obtain contraceptives. Before the pill most women had been reluctant to seek contraceptive help from their physicians, preferring instead to use non-medical techniques. The necessity of a prescription for the oral contraceptive, however, meant that now women increasingly had to confront their doctors directly for contraception.[15]

The increase in the demand for the pill had major implications for the attitudes of the medical profession to contraception more generally. Focusing on Britain and the United States, chapter 5 shows that the response of the medical profession varied between places and was shaped by social and medical attitudes towards women's health that predated the pill. The oral contraceptive, because it was a prescription drug, was unlike the contraceptives medical practitioners had previously encountered. Prior to the pill the main contraceptive issued by doctors had been the diaphragm, but many had disliked distributing the device because it required careful fitting and this was widely regarded as falling outside the medical remit. The pill, however, was very different. Not only did it require medical prescription, but the fact that it interacted with the physiology of the body and that it needed to be taken by healthy women over long periods of time also meant that it necessitated greater medical supervision.

In addition to turning contraception into a legitimate medical activity, the drug promoted a new form of preventive medicine. Requiring regular medical check-ups, such as breast examinations and cervical smears, the pill allowed medical practitioners more scrutiny of their female patients than ever before. This was particularly useful at a time of increasing emphasis on preventive medicine and the rise of cancer screening programmes.

While the medical profession was coming into increasing contact with women as a result of the pill, the type of woman taking the drug was also changing. As chapter 8 makes clear when the pill was first released in the United States and Britain it was directed towards the older married woman who already had children. Within a short time, however, the pill had become a contraceptive preferred by the young married woman with no children. For these women the drug allowed the means to plan their families while continuing their education and starting a career. From the early 1960s single women also began to join the ranks of those taking the pill, many of them gaining access either through their university health clinics or by feigning to be married. By the 1970s lack of marital status no longer posed an obstacle to access, and the consumer was becoming steadily younger. From the mid-1970s young teenage girls began to swallow the pill in increasing numbers. Such changes in the type of woman taking the pill reflected a more general trend in society whereby public debate about sex had become more open and there was greater access provided to birth control. To some extent it might be argued that the pill merely accelerated a trend begun long before its arrival.

As an innovation it is not surprising that the pill initially attracted women from the younger, better educated and wealthier sections of society. From the early 1970s, however, the socioeconomic profile changed, with less educated and poorer women making up an increasing proportion of those taking it. Part of this reflected easier access to the product as a result of growing governmental and charitable sponsorship of family planning services. It also highlighted the fact, however, that women from the higher socioeconomic and educated groups were the first to abandon the pill once its health hazards were publicized.

What is most striking about the history of the pill is the fact that such large proportions of women, particularly in developed countries, have taken it at some point in their lives. In 1985 a survey of sexually active British women aged 16 to 29 undertaken by the Royal College of General Practitioners, for example, indicated that only 5 per cent had never used the contraceptive.[16] Even in less developed parts of the world where the pill has been less popular, it has become a very familiar technique. Conversations from 1977 to 1983 between an anthropologist and the Zhutoasi, hunter-gatherer people residing in the Kalahari Desert of Botswana, revealed that word of the pill had reached even those living in one of the least industrial parts of the world.[17] An international survey in 1994 indicated that, apart from the condom, no other method was so widely available and used in so many countries around the globe.[18]

Despite its widespread diffusion, the response to the pill around the world has been complex and has changed over time. Women's decisions to take the pill have been greatly dependent on their age, class, marital status and the kinds of relationships they have with men, as well as on where they live. Their decisions have also been shaped by the types of contraceptive they used before the appearance of the pill, as well as by the changing knowledge about its safety and their own understanding of such complications. These factors have also had an important influence on men and the ways in which they have received the oral contraceptive. While some men initially saw it as a threat and resented the control it gave women over their fertility, others became enthusiastic about the freedom it gave them from the responsibility for contraception, and the spontaneity it allowed to intercourse.

The multiple responses to the oral contraceptive among women and men around the world highlight the complex social, political, economic and religious climates in which it was introduced and used. Today the words 'the pill' have become an everyday part of speech, often used in conjunction with a remarkable freedom to speak about sex and contraception.

This could not be more of a contrast with the situation when the pill first arrived, when contraception itself was considered a dirty word in most households around the globe. Indeed it was something that was usually only mentioned in a whisper. Pharmaceutical companies were themselves afraid of touching anything associated with it for fear of a backlash. During the 1950s contraceptive research and sales were still highly illegal in many parts of the world. In this book I examine how this attitude changed and the degree to which the pill, together with a rising concern about world population growth, contributed to an increasing frankness in talking about sexual matters and contraception.

One of the most dramatic episodes in the history of the oral contraceptive was the reaction of the Catholic community. For many within the Catholic establishment the appearance of the pill provoked one of the most bitter disputes they had encountered since the time of Galileo and his promotion of the idea that the earth revolved around the sun. Swallowed at a time separate from intercourse, the oral contraceptive was unlike any other artificial contraceptive the establishment had ever debated. Scientifically and socially it challenged many of the traditional theological teachings on marriage and the role of contraception. Arriving in a period when the church was undergoing a radical transformation and beginning to reach out to its lay members, the pill became a vital symbol in the fight for modernization.

Three Catholics were at the forefront of the development and approval of the pill. The first was the lapsed Catholic, Margaret Sanger (1879–1966), who had watched her pious and religious mother deteriorate and die prematurely after bearing 11 children. Best known for her tireless campaigns over half a century for legal access to contraception in the United States, it was she who prompted scientists to begin the research into a hormonal contraceptive pill. The second was the obstetrician and gynaecologist Dr John Rock (1890–1984), who conducted the first human trials on the drug; and the third was Dr Pasquale DeFelice, who reviewed and approved it for the American regulatory body, the Food and Drug Administration. Rock, with five children and 19 grandchildren, and DeFelice, with ten children, were both devout Catholics who were deeply steeped in Catholic philosophy.[19] Of these three, it was Rock who was seen as the greatest threat to the church and its teaching on contraception.

The interaction between Rock and the Catholic church is but one story among the many that can be told about the history of the oral contraceptive.

Many myths in fact surround the pill and its origins. One such legend is that three 'fathers' created it: Gregory Pincus (biologist), Carl Djerassi (chemist), and John Rock (obstetrician-gynaecologist).[20] In a recent paper Djerassi calls himself 'The mother of the pill'.[21] Such mythology partly stems from the fact that much of the early history of the oral contraceptive was written by the scientists and medical experts involved in its initial development, who had an interest in promoting themselves as its inventors.[22] Scientists have not been the only ones to eulogize their efforts, however. In 1965, for instance, Dr Anne Biezanek, an English Catholic convert who had seven children and was renowned for her public protest against the Catholic church and its stand on contraception, noted:

Of all the great works that men have undertaken for women, [the pill] must surely rank amongst the noblest. The work was instigated at a time when financial reward was very slight and the risks considerable. It was done in the teeth of social disapproval and in the teeth of great apathy on the part of the medical profession at large. The first men who devised those things at such risk to themselves must one day be named and honoured by all women as 'the instigators of the revolution'.[23]

Such enthusiasm for the work of these scientists began to fade after 1970, however, once the drug began to be associated with serious side-effects. In recent years much of the history of the pill tends to attack the original investigators for inadequately testing the product before releasing it on to the market. In this context the pill is seen as a product developed primarily by male scientists to control women, and women are frequently depicted as having been used as unwitting guinea pigs.[24] This criticism not only ignores the historical context in which the pill was developed,[25] but reinforces the idea that it arose out of the work of individual male scientists. Yet, as this book shows, the research on the pill was both initiated and funded by women.

Using an array of new primary sources and oral interviews with some of the key participants in the history of the pill, the following chapters show that the oral contraceptive cannot be seen as a pure triumph for science; neither should it be seen as solely the invention of male scientists. These perspectives miss the complex social context in which the pill was developed, as well as the extensive network of people and skills needed for its emergence, and the political climate in which it was first adopted. The making of the pill was dependent on the expertise and knowledge of a variety of people – men and women – from a multitude of disciplines and backgrounds. One of the most interesting features of these individuals was that many of them remained on the periphery of society and their work was often viewed with great suspicion, reflecting the sensitive nature of contraceptive research in the first half of the twentieth century.[26] Only once the pill had become an accepted part of life were they celebrated.

1
The Population Problem and the Pill

In 1950, five years after the Second World War, Margaret Sanger, leader of the American birth control movement and chief promoter of the development of the oral contraceptive, forecast 'that the world and almost all our civilization for the next twenty-five years is going to depend upon a simple, cheap, safe contraceptive to be used in poverty-stricken slums and jungles, and among the most ignorant people'.[1] Echoing this view four years later, the Catholic obstetrician-gynaecologist John Rock, who ran some of the early clinical trials of the first oral contraceptive, declared that such a pill would be the leading weapon against starvation and war: 'If it could be discovered soon, the H-bomb need never fall.' Rock saw such an oral contraceptive as providing the 'greatest aid ever discovered to the happiness and security of individual families – indeed of mankind'. According to Rock, 'the greatest menace to world peace and decent standards of life today is not atomic energy but sexual energy'.[2]

Spoken at a time when the Cold War (1945–91) was intensifying, both Sanger's and Rock's statements highlight the political and economic context in which the pill was initially developed. The years between 1948 and 1953 had been a time of particularly grave tensions between the United States and the Soviet Union. During this period not only had the Soviets attempted unsuccessfully to blockade the Western-held sectors of Berlin (1948–9), but the United States and its European allies had formed the North Atlantic Treaty Organization (NATO) in 1949, a military alliance designed to curb the Soviet presence in Europe. The Soviets had also managed to explode their first atomic bomb, ahead of the time predicted by the West and ending the American monopoly on this weapon. In addition,

Chinese communists had taken power in mainland China (1949) and the Soviet-supported communist government of North Korea had invaded American-supported South Korea (1950), launching a bitter war that was to continue until 1953. Elsewhere in Africa and Asia, pressures were also growing for independence from the imperial powers of Britain, France, the Netherlands and Belgium. Two of the most populous nations in the world, India and Indonesia, had achieved independence in 1947 and 1949 respectively, after long and bitter struggles. Moreover, it was unclear what political and economic direction these newly formed states would take, and many within the Western bloc feared they would adopt communism and become allies of the Soviet Union.

For those living through the 1950s the stability and future of the world therefore seemed far from secure. Not only were tensions increasing between the United States and the Soviet Union, anxieties were intensifying about the growth of population around the globe. At the heart of the concern was the noticeable increase of population in less developed parts of the world. Population growth in parts of Africa, Asia and Latin America, for instance, appeared not only to be accelerating far more rapidly than in many developed countries, but seemed far more rapid than that experienced in any part of the world prior to 1950.[3] Representing more people to feed, clothe, shelter and later to provide work for, the babies being born to the poorest and most impoverished women in the world appeared to many, such as Rock and Sanger, a potential threat to world stability. What they feared most were the pressures population growth would put on developing nations, providing ammunition for discontent and communism.[4]

Anxiety about excessive fertility was not confined to what was happening in the developing world. Much concern was also expressed about the high birth-rates among the indigent poor within developed countries, which it was feared could fuel economic dislocation and disorder closer to home. By contrast with the poor, the fertility of the upper and middle classes was not seen as a threat; rather it was to be encouraged precisely because it provided people who would uphold the values of the 'civilized' world. What was ultimately at risk was the middle- and upper-class way of life. As one of Sanger's supporters, Mrs Harry Guthman, pointed out in 1950, population increase prevented economic progress and any means of raising the standard of living.[5]

Guthman and Sanger, like many other contemporaries, attributed the recent explosion in population growth to advances in medical science. This had cut the number of deaths and improved the chances of infant survival, while doing nothing about curbing fertility. As Rock put it in 1954, 'The union of Science and Humanitarianism is increasingly successful in the exemplary prevention of premature death which in the evil past restricted populations. Can this same union do nothing now to prevent [the] smothering of mankind by Man, before evils of the past inevitably again take over?'[6] Seeing overpopulation as a menace, he was convinced that the only way forward was for more scientific research into simpler methods of birth control such as an oral contraceptive. Having caused the problem in the first place, science now had to come up with a solution. Yet not everyone was going to agree with the scientific solution adopted. Not only was the oral contraceptive to meet great opposition from the Catholic church on religious grounds; it was also opposed by many communist governments who equated the technology with imperialism and capitalism.

The development of the pill was therefore powerfully intertwined with the politics and rhetoric of the Cold War and the threat of overpopulation. Symbolically it was more than just a tool for contraception. From the start it was linked with science and the hopes that it could curb population growth and bring about world stability. Questions about population growth and its implications for social stability, however, were not new in the postwar era. Indeed, many social reformers and statesmen had been concerned with the links between population and national economic wealth, social order and military strength since the nineteenth century. Yet the nature of this discussion changed radically after the Second World War, shifting from equating large populations with economic and military strength to seeing them as a danger to global security. This debate had a profound effect on the development and adoption of the pill.

The population question and differential fertility

Population size has been a matter of political and social interest for centuries. Some of the most influential ideas on population have been drawn from the writings of the British clergyman-turned-economist Thomas Malthus in the late eighteenth century. Believing that the global population doubled in size every twenty-five years, Malthus feared that population growth would soon outstrip the world's resources. Moreover, he argued that the population had already reached its maximum limit and that a catastrophe was imminent. For him, famine, poverty, pestilence and war were the natural means of keeping population growth in check. Accordingly he argued against the provision of social welfare or food to the poor because he saw it as interfering with a natural process.[7] While gaining great popularity, Malthus's writings were not entirely original, but were partially based on the ideas of the French philosopher Condorcet. Condorcet, however, while pointing to population expansion, had a different interpretation of its implications. Unlike Malthus, he did not believe that population growth had reached its upper limit, and felt that any further increase could be overcome by the intelligent use of science, social reform and human reasoning, as well as contraception.[8] The differing positions of Malthus and Condorcet helped shape population debates in subsequent years.[9]

By the late nineteenth century the focus in Europe had shifted to the problem of fertility decline. Some of the earliest concerns about the decrease in the birth-rate occurred in France which experienced perhaps the most drastic decline in Europe after 1870.[10] The fear of German invasion, reinforced by the French defeat during the Franco-Prussian war (1870–1), haunted French politicians, many of whom equated France's weakness with the country's falling fertility rate. Such anxieties also dominated the politics of other count-ries. Heightened anxieties about the size and health of the population, for instance, dominated British politics in the aftermath of the South African war (1899–1902).[11]

Far more dangerous than unchecked fertility was the apparent class differential affecting its trend. What was most disturbing to many social reformers was that the statistics implied that those who were reproducing least were the better educated and more economically successful middle and upper classes. The poor, regarded as the most ignorant, unhealthy, unfit and immoral members of society, were continuing to procreate at very high rates. In the United States, anxiety focused on what appeared to be the greater reduction in the birth-rate of white native middle-class Americans relative to that of the ethnic immigrant poor. Wherever the debate took place, worries about differential fertility were exacerbated by the wider social and economic upheavals of the day, such as mounting political discontent and radical unionism among the working class, and the escalating costs of social reform, which many saw as inadequate to curb the ominous threat of poverty and discontent. Added to this were accelerating international economic and military competition, the collapse of empires and worsening economic depressions.[12]

Some of the most vocal participants in the population debate were neo-Malthusians and eugenicists. Originally started in Britain and primarily led by upper middle-class, white, Anglo-Saxon, Protestant and educated leaders, the neo-Malthusian and eugenics movements were ideologically complex, and the ways they perceived population issues and the solutions they offered were diverse.[13] Both ideological movements feared that the differential in fertility signified the degeneration of the physical and mental health of the nation. Some neo-Malthusians attributed the problem to the social and economic upheavals caused by rapid urbanization and industrialization. On the other hand, some eugenicists attributed the problem to recent advances in medical science, especially public hygiene, and generous social policies, which they believed had promoted the greater survival of the inherently 'weak' and 'inferior' members of society. For them this represented a disturbance of the natural order of evolution and the survival of the fittest as outlined by Darwin, on whose account their ideas were based. Moreover, some eugenicists saw the higher fertility of the lowest socioeconomic classes not only as an economic burden on the nation, but also as a genetic aberration.[14] Seeing differential fertility in biological terms, eugenicists and neo-Malthusians promoted the idea that fitter members of society should be encouraged to 'breed' in greater numbers, while those deemed less fit should have their fertility controlled. Within this context, human reproduction was to be scientifically managed. Known as selective breeding, this policy was considered vital to the improvement of the 'race' and the health of the nation.

Eugenics and neo-Maltusianism provided a convenient means of explaining and resolving many of the social and economic difficulties of the day, ranging from immigration problems to what was thought to be a deterioration in health and living standards, and a decline in military and economic strength. These ideas attracted support across the political spectrum in both Europe and the United States, gaining the attention of a number of prominent political figures, as well as well-to-do professionals, physicians, social workers, clerics, writers and professors, notably in the biological and social sciences.[15] Not everyone, however, agreed with their ideas and the solutions they proffered. Moreover, the degree to which eugenicists and neo-Malthusians were able to influence policy varied enormously, and was greatly dependent on the politics of individual countries and how well their ideas fitted in with more general perceptions about how to tackle population questions.

Different solutions adopted

By the interwar years various countries in Europe as well as the United States were developing different strategies to address the population issue. One of the most popular was to promote more births among the 'fit' and the healthy within the nation. Indeed, such births increasingly became politically equated with a nation's economic and military survival. Known as 'pronatalism', this policy found some of its most forceful promoters in the fascist countries of Spain, Italy and Germany. Here a range of incentives, including government loans, were provided to encourage higher fertility among the 'fittest' members of society. While less extreme than these totalitarian regimes, many other European governments also adopted pronatalist approaches during these years. In Sweden, for instance, the introduction of maternity relief in 1937 aimed to increase the population. Similarly, in France special government premiums were paid to encourage couples to have more babies.[16] The rise in maternal and child welfare provision during this period in countries such as Britain, France, Denmark, Sweden and the United States was essentially part of a pronatalist programme.[17]

In Europe as well as the United States the emphasis on pronatalism thwarted attempts to legalize abortion and increase access to contraception during the interwar years. Many politicians and social reformers saw abortion and contraception as the equivalent of national suicide.[18] In 1920 France passed a law which prohibited the sale of contraceptives. During the Second World War, with the German occupation of France, the collaborationist French Vichy government also passed laws declaring abortion to be a 'crime against society, the state and the race – an act of treason punishable by death'.[19] Similarly, in 1941 Franco's regime in Spain elevated abortion to a crime against the state and severely restricted access to contraception.[20]

The advocacy of pronatalism, however, should not be equated with an argument for the reproduction of children at any cost. In the case of Nazi Germany, pronatalist policies were intrinsically tied to questions of antinatalism, the prevention of births deemed 'unsuitable'. An instruction put out by Goebbels's Ministry for Propaganda highlights the belief of many pronatalists during these years: the goal is not 'children at any cost', but 'racially worthy, physically and mentally unaffected children of German families'.[21] Germany was not the only country to twin antinatalism with its pronatalist policies. During the early twentieth century, while many governments across Europe and in the United States were making increasing provision for mothers and their infants and encouraging motherhood, compulsory sterilization was also gaining increasing ground.

Some of the earliest antinatalist measures were undertaken in the United States, where 3,233 people were compulsorily sterilized between 1907 and 1920. Among these were epileptics, the insane, and habitual or confirmed criminals who had been incarcerated for drug addiction or sexual offences, such as rape.[22] By the 1920s the average rate of sterilization had reached between 200 and 600 per year. This shot up to 2,000 to 4,000 per year after 1930. Such policies had mass appeal around the country. In 1937 the American magazine *Fortune* reported that 37 per cent of citizens in the United States endorsed compulsory sterilization of habitual criminals and 66 per cent were in favour of sterilizing those regarded as 'mentally defective'. In 1941, 36,000 people were sterilized, and, many families facing the prospect of going on welfare feared they would be sterilized.[23]

Sterilization was not a project confined to the United States. Sweden, for example, pursued a rigorous sterilization policy from the interwar years right up to the 1970s, leading to the sterilization of 60,000 people in total. Most were those classified as mentally defective, but this category was loosely defined so that a very wide range of people were sterilized, including those who were considered to be 'displaying undesirable racial characteristics', to have poor eyesight, or to be living a vagabond life. Single mothers and habitual criminals were given no right of appeal against sterilization. Other countries also attempted to institute the practice. Britain, for instance, tried but failed to pass sterilization laws in 1913 in association with its policies related to mental deficiency. During the 1930s Norwegian socialists also favoured the use of sterilization, seeing it as part of a planned socialist society.[24]

Taken to even greater and more horrific extremes were the sterilization measures implemented in Germany under National Socialism. In 1933 the Nazi regime passed a Eugenic Sterilization Law which was based on the Model Sterilization Law developed by the Eugenics Record Office in the United States. The German law, however, went far beyond the policies implemented in the United States. By 1937, 225,000 people had been sterilized in Germany, almost ten times the number sterilized over the previous 30 years in the United States. The brutal sterilization procedure also resulted in the death of approximately 5,000 people, over 90 per cent of whom were women. Over half of those sterilized were categorized as 'feeble-minded' or 'mentally deficient'. Many of the victims included those suffering from 'schizophrenia, epilepsy, blindness, severe drug or alcohol addiction, and physical deformities that seriously interfered with loco-motion or were grossly offensive', or with hereditary defects.[25] By 1939 a policy of euthanasia had replaced sterilization, leading to the shooting of victims and then to the erection of gas chambers. Those killed not only included thousands of inmates from psychiatric clinics and other institu-tions who were considered too old, ill or handicapped to work, but also those considered racially inferior, particularly Jews, gypsies and blacks.[26]

While the zeal for sterilization faded in the light of the Nazi atrocities, it is important to remember how popular ideas of selective breeding were during the interwar years. For instance, although brutal in its impact on women, sterilization was favoured by many feminists during this period. Margaret Sanger, for instance, who championed her cause in the hope of enhancing women's position in society, did not see sterilization as a con-tradiction in her campaign.[27] She advocated the 'national sterilization' of 'certain dysgenic types', whom she saw as destroying the civilized 'way of life'. Like many other social reformers in these years Sanger saw the chief object of birth control as being to produce 'more children from the fit and less from the unfit'.[28] It could be argued that Sanger and her fellow sup-porters were merely utilizing the eugenic rhetoric of selective breeding as a convenient platform on which to build their demands for increased access to contraception. However, for Sanger the eugenic language and the call for sterilization were a powerful means of adding scientific credibility to her calls for greater access to contraception. For Sanger the scientific cri-teria promoted by eugenicists was vital not only in justifying the use of con-traception on social and economic grounds but also in challenging the medical profession's derision.[29]

The eugenicists' call for sterilization was not universally accepted, how-ever. In Britain, for instance, the eugenics movement met great resistance in its attempt to have legislation passed to allow for a comprehensive voluntary sterilisation programme to deal with the mentally 'unfit' . The difficulty they experienced in winning support is particularly interesting given the fact that during the interwar years many prominent British polit-ical figures, such as Lloyd George, Eleanor Rathbone, Joseph Chamberlain, William Beveridge, Winston Churchill and Harold Macmillan, used eugenic arguments for tactical gains. Nonetheless, voluntary sterilization never had much appeal to the medical and scientific community, many of whose members argued against the eugenic premise that mental deficiency was inherited. As a result, individuals who wanted sterilization, particularly vasectomies, as a means of contraception within marriage often found difficulty in finding surgeons willing to undertake the operation in Britain. Many within the working class were also hostile to the idea of voluntary sterilization, seeing it as a measure which was primarily directed at them. In addition the Catholic church was also strongly opposed to sterilization.[30] Clearly, the degree to which antinatalist measures, such as sterilization, could be undertaken depended greatly on the political climate and culture of each country.

The planning of population and national security

By the 1940s the population debate had taken a new turn in the light of the Depression and the Second World War, both of which had encouraged rationalization and economic planning in countries such as Britain and the United States. Within this context fertility became something which many thought should be and was susceptible to planning. Much of the debate around fertility also reflected wider beliefs about science and the rationalization of modern life. One American family planning poster in the early 1940s effectively captured the spirit:

> MODERN LIFE IS BASED ON CONTROL AND SCIENCE. We control the speed of our automobile. We control machines. We endeavour to control disease and death. Let us control the size of our family to ensure health and happiness.[31]

Significantly it was in this period that birth control became known as 'family planning', primarily directed at the prevention of 'unplanned' pregnancies.[32] Within this new thinking there was a new concern about what constituted a healthy family.

It was alongside ideas like these that planned families became intrinsically tied to questions of economic and national security. As one statement drafted by the Planned Parenthood Federation of America (PPFA) in 1940 argued:

> A nation's strength does not depend upon armaments and manpower alone; it depends also upon the contentment ... of its people. To the

extent that birth control contributes to the health and morale of our people, it makes them less receptive to subversive propaganda, more ready to defend our national system.[33]

The intensifying international anxiety with the onset of the Cold War reinforced the equation of family planning with national security in the postwar years. The planned nuclear family increasingly symbolized domestic and national harmony. The nuclear family was perceived as conforming to certain ideals. Anyone who failed to achieve these ideals was regarded with suspicion. They included those bearing children outside of marriage, couples who conceived more children than intended, as well as those who failed to produce children.[34]

Some of the condemnation, however, was targeted at poor women, who, as earlier in the century, were considered too illiterate, ignorant and feckless to plan their families. Now, however, the obsession of some policy-makers extended beyond an internal preoccupation with social problems caused by the high birth-rate of the poor on the home front, to an international anxiety about the high fertility rates in the socioeconomically disadvantaged parts of the world. Such apprehension was reinforced by statistics released by the United Nations in the 1950s which indicated that the population of the 'underdeveloped' world was growing twice as fast as that of more 'advanced' countries. As tables 1.1 and 1.2 indicate, the size of the population had indeed increased substantially worldwide between 1900 and 1950, most notably in Africa and Asia, where the numbers had more than doubled. Papers in New York in 1954 blazoned headlines such as: 'UN sees population of 4 billion by '84 causing food crisis.'[35] Moreover, the figures showed that within 40 years three-quarters of the population of the world would be living in the least developed areas. While historically the actual percentage distribution of population around the world had not changed very substantially since the eighteenth century (table 1.3), the dramatic increase in population size in areas like Africa and Asia was seen to be particularly alarming. Perceived to hinder the economic development and prosperity of the 'underdeveloped' world, such an unprecedented rise in population was seen as a threat to the world's social and economic order and the destruction of Western culture and ideals.[36]

These statistics were particularly disturbing to politicians and social reformers in the wake of the mass starvation and upheaval in the aftermath of the Second World War. Indeed, some attributed the problems they faced to the slow pace of industrialization and the dramatic rise of population in

Table 1.1   Population size for world and major areas, 1750–1998 (millions)

	1750	1800	1850	1900	1950	1998
World	791	978	1262	1650	2521	5901
Africa	106	107	111	133	221	749
Asia	502	635	809	947	1402	3585
Europe	163	203	276	408	547	729
Latin America and the Caribbean	16	24	38	74	167	504
Northern America	2	7	26	82	172	305
Oceania	2	2	2	6	13	30

Sources: UN, *The Determinants and Consequences of Population Trends*, vol.1 (New York, 1973); UN, *World Population Prospects: The 1998 Revision* (New York, 2000).

Table 1.2   Average rate of increase in population in world and major areas, 1750–1998 (per cent)

	1750–1800	1800–1850	1850–1900	1900–1950	1950–1998
World	24	29	31	53	134
Africa	1	4	20	66	239
Asia	26	27	17	48	156
Europe	25	36	48	34	33
Latin America and the Caribbean	50	58	95	126	202
Northern America	250	271	215	110	77
Oceania	0	0	200	117	131

Sources: UN, *The Determinants and Consequences of Population Trends*, vol.1 (New York, 1973); UN, *World Population Prospects: The 1998 Revision* (New York, 2000).

Table 1.3   Percentage distribution of population for major world areas, 1750–1998

	1750	1800	1850	1900	1950	1998
Africa	13	11	9	8	9	13
Asia	64	65	64	57	56	61
Europe	21	21	22	24	22	22
Latin America and the Caribbean	2	3	3	5	7	9
Northern America	0.3	0.7	2	5	7	5
Oceania	0.3	0.2	0.2	0.4	0.5	0.5

Sources: UN, *The Determinants and Consequences of Population Trends*, vol.1 (New York, 1973); UN, *World Population Prospects: The 1998 Revision* (New York, 2000).

the 'underdeveloped' world. What they feared most was that such areas would become a ready breeding ground for communism. As John Rock put it, overpopulation and communism were 'more than synchronous'.[37] These perceptions were reinforced in 1949 by the revolution in China and by Indian and Indonesian independence, and strengthened by the rise of independence movements in Africa and economic nationalism emerging in Latin America in the early 1950s.[38] Some of the sentiments of the era can be seen from an article by the American journalist Robert Coughlan in 1959. In reflecting on the rise in world population, he asked:

> What kind of life can these new billions have? The living standards of the present generation are miserably low, and there is heavy pressure on native political leaders to try to raise them. But it takes time to create the means of production, especially in retarded countries and more especially by democratic methods. ... What is almost certain to happen instead unless birth rates fall, is a lowering of standards until human misery finally puts a brake on breeding – probably not, however, until democracy has been chucked overboard in favor of some form of dictatorship. The likely choice is Communism.[39]

Communism was not the only threat envisaged. Some, like Rock, also pointed to the devastation of the earth's resources by overpopulation, drawing on the old Malthusian concerns about population growth outstripping the world's ability to feed itself.[40]

As had been the case in the earlier debates, some people not only feared a depletion of resources, but the collapse of social and political order, which ultimately protected the more privileged individuals and countries. The United States played a leading role in the debate. As the dominant world power after the Second World War, the country had a vested interest in maintaining political and economic stability. For Americans, population growth was equated with instability and ultimately with their worst foe – communism.[41] Much of the American debate was couched in terms of the struggle of democracy against the rise of the totalitarianism of communism.[42] A quotation from an invitation to attend a fund-raising event in 1960 to combat population growth sums up the argument:

> Throughout most of the world today there is a race between living standards and exploding populations. The whole future of freedom depends on the outcome. India, Pakistan, Indonesia, Malaya, the

Philippines, Taiwan, and Ceylon in Asia, together with large sections of the Middle East and, in this hemisphere, parts of South and Central America and almost the entire Caribbean area are affected by a geo-metrical population increase which devours their resources and beggars and embitters their peoples. With the Communists capitalizing on this situation, we in the industrialized West are threatened with loss of raw materials essential to our way of life – and in fact vital to our defence.[43]

Such views were not confined to the United States. British parliamentary debates and newspaper articles showed similar concerns during the 1950s and 1960s, reflecting British concerns over the break-up of the empire and demands for independence from former colonies. In 1955 a debate in the House of Commons indicated that politicians feared that population growth would undermine any welfare and development aid they provided for Britain's colonies. As one British MP, Thomas Reid, put it, unless birth control was established in the colonies, all British efforts 'would be doomed to failure'. He went on to argue:

It is impossible to expect over 50 million of us, who practise birth control and have only small families, to bring up our own families, and vote £1,600 million for our own and our Dependencies' defence to save the world from Communist imperialism and, at the same time, provide for the families of those who refuse to limit their numbers.[44]

For Britain the question of population control was intertwined not only with external concerns about empire, but also with questions relating to manpower for the internal economy. During the 1950s Britain had actively encouraged the arrival of immigrants from commonwealth countries to help with its labour shortages, particularly transport and construction work. By the mid-1960s, however, when there was no longer such a scarcity of workers, immigration, frequently associated with population growth in the 'underdeveloped' world, was increasingly feared. Fierce debates raged over whether Britain would be able to provide jobs and enough living space for its citizens in the light of the number of people arriving on its shores. As the MP David Renton put it in 1966,

The UK is one of the most densely populated countries in the world: we have 570 people per square mile, which is a higher density than any-where else in the world except Formosa, Belgium and Holland, and

Hong Kong. The UK has a far higher density than India, Pakistan and Jamaica whose countries have been sending so many people here in recent years.[45]

Within this context, contraception came to be seen as an urgent priority for government policy.

Population initiatives

From the early twentieth century many individuals and organizations sponsored schemes to deal with the issue of fertility. Most notable were the powerful feminist advocates of birth control, such as Margaret Sanger in the United States and Marie Stopes (1880–1958) and Margery Spring-Rice (1884–1970) in Britain, who established a wide network of birth control clinics as well as research programmes to investigate more effective means of fertility control. In addition to their efforts, a number of philanthropic organizations also established research programmes to investigate demographic trends and sponsored biomedical studies of reproductive behaviour and fertility control. One of the most active organizations on this front was the Rockefeller Foundation, the American philanthropic organization which from 1911 helped sponsor birth control clinics, the adoption of contraception by the medical profession, and research in endocrinology, biomedicine and sexual behaviour. Studies in population, including fertility and the use of contraception, were also financed by American organizations such as the Scripps Foundation and the Milbank Memorial Fund in the interwar years.[46]

Such schemes were extended during the postwar era. Seen as the medicine for curing poverty and promoting economic development, many of these programmes and policies reflected the ideas of the early twentieth century. Now labelled 'population control', the prime purpose of such work was to reduce the birth rate in 'underdeveloped' nations and among the poor in the more developed world. Much of this policy was influenced by ideas beginning to develop among leading demographic social scientists, which emphasized the link between population growth and national economic development. Two of the key figures in this discussion were Frank W. Notestein, director of the influential Office of Population Research,[47] based at Princeton University, and Kingsley Davis, a senior researcher at the same institution. During the mid-1940s both men published articles on the topic of demographic transition. Both traced the earliest and strongest population growth to the time of industrialization which had improved food supplies, agriculture, transport, sanitation and medicine, and had raised the overall standard of living. This had resulted in a decline in previous high rates of mortality. Fertility, on the other hand, had remained high and unaffected during this period of modernization, only falling once full-scale industrialization had been established and new aspirations of individualism and consumerism had taken hold within society. Couched in terms of demographic evolution, the argument was that European countries had gone through the transition earliest and were now reaching a state of equilibrium. By contrast many countries in less developed parts of the world, where industrialization had not even begun, were considered not to have even started the demographic transition.[48]

At the heart of the analysis was the belief that in order to progress economically all countries needed to pass through the various stages of the demographic transition. Promoted as part of the economic planning initiatives after the Second World War, these ideas were to become increasingly popular in the following years. During the 1950s Notestein and Davis became advocates of government-sponsored family planning as an urgent policy for those countries which had not yet begun the demographic transition.[49] As the historian Elizabeth Watkins has pointed out, 'instead of allowing social and economic change to lead people to voluntarily control their fertility (as had been the case in Western Europe and the United States), the experts wanted to introduce birth control before modernization and industrialization had taken place.'[50]

By the early 1950s new population control initiatives had been launched. This included the founding of the International Planned Parenthood Federation (IPPF) which was established by Margaret Sanger and others in 1952 to coordinate family planning programmes on an international scale;[51] the creation of the Population Council in 1952 by John D. Rockefeller III to fund biomedical and scientific research into contraception and other means of limiting population growth; and the investment by the Ford Foundation in research and training in fundamental and applied reproductive science. Until the late 1960s the Ford Foundation was the principal private donor in the population field, sponsoring not only activities of its own, but also those of the IPPF and the Population Council. Approximately half of the Population Council's expenditure in the years between 1954 and 1971 was financed by the Ford Foundation, totalling $45 million. Much of the work of the Foundation and the Council focused on academic training and scientific research.[52] In choosing to promote academic research and training, the Ford Foundation and the Population Council set themselves apart from other workers in the field, such as family planning activists, who focused on ameliorative action.[53]

Alongside these activities were also the propaganda initiatives undertaken by private businessmen. One of the most notable and active was Hugh Moore, the Dixie Cup magnate. In 1954, Moore financed the publication and distribution of a pamphlet entitled *The Population Bomb* to 10,000 influential Americans. Deliberately alarmist and anti-communist in tone, the pamphlet aimed to stir up immediate action to combat overpopulation, which Moore saw as the greatest fuel for communism and threat to world peace. As the pamphlet stated,

Today the population bomb threatens to create an explosion as disruptive and dangerous as the explosion of the atom, and with as much influence on prospects for progress or disaster, war or peace.

But while the atom bomb is only being stockpiled, the fuse of the population bomb is already lighted and burning. *Every day* adds more than 100,000 people to the population of this planet.[54]

A letter widely circulated in 1956, signed by Moore, revealed his motivations for the campaign: 'We're not primarily interested in the sociological or humanitarian aspects of birth control. We *are* interested in the use ... which the Communists make of hungry people in their drive to conquer the earth.'[55]

Many family planners and population experts were highly critical of Moore's brash and aggressive style, fearing it would threaten the foundations of international cooperation in birth control, and fuel opposition. Nonetheless, Moore was a key supporter of their work, financially aiding organizations such as the Planned Parenthood Federation of America, the International Planned Parenthood Federation and the Population Reference Bureau.[56] Moore was also instrumental in swaying the American government in favour of population control. In 1958 he telegraphed Major-General William H. Draper Jr, who chaired the President's Committee to Study the United States Military Assistance Program, stating, 'If your committee does not look into the impact of the population explosion you will be derelict in your duty.'[57] Set up to explore overseas assistance programmes, Draper had been appointed to the chair by President Eisenhower with the explicit brief not to forget the question of population.[58] Moore found a powerful ally in Draper. As a result of his work on the committee, Draper became a strong proponent of population control for, as he saw it, the population question was a major obstacle to the American 'aid program and to the progress of the world'.[59] In accordance with this, Draper advocated that the committee recommend birth control assistance alongside economic aid.[60]

While failing to gain overt US government support to provide contraception alongside economic assistance, the publicity surrounding the Draper Committee transformed the population cause from a relatively minor social movement into a major geopolitical issue. The committee's report spurred the establishment of a World Population Emergency Campaign (WPEC) which raised funds and promoted consciousness-raising activities. In 1962, Eisenhower and Truman were honorary sponsors of the WPEC. It used a wide range of media, including newspapers, radio, television and films, to expand its audience.[61] Private philanthropic funding of population activities rose 30-fold between 1962 and 1970.

By the late 1960s, the American government had become much more willing to support the population cause. The reasons for this shift are partly captured by the words of President Lyndon Johnson who, in 1965, during the twenty-fifth anniversary of the United Nations, declared that 'less than five dollars invested in population control is worth a hundred dollars invested in economic growth'.[62] Two years later he announced, 'next to the pursuit of peace the really greatest challenge to the human family is the race between food supply and population increase. That race ... is being lost.'[63] This marked the beginning of federal sponsorship of family planning within the United States, as well as overseas. Between 1965 and 1968 funding for family planning on the domestic front increased from $8.6 million to $28.2 million; by 1969 the sum had risen to $56.3 million. At least 6 per cent of special grants for maternity and child welfare were also earmarked for family planning. Much of this spending was intended to make family planning accessible to the estimated 5.2 million poor women in America in need of birth control. Twinned with the campaign 'War on Poverty', this sponsorship was based in part on the assumptions that a reduction of births was the key to ending poverty among the poor and to ending the wider social problems of urban decay, welfare dependency and the increase in extramarital births.[64] Similarly, on the international front the American government began to fund population and family planning programmes in 'developing' countries. Spending in this area jumped from

$2.1 million to $34.7 million between 1965 and 1968. By 1968 the United States was providing $131.7 million for the population work undertaken abroad by the US Agency for International Development (USAID) and the National Institute of Health.[65] By the end of the 1960s, therefore, family planning had not only become respectable but was also seen as a political and economic necessity.

Philanthropic and government sponsorship of contraception was not confined to the United States. In 1957, for instance, a British umbrella body, called the Oliver Bird Trust (OBT), was set up to advance fertility control through education, research and clinical investigation. The trust was funded by a £10,000 donation from Captain Oliver Bird. Originally a businessman in the food industry and a Conservative Member of Parliament, Bird had a strong interest in family planning and sexual matters.[66] He was keen to fund research that would help develop a simple and effective contraceptive that could be used to curb population growth, which, like Moore and others, he saw as endangering world peace.[67] The OBT included leading family planning activists, such as Margaret Pyke (1893–1966), as well as experts in the reproductive field such as the biologist Alan Parkes (1900–90), and medical practitioners interested in fertility control, such as Gerald Swyer (1917–95) and Margaret Jackson (?1899–1987).[68] The aims of the OBT were to encourage the 'production of healthy children by parents who have the health and means to care for such children adequately'.[69] In attempting to get its message across to the British nation, the OBT used many different methods, ranging from the promotion of scientific lectures by high profile experts in the fertility field, to broadcasts on radio and the new medium of television, and journalistic articles. By 1959 the work of the OBT was attracting open debate in the British Houses of Parliament.[70] By 1964 the British government was financing family planning programmes as part of its technical assistance schemes to former colonies.[71]

Action was also being undertaken elsewhere in the world. From the late 1950s the Swedish government, through the Swedish International Development Authority (SIDA), was helping to provide technical assistance in family planning to places such as Sri Lanka (then Ceylon), and pioneering schemes in information, education and communication for family planning in Pakistan. Sweden was also the first nation to subsidize contraceptive supplies to family planning programmes for the 'underdeveloped' world. By the late 1960s similar schemes were being funded by Norway, Denmark and Canada. In 1968 the United Nations also set up a new agency to deal with population issues as a result of increasing pressure from representatives from Sweden, the United States and elsewhere. Called the United Nations Fund for Population Activities, this institution received $178.9 million from 100 nations in 1968. The aim of the organization was not only to stimulate demographic research and training but also to develop a coordinated family planning policy involving all agencies across the world. Under the leadership of Robert S. McNamara (previously US Secretary of Defense), the World Bank also became closely linked with population and family planning policies from 1968.[72] Between 1965 and 1972 worldwide support for contraceptive research rose from $31 million to $110 million, the largest contribution coming from the United States.[73] This was to continue in the following decades. By 1983 the United States was contributing at least 85 per cent of the world's expenditure ($167 million) on basic reproductive research and on the testing and safety of new contraceptives. Of this, 59 per cent was funded directly by the government, 21 per cent by American pharmaceutical companies and 4 per cent by charitable bodies.[74]

Opposition

While the funding of population activities, and particularly family planning, expanded to an unprecedented level by the late 1960s, in the previous two decades few would have imagined that funding could be achieved even on a small scale. During the late 1940s, Prescott Bush, an American Senator from Connecticut, had lost his seat in Congress as a result of campaigning for family planning.[75] Similarly, in 1948 Julian Huxley (1887–1975), the first director-general of the United Nations Educational, Scientific and Cultural Organization (UNESCO), had been greeted with little enthusiasm when trying to raise the problem of overpopulation in relation to economic progress. Again, hostile resistance followed Dr Evang of Norway's attempts to get the World Health Organization (WHO) to set up an expert committee on the health aspects of population in 1953.[76] The reluctance to pursue population policies continued into the following decade. Capturing the spirit of WHO in these years, Brock Chisholm, former director of the organization, stated, 'No person can get anywhere in any agency of the UN who tries to talk frankly about population problems. ... Every committee is under the influence of the Roman Catholic Church, and no delegate from the United States, Canada, France, Britain, and many other countries of Europe is in a position to defy that taboo.'[77] Similar tensions were present in other international organizations.[78]

Pressure from the Catholic lobby also prevented President Eisenhower from agreeing overtly to the recommendations of the Draper Committee in 1959. As he later admitted, 'When I was President I opposed the use of federal funds to provide birth control information to countries we were aiding because I felt this would violate the deepest religious convictions of large groups of taxpayers.'[79] Some idea of the Catholic opposition to population policies can be seen from a statement made by the Catholic bishops of the United States in November 1959 which denounced artificial birth control on the grounds that it was a 'morally, humanly, psychologically, and politically disastrous approach to the population problem'.[80]

Fear of opposition from the Catholic church was not the only reason for the reluctance to promote population measures during these years. In 1949 General Douglas MacArthur (1880–1964), Supreme Commander of the Allied Powers, denied Margaret Sanger a visa to give lectures on birth control in Japan, then occupied by American forces. Leading to outcries in American newspapers, and even a column of protest from the late President's wife, Eleanor Roosevelt, MacArthur's action was believed by many family planning activists to be a sign of his capitulation to Catholic pressure.[81] MacArthur, however, saw the matter differently. As he argued, 'Birth control, with its social, economic and theological sides, is, in final analysis, for individual judgement and decision. The more basic problem of population is long range and world-wide and certainly not within the purview of prescribed Allied policy or the defined scope of Supreme Commander's responsibility or authority.'[82] Regarding matters of fertility as a question for the Japanese to settle for themselves, MacArthur viewed Sanger's proposed lecture tour as potentially explosive politically, fearing that any American interference in this area would be viewed as 'genocide'.[83]

In the 1950s population control advocates had to be cautious because many less developed countries were suspicious of population policies, believing that rich nations were using the issue of overpopulation in order to blame them for their poverty and to avoid responsibility for providing aid for the development of former colonies. Moreover, Reed claims that

As the Cold War heated up, communist nations became increasingly hostile toward American efforts to aid economic development in the Third World, and joined with Catholic nations to provide formidable opposition within the United Nations to the inclusion of family planning.[84]

Both the US and British governments were only too aware of this situation. In 1955 the British Secretary of State for the Colonies indicated that birth control was too sensitive an area to fund as part of Britain's development programmes.[85] President Eisenhower refused to endorse the Draper Committee's recommendations for family planning on the same grounds in 1959.[86] During the 1950s the Rockefeller Foundation favoured agricultural research over fertility investigations for similar reasons. Known later as the Green Revolution, this policy was directed at producing more efficient crops to feed the growing population, a policy which was seen as less controversial than controlling population.[87]

In the United States the reticence over contraceptive policies was combined with the more general fears of the McCarthy era. Ironically, while many of the proponents of population control couched their ideas in terms of the battle against communism, others equated the promotion of contraception with communist ideas. During the first half of the 1950s Joseph McCarthy's campaign to stamp out communism had resulted in the large-scale harassment of many population control advocates and researchers by right-wing commentators and government officials. McCarthyism also generated a political and cultural atmosphere in which any mention of radical birth control measures was treated with suspicion, and which reinforced the taboos around sex research.[88] The hostility of the American press towards the Kinsey Report on sexual attitudes in the 1950s reflected the negative ways in which such research was construed in this period. As the historian James Reed has pointed out, 'During the hysteria of the McCarthy era, sex research and the international Bolshevik conspiracy were linked together.'[89] The purge of academics between 1952 and 1954 meant that many reproductive researchers were alert to the pressures of McCarthy's officials.[90]

In addition to the McCarthy crusade, researchers working on reproduction had to be careful not to contravene legal restrictions surrounding contraception. This was most severe in the United States, where legislation (known as the Comstock laws) passed in 1873 prohibited the publication of any material considered obscene, such as birth control pamphlets. Only repealed in 1971, the Comstock laws also outlawed contraception and any research on this topic in a number of states.[91] In Massachusetts, where much of the initial biological research was undertaken on the pill, the legal restrictions were particularly harsh. Anyone caught providing the means of contraception, which included implements or drugs for abortion, could face up to five years in jail, or two and a half years in a house of correction, or a fine of $1,000.[92] By 1972 contraception was legal for adults in all states (except in Massachusetts and Wisconsin where contraception was only legally available to the married). In reality, however, more than half the states continued to restrict the sale, distribution, advertising and display of contraceptives.[93] Such limitations on the provision of contraception were not unique to the United States. Up to the early 1970s many European countries, including the traditional Catholic countries of Ireland, France and Spain, but also Belgium, Sweden and the Federal Republic of Germany, severely curbed the advertising and selling of contraceptives as well as sexual education.[94]

Obstacles to the development of the pill

In the United States, where much of the development of the pill occurred, the opposition to contraception made work in this area particularly difficult. The reproductive biologist Gregory Pincus and his team at the Worcester Foundation for Experimental Biological Research in Massachusetts, for example, who were the chief developers of the pill, were highly aware of the controversial nature of their project. Pincus was particularly sensitive because of the backlash he had suffered during the 1930s when his research on parthenogenic (fatherless) rabbits had provoked an outcry in the national press, resulting in his being caricatured as the evil fictional biologist, Bokanovsky, in Aldous Huxley's *Brave New World*. One journalist also equated his 'immaculate conceptions' with the science fiction world of H. G. Wells.[95] In 1937 J. Ratcliff, a reporter writing for *Collier's Magazine*, depicted Pincus as unleashing a force which would allow the 'mythical life of the Amazons to come to life. A world where woman would be self-sufficient; man's value zero.'[96] Combining an attack on feminism with a criticism of biologists interfering with the workings of nature, Ratcliff's attack on Pincus was also anti-semitic in tone. His article caused a sensation in Cambridge, Massachusetts, and probably helped to prevent Pincus from gaining tenure at Harvard.[97]

Undertaking research on the contraceptive pill at the height of McCarthyism, Pincus and his colleagues at the Worcester Foundation were – not surprisingly – anxious about their own welfare.[98] Pincus's son, John, recalled a woman knocking on the door of his father's house one night in the early 1950s, and asking for help because she was unintentionally pregnant. Fearing it was a set-up, Pincus, while being gentle, maintained a careful distance from the woman.[99] The one advantage that Pincus and his co-workers had was that they worked for an independent research institution which was not answerable to an executive board. Financial support for the foundation also came from contributors in the local community, who tended to be liberal. The Worcester Foundation was thus not as prone to the prejudices of the era as other universities and research institutions.[100]

Despite the advantage of working in an independent institution, Pincus and his co-workers could not develop the pill without the help of the pharmaceutical industry. Here the opposition to contraception and explicit discussion of sex matters was strong in the 1950s. In October 1951, for instance, when Pincus asked G. D. Searle, a pharmaceutical company that had funded his previous research, to sponsor his development of the oral contraceptive he met the following response, 'You haven't given us a thing to justify the half-million that we have invested in you ... yet you have the nerve to ask for more research.'[101] Founded in the late nineteenth century by a pharmacist from India, Gideon Searle, the company had established an enviable ethical reputation in the pharmaceutical world. For them the pill represented a significant gamble. On the one hand it might bring the company unprecedented profits, on the other it could lead to ruin. As Searle's representative, James S. Irwin, argued, the company's reluctance to enter the field of contraception reflected the fact that, prior to the pill, contraceptives were commonly associated with disreputable rubber goods usually sold clandestinely in back-street shops. Irwin explained, 'We were a company with an absolutely impeccable reputation ... We were going into absolutely unexplored ground in terms of public opinion.'[102] As he pointed out, even Goodyear Rubber, a company which had a $150 million market in condoms in 1958, was unwilling to publicize its contraceptive trade openly.[103] Searle officials predicted that Catholic wrath alone, given its cumulative influence on patients, hospitals and physician-prescribers, could reduce the company's personnel by at least a quarter.[104] They were thus initially unwilling for its name to be openly associated with Pincus's research on the pill.[105] When a president of another pharmaceutical company, Parke-Davis, heard that Searle was to launch an oral contraceptive, he phoned Searle's chairman, John Searle, to tell him that 'he was crazy to even think of doing such a thing.'[106]

Searle's reluctance to enter the field of oral contraception was shared by many other pharmaceutical companies. Pincus recalled in 1967, 'In the search for an oral progestin we contacted a number of companies indicating that our objective was a contraceptive, and practically all of them refused to co-operate because this was considered a "dangerous field".[107] The small Mexican pharmaceutical company Syntex, for instance, which synthesized the first progestin compound capable of being used for an oral contraceptive but had no marketing organization, was unable to persuade its American collaborator Parke-Davis to market its product. Parke-Davis, which was a long-established and reputable company, regarded the marketing of such a product as too hazardous.[108] The company's fear of a major Catholic backlash was not surprising given that it was sited in an intensely Catholic diocese of Detroit. Charles Pfizer and Co., whose president at the time was an active Roman Catholic, also turned Syntex down for fear of reprisal from the Catholic community and went so far as to insist that the company not handle any agent that could be a potential contraceptive. Eventually Syntex concluded an agreement for marketing its drug with Ortho Pharmaceutical. As an American company already selling contraceptive creams and jellies, Ortho Pharmaceutical had nothing to lose in marketing an oral contraceptive. Nonetheless, even this company had been unwilling to enter the oral contraceptive field until Searle had proved that it was safe to do so.[109]

Turning the tide of opposition

What is so remarkable about the opposition to the development of the oral contraceptive is how quickly it evaporated once it reached the market. The pill's popularity was partly attributable to careful and strategic planning on the part of its developers, and their skilful manipulation of fears about population growth. Long before the emergence of the pill, birth control advocates had used population concerns as a tool for furthering their cause. The urgent political and economic demands arising out of the issue of world population growth in the aftermath of the Second World War provided a crucial backdrop to the campaign to win approval for the pill. Even before the oral contraceptive was seen as a real possibility, birth control advocates and demographers were paving the way for its acceptance through popular articles and conferences.

Such tactics continued to be used by G. D. Searle in the late 1950s. Officials from Searle, for instance, specifically approached journalists at the *Saturday Evening Post* and the *Reader's Digest* to write major articles on the pill so as to canvas support ahead of its launch. Similar articles also appeared in popular magazines such as *Ladies Home Journal* and *Vogue*.[110] Other publicity methods were also used. In 1959, for instance, Pincus toured the world to promote the contraceptive. Coverage of the tour was an enormous success. As Wesley Dixon, the president of Searle, wrote to Pincus, 'The news on Berlin doesn't stand a chance and apparently has been relegated to inside pages in cities where you have been talking ... congratulations on a fine job.'[111] In July 1959 Daniel Searle encouraged Pincus and his co-workers to use the recent publication of the Draper Report to inspire support for the oral contraceptive, suggesting they approach the US Public Health Service and State Department as well as representatives of the 'U.N. and other international organizations that might subsidize and distribute the Pill overseas'. As Daniel Searle put it, 'Perhaps in this way we would not only gain a substantial sales volume for Enovid, but we would also be able to gather even more information about the effectiveness of Enovid under a wide variety of circumstances.'[112]

'Everything is possible in science'

Much of the publicity for the pill harnessed the wider belief in the power of science. One of the basic assumptions underlying the campaign was that science had caused the problem of population growth by reducing mortality rates, and it was therefore up to science to solve the problem. As early as the 1920s, Margaret Sanger had first articulated this view, arguing:

> Ignorance, poverty and vice must stop populating the world. To accomplish this there is but one way. Science must make woman the owner, the mistress of herself. Science, the only possible savior of mankind, must put it in the power of woman to decide for herself whether she will or will not become a mother.[113]

Continuing this line of reasoning much of the rhetoric of the years after the Second World War called for 'scientific birth control' in order to complement 'scientific death control'.[114] The faith that was entrusted to science in the postwar era was summed up by Pincus's announcement to his wife when beginning research into the development of the pill: 'Everything is possible in science.'[115] Within this context, the assumption was not only that science had the power to achieve a solution, but that scientists had a responsibility to do so. Alan S. Parkes, who was active in the organization of British clinical trials on the pill, summed up the feeling of many in those years when he claimed, 'Medical Science is largely responsible for creating the problems of overpopulation, old people, and survival of the unfit, and it can reasonably be expected to take a large share of the responsibility for solving them.'[116]

In line with this thinking, science, rather than social, economic and political factors, was blamed for population growth and the world's tensions. Scientific contraception, such as the pill, rather than the redistribution of resources, was thus seen as the way forward for solving the world's problems. Seeing science as the problem and, as holding the answer, made it easier for policy-makers to manipulate the issue rather than attempt to change the world's economic and social structure. In this debate the pill was seen as a perfect tool for solving the problem.[117] As early as 1951 a report from a conference on population issues, attended by Pincus, highlighted the optimism invested in the pill from the start when it stated: 'The explosive increase in world population could be squelched by a tiny pill.'[118] Years later, in summing up the contribution that G. D. Searle had made in creating the pill, the chairman of the company, John G. Searle, expressed it in similar terms:

> I am sure when the history books are written, our organization's greatest single contribution to mankind will be 'Enovid'. It is a positive answer to a world threatened by overpopulation, and the resulting poor subsistence, poor shelter, and poor education that surplus peoples are forced to endure.[119]

Conclusion

As this chapter has shown, the conceptualization and development of the pill was intrinsically linked to debates over population size and differential fertility in the twentieth century. Enthusiasm for the distribution and development of new contraceptives was severely limited in Western Europe and the United States by the overall equation of large populations with economic and military strength. Fertility control was considered desirable only among those perceived to be the least fit and economically sustainable members of society. State legislation and disapproval by the Catholic church reinforced the taboos connected with contraception further. By the end of the 1940s, however, the debate over population had extended the question of fertility differentials beyond an internal concern with differences in the birth-rate between rich and poor to the external threat now arising from a rapidly increasing population in the least socially and economically developed countries. Such growth, it was feared, would hamper the economic welfare and progress of more advanced nations. Added to this was the intensification of the Cold War and the growing demand for economic and national independence among African, Asian and Latin American countries, which many in Western Europe and the United States feared would fuel the communist cause.

Presented as the scientific solution, the pill promised to prevent the economic and political upheaval many feared the growing population would generate. In this climate all the previous political, social and religious taboos around contraception faded. Even the developers of the pill were surprised by the speed with which it became accepted. As Searle's representative, Irwin Winter, recalled, 'We underestimated the receptivity of the product. ... We were overly cautious. All my experience told me that you could not do this without getting your teeth knocked out – or some of them. And we didn't lose any teeth.'[120]

Sold to the world as the means for peace, the pill was, however, more than an ideological tool. The following chapters show that the ways in which women used the pill went far beyond the expectations of its developers. As we shall see, the rapid acceptance of the pill and its widespread use indicates that for many women it did not necessarily represent a coercive method of control, but rather a means of releasing them from the age-old burden of pregnancy and motherhood. Letters written to Pincus and his fellow workers in the mid-1950s indicate how keen many women were to obtain an effective contraceptive. Some were willing to be guinea-pigs in the clinical trials being set up by Pincus in order to gain access to the product. For many women, the risks involved in taking a pill for which the long-term health consequences remained unknown outweighed the hazards and hardships of an unwanted pregnancy.

Much of the popularity of the pill stemmed from a deep-rooted yearning for contraception quite independent of the hopes initiated by its developers. This did not mean that its promoters were unable to use this desire to their political advantage. Indeed the promotion of the pill by the lobby for population control provided the pharmaceutical industry with enormous business. Between 1972 and 1979, for instance, between 25 and 30 per cent of the $15 million spent by USAID on family planning was spent on oral contraceptives sold by one pharmaceutical company, the Syntex Corporation.[121]

The promotion of the pill as a method of control was therefore double-edged. On the one hand, it could be seen as a useful tool for curbing population growth and a device of the privileged few for maintaining the social and economic order. On the other, for many women the pill represented a liberation from continual childbirth and a means for sexual independence. Nonetheless, as the following chapters show, in practice the distribution and consumption of the pill generated a more complex set of expectations than population experts, developers of the pill or the first women who took it ever envisaged. Conceived as a scientific solution to a problem created by science, the pill and its acceptance could not be disentangled from the social, political and economic context in which it was developed and the ways in which it was used.

2
The Contraceptive Challenge:
The Search for a Pill

As early as 1921 an Austrian physiologist, Ludwig Haberlandt (1885–1932), announced that it was possible to create a hormonal contraceptive pill.[1] The idea of an oral contraceptive was not new. From the time of Hippocrates, various preparations derived from the crocus, the laurel, nettle seeds, peony roots and other mineral sources had been suggested for contraception. What was new about Haberlandt's proposal was that the oral contraceptive could be made from hormones.[3] Such a suggestion represented a radical departure from the kinds of contraceptives then available. Up to that time, most couples had relied on rudimentary forms of contraception such as withdrawal (*coitus interruptus*), abstinence, prolonged lactation, abortion and infanticide. By the late nineteenth century those with money could buy rubber sheaths, diaphragms, syringes and chemical suppositories; the first two of these had become increasingly available with the emergence of new ways of manufacturing rubber.[2] Of all the techniques, barrier methods, such as the diaphragm or the condom, were considered to be the most effective.

Haberlandt's idea of a hormonal contraceptive promised a totally new technique. Picturing the possibility of using hormones to interact systemically with the body's reproductive process, Haberlandt offered the possibility of preventing conception without any mechanical device at the time of intercourse. Until then, all contraceptives necessitated insertion at the time and site of intercourse. The novelty of a hormonal pill was that it might be taken at a time that was totally unrelated to sexual intercourse.

Unlike previous barrier methods, oral contraception demanded an intricate scientific understanding of reproductive physiology. Moreover, knowledge about the human reproductive cycle and the precise mechanics of sexual hormones in the process of fertilization was relatively limited in the early twentieth century. By the 1930s, however, knowledge that had accumulated from animal experiments, together with investigations into the physiology of reproduction and the isolation of different female hormones, made Haberlandt's idea seem more feasible. Indeed, many scientists and medical experts were convinced that they were only a short step away from using hormones for fertility control and the creation of life. In 1932, Aldous Huxley's path-breaking science fiction novel, *Brave New World,* captured these beliefs. Envisaging a future totalitarian society in which babies would be grown in test-tubes, Huxley depicted women swallowing or injecting hormonal extracts to experience substitute pregnancies and people eating sex-hormone chewing-gum to regulate their sexual libido.[4]

While a novel, Huxley's book is a powerful reminder of the interplay between politics, social values and scientific developments. This interaction was to be no less important in the development of the pill in a democratic world. By the start of the Second World War scientists had come remarkably close to finding an effective means of controlling fertility through hormones. Nonetheless, while significant scientific breakthroughs were made during the interwar period, major obstacles remained, one of the strongest being the sensitive nature of work on contraceptives. In many places contraceptive research was illegal. Not only were few willing to invest money in such a project, many scientists and medical practitioners regarded such hormonal research as disreputable. Significantly it was Gregory Pincus, a leading expert in mammalian sexual physiology, who broke this barrier in the 1950s. Attached to an independent institution which had nothing to lose in reputation, he was inspired by the birth control advocate Margaret Sanger and backed by the money of the rich philanthropist, Katharine McCormick (1875–1967). Their efforts not only resulted in the development of an effective oral contraceptive, but proved important in subverting the social values which had posed major obstacles to its development in previous years.

The new magic bullet: endocrinology and the growth of reproductive knowledge

Much of the knowledge needed for the development of the pill is rooted in the emergence of endocrinology in the late nineteenth century. In 1889 a leading French doctor, the 72-year-old Charles-Edouard Brown-Sequard (1817–94), claimed to have rejuvenated himself by injecting testicular extracts from guinea-pigs and dogs into sensitive parts of his body. Attracting widespread attention, his experiment prompted many scientists to explore the properties of other internal organs and their secretions.[5] By 1905 the physiologist Ernest Starling had identified 'messengers' in the bloodstream which stimulated the action of cells. Calling these agents 'hormones', derived from the Greek word meaning 'to incite to activity', he indicated that these were natural chemical substances produced by particular glands in the body.[6]

By the time of the interwar years, sex hormones had become more than simply a subject of intellectual interest. Indeed, they had become the new magic bullet of medicine. Part of this was inspired by the remarkable success achieved during the 1920s in the use of insulin to treat diabetes, and thyroxine to alleviate thyroid deficiencies and metabolic disorders.[7] For many medical practitioners and scientists there seemed no limit to the extent to which hormones could be put to good medical use. Sex hormones, for instance, began to be used to treat gynaecological disorders, such as menstrual irregularity, infertility and menopausal complaints, as well as to treat various forms of cancer.[8] By the interwar years, research into the clinical and commercial applications of sex hormones had therefore become widespread. The League of Nations itself recognized their importance, arranging scientific and medical meetings to establish biological standardization that could be used on an international scale.[9]

It was not only scientists and doctors who took advantage of this new discovery of hormones. By the early twentieth century people had access to a diverse range of hormonal extracts, or 'organotherapies' as they were then called, without a doctor's prescription. While doctors were disdainful of these products, regarding them as 'nostrums' sold by quacks, organotherapies were not only widely advertised in the public press, but were also sold on a large scale through chemists' shops. Made from organs of animals discarded as abattoir waste, organotherapies promised cures for a variety of conditions, including hair loss and baldness, premature greyness, sterility, feminine troubles, general ailments such as high blood pressure, indigestion, allergies, anaemia, skin problems and addictions such as alcohol and smoking. A number of organotherapies were also marketed on the basis that they improved sexual virility. In many cases sex hormones were grouped together with vitamins and marketed on the grounds that they improved the growth and development of the body's tissues. Part of the popularity of organotherapies might also have stemmed from the influence of meat traders, particularly in the United States and continental Europe, who quickly realized that organotherapies could provide a lucrative sideline to their main business.[10]

With this surge of interest in hormones came new ideas about the reproductive system. Some aspects of reproductive physiology had been documented for centuries. Castration, for instance, was known to cause feminization. During the nineteenth century animal experiments had also shown sexual characteristics to be determined by internal secretions produced by male and female reproductive organs. More importantly, by the late nineteenth century, gynaecologists had determined that it was women's ovaries rather than their nervous systems which regulated their reproductive cycle. Nonetheless, many questions remained unanswered.[11] Until the 1930s, for example, little was understood about ovulation and fertilization and the specific hormones, progesterone and oestrogen, which activated these processes. Understanding these mechanisms was vital for the development of hormonal contraceptives.

Today contraceptive pills prevent pregnancy primarily through the suppression of ovulation. The mechanism causing the inhibition of ovulation was first elucidated in the late nineteenth century by John Beard at Edinburgh University and the French histologist Auguste Prenant in Nancy. Investigating the ovaries of animals, they observed that no ovulation took place during pregnancy. Their work, together with work by Professor Zschokke in Zurich, led to the discovery of a yellow substance (corpus luteum) in the ovaries produced by ruptured egg sacs. From this it was deduced that the corpus luteum contained something which prevented ovulation during pregnancy.[12] During the 1920s and 1930s a number of European and American scientists transplanting ovaries from pregnant animals to non-pregnant animals confirmed that corpus luteum was an effective inhibitor of ovulation. In 1934 progesterone was isolated as the specific hormone in the corpus luteum which stopped ovulation. Between 1937 and 1939 animal experiments confirmed progesterone to be an effective suppressant of ovulation.[13]

Progesterone was not the only hormone discovered to be an effective regulator of ovulation. Other experiments with ovarian extracts in the early twentieth century provided evidence of a further female hormone, oestrogen, which also affected ovulation. In 1912 and 1913 scientists in Paris and Vienna obtained ovarian extracts which produced sexual changes in castrated animals. In 1923 the American scientists Edgar Allen (1892–1943) and Edward A. Doisy (1893–1986) detected a pure oestrogenic hormone within the ovaries. This, they discovered, could induce ovulation in rats.[14] During the late 1920s a gynaecologist based in Vienna, Otfried Fellner, succeeded in producing an oral preparation he called 'feminin', which contained oestrogenic hormones. He discovered 'feminin' could cause sterility in rabbits and mice. From this it was clear that oestrogen as well as progesterone could inhibit ovulation and thus prevent pregnancy.[15] Research carried out on guinea-pigs by scientists in St Louis further confirmed these findings. By 1935 Doisy and others, including the German biochemist Adolf Butenandt (1903–95), had isolated oestrone as the specific oestrogen compound active in this process.[16] Another female oestrogen, oestriol, had also been isolated five years previously by an English researcher, Guy Marrian (1904–81), from the urine of pregnant women. This was found to be an important analogue of oestradiol, the most active of the naturally occurring oestrogens.[17]

Investigations into progesterone and oestrogen not only provided the clues for the inhibition of ovulation during these years, but also the key to understanding the full menstrual process. One of the major breakthroughs in understanding the female reproductive cycle was achieved by the American scientist George W. Corner in the late 1920s. He showed that menstrual bleeding was prevented in the first half of the month by oestrogen produced in the ovaries, and stopped in the second half by progesterone secreted from the corpus luteum. Corner also pointed out that menstrual bleeding occurred with the decline of corpus luteum and the discontinuance of progesterone. This discovery was crucial in refuting the long-held belief that ovulation coincided with menstruation. Scientists and medical experts now came to the critical realization that ovulation occurred mid-cycle.[18] Equipped with such information, scientists now had a much clearer idea about when to intervene in the reproductive process and which hormones to use as a contraceptive for preventing ovulation.

Steroidal hormones and early searches for an oral contraceptive

At the same time that knowledge about the reproductive cycle and the mechanism of hormones was deepening, a small number of scientists were beginning to apply this information to developing an oral contraceptive. Scientists in various countries began to undertake investigations into a range of substances. Such research was not easy. One of the problems was to find cheap supplies of hormones. Most hormones in the interwar years were derived from vast quantities of animal organs or by-products and the process of extraction was long and expensive. In order to get their hormonal supplies, scientists were dependent on an intricate network linking abattoirs, hospitals and stud farms.[19] Moreover, much of the investment in hormonal research and production during this period was focused on treatments for gynaecological and obstetrical disorders and not contraception. Few companies were willing to invest in the contraceptive aspects of hormones for fear of social disapproval. In 1933, for instance, the Dutch company Organon refused to test a female hormonal preparation, Menformon, for contraceptive purposes. Yet they had been perfectly willing to test the product as an alleviation of menstrual complaints. Company officials saw its use as a contraceptive as a venture that would spark hostility not only among the public but also among Dutch clinicians and general practitioners, who saw oral birth control as dangerous to women's health.[20]

Similar reservations occurred in Britain in the case of a non-steroidal oestrogen compound called stilboestrol (diethylstilboestrol in the United States). This had been developed by the eminent biochemist Sir Charles Dodds (1899–1973), while he was working at the University of London. Financed by the Medical Research Council (MRC), a government-sponsored institution, stilboestrol proved to be two and a half times more potent than the naturally occurring female oestrogens. Described by contemporaries as a 'brilliant achievement of modern chemistry', stilboestrol had attracted attention in the British medical press by the late 1930s for its ability to cause temporary sterility.[21] While MRC officials were initially proud of the development of stilboestrol, they were less than enthusiastic about its use as a contraceptive. Not only did they see this as an unprofitable venture, but also more importantly they feared that the drug, because it could also be used to prevent the implantation of a fertilized egg, might be used for the highly illegal alternative purpose of abortion, which was regarded as a major social problem during these years.[22] For this reason stilboestrol was placed on the British official list of poisons in 1939.[23]

Reservations about the use of hormones for contraceptive purposes, however, were not universal. Those campaigning for the extension of sterilization of the 'unfit' in Europe and the United States, for example, were enthusiastic about their use. For such people, hormones represented a way of finding a non-surgical method of sterilization. In the United

States, for instance, where some of the earliest compulsory sterilization measures had been implemented, Raphael Kurzok highlighted oestrone as a possible means of inducing temporary sterilization when he addressed a conference in New York in 1936. Four years later K. J. Karnasky in Texas also identified stilboestrol as a potential method of sterilization. Neither Kurzok nor Karnasky, however, followed up these ideas.[24]

However, the Austrian physiologist Ludwig Haberlandt, based at the University of Innsbruck, was one researcher who pursued the contraceptive significance of hormonal agents further in the interwar years. From his perspective this project was important for addressing socioeconomic and political conditions in Austria and German-speaking lands in the immediate aftermath of the First World War. Like many social reformers in this period, Haberlandt was acutely aware of the economic plight of many large families as a result of demobilization, severe unemployment and supply problems. Part of his aim was to find a hormonal contraceptive which the medical profession and government could use for sterilization. Haberlandt's ideas, however, reflected a more general shift in social opinion that was beginning to favour contraception.[25] One of his motives in developing a hormonal contraceptive was to enable women to space their births, reduce family size and gain a temporary respite from pregnancy when they suffered from ill-health. For him contraception would pave the way to human happiness.[26]

Whatever Haberlandt's motivations, he had successfully conducted a series of animal experiments by 1927, proving the contraceptive value of ovarian and placental extracts.[27] By the late 1920s he was negotiating with the German-based pharmaceutical firms E. Merck and I. G. Farben to produce a progesterone-based hormonal contraceptive. Neither of these companies, however, were willing to take on the project. Despite the increasing use of contraception among couples in these years, research into contraception remained highly taboo. Haberlandt himself was denied promotion in his own academic institution because of the hostility of the Catholic lobby to his contraceptive work. Despite these difficulties, in 1928 Haberlandt secured an agreement to develop his hormonal contraceptive with Gedeon Richter, a Hungarian company producing hormones, based in Budapest. By 1930 the company had commercially registered a compound called Infecundin. Haberlandt faced problems getting the product tested on humans because he was not a clinician. Although he approached a number of physicians to try out the drug as a hormonal contraceptive in women, no one was willing to support it.[28]

Though Haberlandt himself died prematurely in 1932, his product was tested at a women's hospital in Innsbruck in 1934. The results of this research were never published. The drug, however, had its commercial registration renewed in 1940 and 1950. Infecundin, or a similar substance called Profecundin, is also rumoured to have been promoted in Germany during 1942. What it was used for remains unknown. Employers at Gedeon Richter deny ever having marketed the product as a contraceptive during the 1930s and 1940s. Nonetheless, in 1966 Gedeon Richter, by then a state-owned company, promoted Infecundin as the first Hungarian contraceptive pill. This might have been a derivation of the original substance.[29]

While Haberlandt experimented with natural hormones, others were beginning to investigate the possibilities of synthetic steroidal hormones. One of these was the orally active progestational agent developed in 1938. Produced by Hans H. Inhoffen (b. 1906) and other scientists working for Schering laboratories in Berlin, this substance proved (in tests on rabbits) more potent when taken by mouth than pure progesterone. Trials with women showed that, when swallowed, it was six times more potent than injections of pure progesterone.[30] Inhoffen also synthesized two compounds which had high oestrogenic potency. The first was 17α-ethinyloestradiol which had a high oestrogen activity when taken by mouth. The second was 17α-ethinyltestosterone, generically known as ethisterone. Developed from the male hormone testosterone, ethisterone exhibited unexpected progestational (female) characteristics. Yet, while such oestrogenic compounds were recognized as early as 1945 for their contraceptive value, it was to take another two decades before they were officially used for this purpose. Ethisterone, for instance, became a key oestrogenic component of oral contraceptives in later years.[31]

Hormones were not the only substances investigated for their oral contraceptive value. In 1935 N. C. Nag had found that injecting rats with oil from a plant called the *Pisum sativum linn*, a common field pea in India, prevented or greatly reduced pregnancy. Metaxylohydroquinone was discovered to be the active ingredient in this process. By 1949 S. N. Sanyal, an Indian scientist based at the Calcutta Bacteriological Institute, had manufactured a pill from metaxylohydroquinone. In June 1953 the pill began to be tested on women enlisted at Baleodas maternity hospital in Calcutta. Most of these women came from low income groups and had minimal education. Few had used contraception before. Running for two years, the trial included a total of 727 women. Most of these subjects were divided into two groups: 427 patients who visited the hospital clinic, and 232 patients who were visited by health visitors in their own home. Each patient was expected to take the pill on certain days before the expected onset of menstruation. Reported in the international medical press, the research showed the drug to be between 50 and 75 per cent effective in preventing pregnancy, and to have no adverse effects.[32] Later the Indian government also sponsored a trial with the substance under the auspices of the All India Institute of Hygiene and Public Health, Calcutta. Results from this research were similar to those of the trials carried out at Baleodas hospital.[33] Despite its promising results, however, the pea pill never became a marketable oral contraceptive, both because of its low rate of efficacy and its difficulty in attracting international funding.

Another plant explored for its contraceptive properties was *Lithospermum ruderale*. Bearing white-petalled flowers and coming from the same family as the forget-me-not, the plant was known to grow in the American desert as well as in English hedgerows and cornfields.[34] Interest in the plant had been awakened because Shoshone Indians, a tribe living in Nevada in the United States, were known to use it for preventing pregnancy. In 1949 Dr B. P. Wiesner, a human fertility specialist, together with the physiologist Professor John Yudkin, began to experiment with the plant on mice. Conducted at London University these investigations showed the plant to be 100 per cent effective in inhibiting the oestrus cycle in mice.[35] In 1952 the drug was tried on four British housewives for one menstrual cycle, and showed itself to be an effective suppresser of ovulation. With such promising results, Yudkin and Wiesner began to look for ways to cultivate and synthesize the plant on a larger scale. Joining in on the venture was the company Stafford Allen and Co. Ltd.[36]

Lithospermum extracts also sparked great interest in the Medical Research Council in the UK, which provided laboratory facilities for a chemist, De Laslo, to investigate its contraceptive properties. This support is particularly striking when we recall the MRC's reluctance to push stilboestrol as a contraceptive in the 1930s.[37] *Lithospermum* extracts were just one of a number of other possible contraceptives explored by the MRC in the 1950s. Part of this reflected the increasing anxiety about population growth during this decade. A number of MRC officials expressed a desire to 'find a method of contraception that might be acceptable and practicable in backward and overpopulated countries'.[38] Nothing, however, came of *Lithospermum*, or the other compounds investigated by the MRC in these years. This partly stemmed from the reluctance of the MRC to pursue such research openly. Despite their desire to help with the population question, MRC officials did not want the institution's name associated with such a venture for fear of its social and political consequences. In 1953 an MRC representative, Himsworth, admitted to the reproductive biologist Alan Parkes: 'a public body like the Council must proceed with considerable circumspection in promoting work in a subject like the control of fertility.' He stressed:

> To you and me the objections that might be raised may appear irrational. But I think it would be a mistake to underrate them and so run the risk of exposing scientific work on the whole subject of fertility to obstruction and possibly interference. For this reason, much as I dislike doing so, I should refrain from advertising any work in this field even when, as is the case, the probability is strong that the substances alleged to have relevant actions will be introduced for human use, and we have ample justification for investigating in animals their possible modes of action and dangers.[39]

Overall the MRC regarded contraceptive research as 'an occasional sideline' rather than central to their research programme.[40]

Another substance explored for its contraceptive properties was a soluble form of hesperidin, a chemical product derived from a fruit that resembled the structure of an orange. Explored orginally for its anti-haemorrhagic effect, phosphorylated hesperidin was discovered in the late 1940s to have potential as a contraceptive in men and women. Between 1949 and 1952 animal and human investigations were carried out in Massachusetts. This included a clinical trial of 300 couples with the substance for a period of 30 months. These were married couples of varying ages with proven fertility. While the substance was found to have some contraceptive effect, it was regarded as unreliable and was never adopted as a contraceptive.[41]

Initiating and funding research for the first marketable contraceptive pill

While it is clear that researchers were conducting tests to discover an oral contraceptive from the late 1940s into the 1950s, many found it difficult to obtain money to do such research. The hesitation of the MRC indicates the general difficulties investigators faced during this period. Although research money existed for basic scientific research into endocrinology and reproductive physiology through philanthropic organizations such as the Rockefeller Foundation, little investment was available for exploring how this research might be applied to practical contraceptive technology.[42]

Significantly it had been an individual American philanthropist, Clarence Gamble (1894–1966), and not a government body, who had initiated and funded the clinical trials with the Indian field pea, *Pisum sativum linn*. Inheriting a fortune from Proctor and Gamble Company, the manufacturer of Ivory soap, Gamble had little to fear in terms of his social status. Originally trained as a physician, from 1925 he began to deploy his money in testing the efficacy of new contraceptives around the world. From his perspective, such research was crucial for making birth control medically and socially respectable. His sponsorship of the trials in India was one of many initiatives he undertook in the contraceptive field.[43]

It was to be the enthusiasm and drive of Margaret Sanger which proved critical to the development of the first marketable pill. As early as 1912 Sanger had expressed the hope of finding a 'magic pill' for contraception.[44] This was part of her long-term strategy to improve access to birth control. Sanger's zeal for this quest had been awakened by her own personal experiences. The sixth of eleven children, she was born in Corning, New York in 1879. Her parents were first generation Irish-American Catholics, who had been uprooted from County Cork by the great famine. She had grown up in the midst of a large and devout Catholic Irish immigrant community, and was baptised at the age of 13. Her first real friendships were formed with churchgoing Catholic girls who, even as they attended Mass every Sunday, would ridicule the frocked parish priests. Her father Michael Higgins, a stonemason by trade, preached socialism and was contemptuous of religious authority, and he had a continuous struggle to gain work given that most of it depended on cutting gravestones for church cemeteries. By contrast her mother, born Anne Purcell, was a pious Catholic, whose religious faith helped her keep the family together in the face of eviction and deprivation. Margaret remembered her mother constantly coughing in terrible pain because of chronic tuberculosis and wasting away as a result of constant pregnancies that weakened her resistance to the disease. She died at the age of 50. Later on Margaret was to blame her parents' ignorance about contraception for the harsh life her mother had experienced, as well as her premature death. Margaret dedicated her first book to the memory of her mother, 'who gave birth to eleven living children'.[45]

Originally wishing to be a doctor but finding it difficult to enter medical school because of sexual discrimination and educational and financial constraints, Sanger enrolled in training to be a nurse shortly after her mother's death in 1899. Married in 1902, Margaret soon experienced some of the health problems she had witnessed in her mother. Having suffered tuberculosis herself, and pregnant within six months of marriage, she quickly deteriorated physically and mentally. Advised against a further pregnancy on health grounds, Margaret and her husband faced the dilemma encountered by young and passionate couples at a time when access to reliable contraception was still limited. Her distaste for condoms and the withdrawal method in later years might indeed have come from the personal frustrations she experienced during this time. After she bore two more children in 1908 and 1909 Margaret and her husband soon faced the financial hardships that forced her to take up nursing again to support the family. Working on the Lower East Side of New York, where she witnessed the ill-health and deaths of many women who resorted to illegal abortion to cope with constant childbearing, she became even more resolved in her fight for greater access to contraception and began to envisage a contraceptive pill. In mounting this campaign, she argued against the Catholic doctrine forbidding contraception, charging the church with aligning itself 'on the side of ignorance against knowledge, of darkness against light'.[46]

By the end of her life Sanger had married twice and openly admitted to having had at least four lovers. Her diary entry of 1914 captures her delight in and enjoyment of sex: 'I love being ravaged by romances.'[47] Years later a friend, Mabel Dodge, recalled that Sanger was 'the first person I ever knew who was openly an ardent propagandist for the joys of the flesh'.[48] Sanger's campaign for contraception, therefore, was not only bound with up with a fight to improve women's health, but also to give women the sexual freedom already enjoyed by men. Despite facing a jail sentence in the early 1900s, and a great deal of opposition throughout the early twentieth century, by the time of her death Sanger had established a number of birth control clinics in the United States and an international organization, together with several journals, to promote scientific efforts to improve contraceptive methods.[49] Moreover, it was Sanger who provided the impetus for developing the first contraceptive pill.

For Sanger it was vital to find a contraceptive technique that would grant women full control over their fertility without the cooperation of the male as was necessitated by barrier contraceptive methods. Ideally she saw this as something that could be taken by mouth and not at the moment of intercourse. Writing to a friend in 1946, she summed up the strength of her feelings on the matter: 'I was feeling more and more despondent as I saw and realized more than ever the inadequacy of the diaphragm reaching millions of women who need and should have something as simple as a birth control pill.'[50]

In looking to boost contraceptive research, Sanger found a powerful ally in Katherine Dexter McCormick. Born into an aristocratic family in Michigan in 1875, Katherine was the second of two children of Writ Dexter, one of Chicago's most successful lawyers, and came from a family which had long ties with Harvard and Harvard Law School. In 1904 she became the second woman ever to graduate from Massachusetts Institute of Technology, majoring in biology.[51] That same year she married Stanley McCormick, heir to the fortune of Cyrus McCormick, inventor of the reaper and founder of the International Harvester Company. Having married into wealth, however, Katherine found herself trapped with a man who, within two years, turned out to suffer from schizophrenia.[52] In 1909 she won legal control of her husband's estate when Stanley was declared legally insane, and she began to immerse herself into the woman's suffrage issue, becoming the vice-president and treasurer of the National American Woman's Suffrage Association, an organization which in 1919 helped to secure women's right to vote in the United States.[53]

After meeting Sanger in 1917, Katherine Dexter McCormick also began to invest some of her time in birth control issues, becoming one of the European travellers who smuggled diaphragms into the United States during the 1920s in order to supply Sanger's contraceptive clinics. Like Sanger, McCormick saw contraception as the key to improving women's position. Part of her interest in contraception might have stemmed from her own marriage and a desire to prevent conception of children who risked inheriting the same affliction as her husband. Moreover, her decision not to have children had to be balanced against constant sexual demands from her husband.[54] Significantly, in 1958 McCormick remarked that she 'didn't give a hoot for a male contraceptive', and all that concerned her was a female one.[55] Four years after the pill was officially launched McCormick reiterated her desire for a contraceptive which met the needs of women. As she wrote,

The oral contraceptive inaugurated and maintains a new era of sex relations for mankind, – fundamentally it is a sex revolution for human beings ... The oral contraceptive vitally concerns women and their bodies. I think that women do not care to have mechanical gadgets of one kind or another introduced into the innermost parts of their bodies, and that is solely a man's point of view that they do not object to this procedure.[56]

Like Sanger, McCormick saw a 'fool-proof' contraceptive as an important weapon in the fight against population growth.[57]

For twenty years McCormick corresponded with Sanger about furthering contraceptive research. Since she was trained in biology, McCormick had the necessary scientific background for understanding the research needed to achieve a contraceptive pill. Her marriage to Stanley McCormick also provided her with vast financial resources. In the words of John Rock, the obstetrician who planned the human trials of the first marketable pill, McCormick was 'as rich as Croesus. She had a *vast* fortune ... she couldn't even spend the interest on her *interest.*'[58] Prior to her husband's death in 1947, however, McCormick was restricted in the amount she could devote to contraceptive research because much of her fortune was invested in neuropsychiatric investigations in an effort to find a cure for schizophrenia to help her husband.[59]

In 1950 McCormick began to consult Sanger in earnest about the best way to invest her money in contraceptive research. Sanger recommended the distribution of $100,000 a year to several university laboratories to promote contraceptive projects.[60] Bureaucratic procedures involved in settling her late husband's estate, however, temporarily prevented McCormick from pursuing this line. In March 1952 Sanger alerted McCormick to the possibilities of funding a new avenue of research. This was the work of Gregory Goodwin Pincus.[61] Sanger had met Pincus through Abraham Stone, an associate of the Planned Parenthood Federation of America and director of the Margaret Sanger Research Bureau in New York. During this meeting she had managed to persuade Pincus to consider directing his work towards contraception.[62] Pincus was later to acknowledge that he 'invented the pill at the request of a woman'.[63]

Nicknamed 'Goody', Gregory Pincus was born in Woodbine, New Jersey in 1903 to Jewish parents who had migrated to the United States from Russia in the nineteenth century. The oldest son of a teacher and editor of a farm journal, and nephew to a dean of the agricultural college of Rutgers University, Pincus had originally wanted to become a farmer. Starting his studies at Cornell University in the 1920s he set his sights on becoming a pomologist, an apple specialist. Soon, however, his studies in biology and his intellectual interests took him into the field of genetics and embryology. One of his colleagues attributed Pincus's fascination with genetics to the fact that he was colour-blind, a condition that is inherited. Blessed with a photographic memory, Pincus could digest information very fast.[64]

Gaining an undergraduate degree at Cornell and then a doctorate at Harvard, Pincus soon made a name for himself as an expert on the process of reproduction. As we have seen (p. 34 above), prior to meeting Sanger, he had already courted controversy and attracted media attention with his work to create 'fatherless rabbits'. By the time Sanger met Pincus in 1950 he had managed to co-found and become co-director of the Worcester Foundation for Experimental Biology. Established in 1944, and based in Worcester, Massachusetts, this institution specialized in steroidal research and was a key clearing centre for testing the physiological effects of new steroidal compounds produced by pharmaceutical companies. Pincus himself had become a consultant for several of the pharmaceutical companies, including G. D. Searle in Chicago and Syntex in Mexico.[65] Much of the investigation into the compounds sent by the pharmaceutical firms was to see whether they could be used to treat diseases such as cancer and arthritis, and other nervous and mental conditions such as schizophrenia.[66] Under the direction of Pincus, investigations were also conducted on the process of fertilization in order to find ways of preventing spontaneous abortion and menstrual disorders.[67]

Pincus thus had access to many of the latest discoveries in steroid chemistry, placing him in an ideal position to carry out the hormonal contraceptive research proposed by Sanger. Moreover, the fact that the Worcester Foundation was an independent, non-profit, tax-privileged educational and research institution allowed him much greater freedom to explore the controversial issue of contraception – as we have seen, it would not have been so easy had he been based within a university or government-sponsored establishment.[68] For Pincus, Sanger's contraceptive project also represented a potentially lucrative source of funding for the Foundation.

Spurred on by Sanger, Pincus managed to get $6,500 (equivalent to $43,000 today) from the PPFA between 1951 and 1952 to study hormonal contraception.[69] This allowed Pincus and his colleagues to study the oral administration of progesterone in animals. From these studies it seemed feasible that Pincus could develop an oral contraceptive. Despite its promising results, however, the PPFA was reluctant to fund the project further.

From their perspective the research did not differ from animal experiments being conducted elsewhere, such as those at the National Drug Company in Philadelphia.[70] Within the PPFA Pincus's work was also viewed with suspicion because it did not conform to the organization's 'accepted social code', which involved research into existing methods of birth control or projects undertaken by medical doctors in clinical settings. In the eyes of PPFA officials, the development of a pill was too risky in terms of its potential side-effects and ineffectiveness. Any flaw in the project would, they feared, backfire badly on the organization and the family planning movement as a whole.[71]

While the PPFA was reluctant to fund Pincus further, McCormick was excited about his work. She had never met Pincus, but was familiar with the Worcester Foundation, having collaborated with its other co-director, Hudson Hoagland, through her sponsorship of research into schizophrenia.[72] In May 1952 McCormick, then aged 76, moved from Santa Barbara to Boston with the intention of following Pincus's work. By June 1953 she had agreed to pay $10,000 a year towards the pill project.[73] This sum was subsequently increased to meet whatever expenses Pincus incurred, including $50,000 to build a new animal house and funds for extra building space to expedite the human trials.[74] McCormick saw this money as crucial in freeing Pincus from what she saw as the frustratingly bureaucratic red-tape of the PPFA.[75] By 1960 McCormick had provided over $1 million for clinically testing the drug. Data from these trials provided the basis on which the US Food and Drug Administration (FDA) approved the first pill.[76] McCormick's funds were not only vital to the development of the pill, but also necessary to the overall financial well-being of the Worcester Foundation. For the remainder of her life McCormick gave the foundation donations of between $150,000 and $180,00 a year. She also left the foundation $1 million in her will. Overall, her contribution to the pill project amounted to over $2 million (equivalent to $12 million today).[77]

One of the most important facets of McCormick's funding was its flexibility and her ability to contribute money at short notice.[78] Moreover, McCormick's financial support started at a significant moment, in 1953, when insufficient funds threatened to halt Pincus's work.[79] Not only was Pincus failing to get money from the PPFA, but few pharmaceutical companies were willing to help him in his research.[80] One of the most pressing problems at this time was finding a sponsor for human clinical trials, which were costly to set up and run. The overall illegality of contraceptive research made this difficult. In 1953, for instance, a philanthropist withdrew previously promised money for the human trials of Pincus's project on discovering that they were to be conducted in Massachusetts where the Comstock laws still forbade contraceptive research.[81] This problem, however, never prevented McCormick's sponsorship.[82]

McCormick not only stands out because of her financial support, but also because of her highly active interest in the day-to-day running of the project. She moved from the warmth of Santa Barbara, California, where she had originally been based to Boston, in order to keep an eye on Pincus and his work. Her words 'freezing in Boston for the pill' written in 1955 capture the essence of her commitment.[83] As had been the case with all her previous charitable contributions, McCormick was scrupulous about following the progress of the pill. Heavy-set and formidable in appearance, McCormick was not a figure to be dismissed easily. As Pincus recalled, she was not an 'insignificant nothing, she was tall and carried herself like a ramrod. Little old woman she was *not*. She was a grenadier.'[84] If a project did not meet her expectations, McCormick was quite capable of withdrawing her interest and financial support forthwith.[85]

McCormick not only paid meticulous attention to the details of the pill research but took a keen interest in trying to solve problems. In doing this she was careful to listen to the advice of others and would spend hours 'over every aspect of each problem to make sure that the ultimate result, regardless of time and expense' measured up to her objectives.[86] From 1954, when Pincus began to set up the initial human trials with the obstetrician John Rock, through to 1960 when the first pill was officially marketed, McCormick was in regular contact with Pincus. She was constantly giving constructive criticism, some of which was acted upon. Pincus, for instance, looked seriously into McCormick's suggestions for employing particular personnel.[87] McCormick's letters indicate that she understood the complicated scientific nature of the experiments and clinical trials. Part of this stemmed from her biological training at university. In addition to examining the minutiae of the scientific and clinical methodology to be used in the laboratory, and consultation on staff, she helped evaluate the sites for the trials as well as the types of patients who were suitable.[88] The high esteem in which Pincus held McCormick can be surmised from the dedication to her in his book, which read, 'to Mrs Stanley McCormick because of her steadfast faith in scientific inquiry and her unswerving encouragement of human dignity.'[89] Sanger, by contrast, did not always grasp the fine mechanics of the science involved in the research. For this she relied on McCormick.[90]

Conclusion

By the Second World War not only had scientists gained a better understanding of reproductive physiology, they had come closer to understanding the precise mechanism that could prevent human pregnancy. In 1945 Professor Fuller Albright (1900–69) of Harvard University, who had been conducting research into menstrual cycles and ovulation during late 1930s and 1940s, argued that fertility could be controlled by a combination of oestrogen and progesterone. Juggling with oestrogen and progesterone, scientists would be able not only to suppress ovulation but also to determine the timing of a woman's menstruation. The medications he suggested were stilboestrol with progesterone.[91] Albright's proposed formula for birth control was remarkably similar to the one later used in developing the first marketable pill.

What is surprising about Albright's idea is that it was not taken up during these years. After all, both stilboestrol and progesterone were available at that time. Stilboestrol, for example, while never patented or sold commercially in Britain, had been seized on and marketed by non-British pharmaceutical companies. By the 1940s the drug was being widely prescribed in the United States and the Netherlands for the prevention of miscarriage and was also being fed to farm animals. However, researchers were wary about using stilboestrol for contraceptive purposes. Part of this caution was linked to the fear that it might produce cancer in humans if taken for long periods.[92] Enthusiasm for using progesterone for contraceptive purposes was also thwarted by the fact that during these years natural progesterone had a low effectivity when taken orally. When given intramuscularly progesterone also frequently caused a severe reaction at the site of the injection.[93]

Lastly Albright's suggestion appeared 'in an obscure journal and in a book with limited readership'.[94] In many ways this reflected the lack of value attached to contraceptive research overall. Despite promising compounds and advances in reproductive endocrinology, few scientists were willing to look for a contraceptive pill for fear of losing their scientific reputation. Those who were willing to take the risk had little institutional or financial support to undertake such a venture.

Katharine Dexter McCormick's investment in Pincus's research marked a turning point in the long search for a contraceptive pill. Writing in 1956, nine months after the launch of the first large-scale clinical trials, Sanger summed up the significance of McCormick's contribution:

Dear Kay, You must, indeed, feel a certain pride in your judgement. Gregory Pincus had been working for at least ten years on the progesterone of reproductive process in animals. He had practically no money for this work and Dr Stone and I did our best to get a few dollars for him and I think that that amount we collected went to pay the expenses of Chang [senior scientist, Worcester Foundation]. Then you came along with your fine interest and enthusiasm – with your faith and wonderful directives – [and] things began to happen and at last the reports ... are now out in the outstanding scientific magazine and the conspiracy of silence has been broken.[95]

It remained to be seen, however, whether McCormick's investment and faith would achieve the safe and effective pill she and Sanger so desired.

3
Sexual Chemistry

In accepting the challenge of Margaret Sanger and Katherine McCormick to develop a contraceptive pill, Gregory Pincus like his predecessors needed to find a compound that would be cheap and effective. The interwar years had witnessed a significant growth in the number of compounds and hormones available for research. Many of the hormones available at this time, however, were very expensive and largely ineffective unless administered in very large doses. This remained a major stumbling block to the development of an oral contraceptive. By the early 1950s, however, when Pincus began to look for a suitable compound to develop a pill, there had been a major breakthrough in steroid chemistry. The source of this revolution was a species of wild yam found growing in the heart of Mexico. Providing chemists with a rich source for manufacturing cheaper synthetic hormones, the yam provided the key to a cheaper hormonal contraceptive than could have been possible before its discovery. Many stages, however, had to be passed before the precise compound was found.

While initially marketed and branded as an American product, the pill was the result of expertise of many chemists throughout the world. Its chemical evolution was strongly intertwined with the rise of a lucrative European sex hormone industry in the early twentieth century, and the migration of many European refugee chemists to the United States and Latin America in the wake of Nazism and the Second World War. The development of the pill was also closely linked to the rising interest in corticoids during the Second World War as a means of reducing stress among pilots, and the discovery of the anti-arthritic drug cortisone in 1949.

In fact, the pill's development profited from the rush to devise better and cheaper ways to synthesize cortisone.

The sex hormone industry in the interwar years

When scientists began in the early twentieth century to investigate the possibility of a hormonal contraceptive pill, the chief source of sex hormones was animal organs and by-products. The proportional amount of hormone yielded was minuscule, however. Scientists therefore needed a vast number of organs and animal by-products, such as urine and bile, before they could produce large quantities of sex hormones. In 1930, for instance, the ovaries of 80,000 sows were required to extract even a tiny fraction of oestrogen. Similarly, in 1931 the German biochemist Adolf Butenandt had to collect 25,000 litres of men's urine in the police barracks of Berlin in order to isolate a mere 50 mg of pure androsterone, one of the male hormones. Given the need for the massive number of organs to supply the hormones, it is not surprising that some of the first companies to provide hormones had strong ties with the meat industry. The Dutch firm Organon, for instance, which was one of the pioneering companies in this area, and later in the manufacture of the pill, was jointly established in 1923 by a pharmacologist, Ernest Laqueur, and an abattoir owner, Saal van Zwanenburg.[1]

Most of the hormonal products available in the interwar period also had to be taken in large quantities orally in order to be effective. Hormones were thus expensive to manufacture and very limited in supply. Progesterone, for example, which scientists first looked at with an eye to developing an oral contraceptive, was so expensive during the 1930s that its use was confined to the highly profitable business of improving the fertility of world-class racehorses.[2]

By the 1930s scientists across the world were intensifying their search for a new means of manufacturing larger and cheaper quantities of sex hormones. One way of doing this was to find ways of synthesizing the hormones. The major advantage they had was that sex hormones are relatively easy to manipulate in the laboratory. Chemically, sex hormones are steroids, which means that they are organic molecules that share a common structure. All steroids have a common honeycomb-like structure consisting of carbon and hydrogen atoms, usually oxygen, and sometimes one or two other elements.[3] These atoms are arranged in four fused rings.

A representation of the basic steroid nucleus of a hormone is shown in figure 3.1 below.

Thousands of hormonal compounds are based on the basic four-ring steroid skeleton. This includes not only sex hormones, but also adreno-cortical hormones (also known as corticosteroids and corticoids), which are crucial for regulating the body's metabolism. Very minor variations in this skeleton, such as switching the double bonds within and between the four rings, determine both the chemical properties of individual compounds and their biological effects, ranging from mineral glucose and protein metabolism to reproduction.[4] Female hormones such as progesterone and oestrogen, for instance, are not that dissimilar in chemical structure from the male hormone testosterone. The simplicity of the structure of steroids therefore makes it relatively easy to modify them chemically; all that is needed are minor changes in the steroidal molecular structure. Indeed this process is constantly occurring. Within the human body, for instance, cholesterol is transformed into progesterone (pregnancy hormone) when in the corpus luteum, and while in the testes progesterone is transformed into testosterone (male hormone). Similarly, in the ovaries testosterone is converted into oestradiol. As figure 3.2 shows, the steroid cholesterol can therefore be made into the female hormone oestradiol, having been already converted into first the progesterone intermediary and then the testosterone intermediary. It can also be used to make cortisone, having originally been transformed into progesterone. By the 1930s chemists had devised a way of mimicking these natural bodily processes to make synthetic hormones. With just a few chemical steps, they were able to change male

Figure 3.1 Basic steroid structure

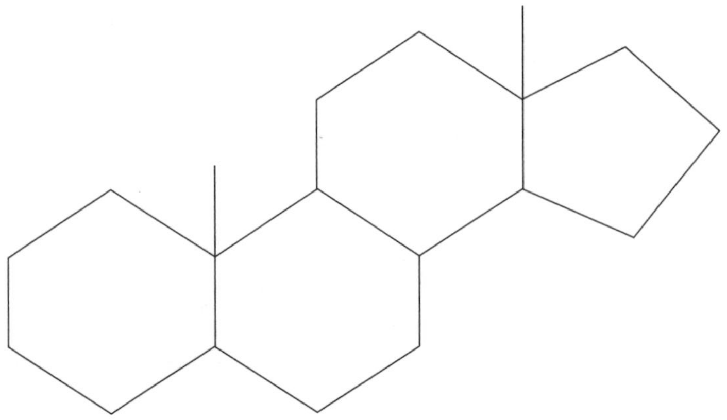

Figure 3.2 Steroid structure of cholesterol, cortisone and three sex hormones, and how they are metabolized and changed in the body

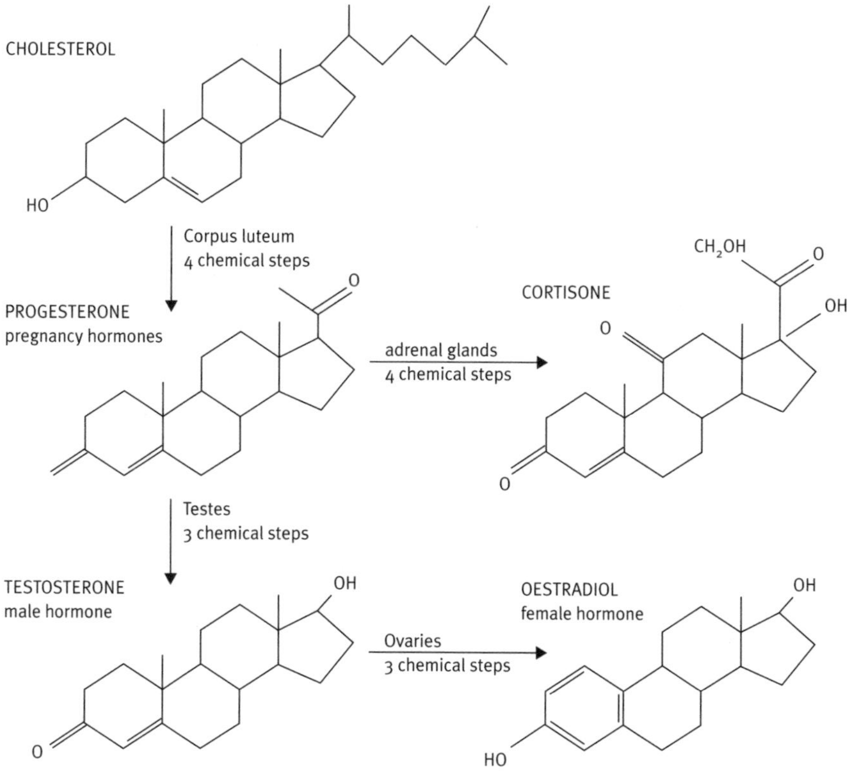

CHOLESTEROL

HO

Corpus luteum
4 chemical steps

PROGESTERONE
pregnancy hormones

CORTISONE

CH_2OH

adrenal glands
4 chemical steps

Testes
3 chemical steps

TESTOSTERONE
male hormone

OH

OESTRADIOL
female hormone

Ovaries
3 chemical steps

HO

OH

Source: L. J. Kaplan and R. Tong, *Controlling our Reproductive Destiny* (Cambridge, Mass., 1994), 68, fig. 4.2.

hormones into female hormones and vice versa. They also discovered a way of converting corticosteroids into sex hormones.[5]

By the 1930s chemists and biochemists working in close collaboration with clinicians had managed to manufacture a number of synthetic hormones in the laboratory which had similar actions to natural hormones. Between 1929 and 1938 a number of sex hormones, such as progesterone, had been isolated in their pure form. Scientists had also found ways of making corticoids. Together with these achievements they were also expanding their ability to synthesize new hormonal compounds. In doing this work they were helped by the fact that steroids can be found abundantly in nature. Indeed, there was an explosion of chemical research into steroids during the 1930s and 1940s.[6]

As the research increased so the pressure grew to find new ways of manufacturing steroids. While many of the first sex hormones were initially isolated from tons of sows' ovaries, bulls' testes, and the urine of animals and humans, by the 1930s scientists were using other raw materials as their starting base. One of the first of these raw materials exploited for developing synthetic sex hormones was cholesterol.[7] By chemically modifying the steroidal structure of cholesterol, scientists found that they could synthesize the female and male hormones. This was quite different from the extractive methods used in isolating hormones from animal organs and by-products. Cholesterol also had the advantage in that it was in plentiful supply. It could be found in fish oils and in animal fats, such as the brains and spinal cords of cattle.[8]

Nonetheless, despite its abundance, the modification process of cholesterol took a long time, making production costs high. The price of hormones synthesized in this way was thus prohibitive. Even once large-scale production was established, synthetic sex hormones were extremely expensive. The price of progesterone, for instance, was $1,000 per gram during the 1930s. Part of this stemmed from the huge quantities of raw materials needed. Butenandt, for example, required a ton of cholesterol, acquired from bovine brains and spinal cords, and the grease of sheep's wool, in order to make 20 lb of the starting material to produce commercial quantities of progesterone.[9] The high cost of synthetic sex hormones was also attributable to the fact that three European companies, Organon, CIBA and Schering, held the key patent rights for synthesizing sex hormones.[10]

The arrival of the Mexican Yam: *Dioscorea*

By the late 1930s pharmaceutical companies across the world were sponsoring academic scientists to find an alternative raw material to cholesterol. A number of researchers had discovered that steroidal compounds found in plants (sapogenins) resembled the chemical structure of cholesterol. One particularly important sapogenin, for instance, later used in the development of the first marketable pill, was diosgenin, isolated by Japanese chemists in 1936 from the plant *Dioscorea tokoro*.[11] Roots from the lily family (including the sarsaparilla root, yucca, agave and true yam) were also known to contain large quantities of sapogenins.[12]

A key pharmaceutical company exploring plant steroids during the 1930s was Parke-Davis, which was keen to defend its position as the leading producer of hormones in the United States against increasing competition from European companies. One of the main scientists they supported in this field was Russell Marker, an American organic chemist based at Pennsylvania State University in Philadelphia. Brilliant, yet volatile, Marker was particularly adept at constructing chemical methods which were efficient at producing high yields of pure crystalline substances from complex organic materials. During the late 1930s Marker achieved a major breakthrough in synthesizing sex steroids while working with the sarsaparilla root. By 1940, he had developed a five-stage chemical process for the conversion of sapogenins into progesterone, which, taken three stages further, produced the male hormone testosterone.[13]

Armed with this process, Marker began to look for new plants that contained larger quantities of sapogenins. Funded by Parke-Davis, Marker led expeditions in the summer of 1940 in the south-west of the United States (Texas) and Mexico to collect different plants in order to screen them for their sapogenin content. With the aid of 17 American and Mexican botanists, Marker collected more than 400 different species.[14] Of all the plants investigated in his laboratory, Marker found that the wild Mexican yam *Cabeza de negro* yielded the highest amount of the sapogenin diosgenin, which he then used to synthesize progesterone.[15] Marker realized that *Cabeza de negro*, when converted with his five-stage process, provided the long-sought alternative raw material needed for the cheap production of sex hormones.

Above all, Marker understood that this plant could provide the means to break the European monopoly in hormone production. Up to this point, five European-based companies, CIBA (Basel), Schering AG (Berlin), Bohringer (Mannheim), Roussel (Paris) and Organon (Amsterdam), had dominated hormonal investigation and production.[16] These companies not only had a strong hold on patents, but were the main suppliers of the female hormones progesterone and oestrone, and the male hormone testosterone. Testosterone was important because it could be manipulated to make analogues of female hormones. In 1937 the five major European companies drew up a joint agreement which allowed them to deploy each others' inventions.[17] American companies were unable to break this monopoly because they were less advanced in steroidal hormone research and held fewer patents. The only steroidal hormone produced in the United States was the female hormone oestrone which was supplied by Parke-Davis.[18]

Entrepreneurs, refugee scientists and the establishment of a Mexican steroid industry

Russell Marker could not break the European cartel alone, neither could he do it from his base in Pennsylvania. From his perspective the only way forward was to set up an industrial laboratory in Mexico. His original funder, Parke-Davis, was unwilling to finance such a project, however. From the company's point of view the initial investment outweighed the potential profits that could be recouped. Alternative sources for steroids were developing during this period and Parke-Davis officials felt these were easier to exploit. Soya beans, for instance, which could be grown in the United States under conditions that could be more closely controlled than in Mexico, were considered a more promising raw material. Other methods for synthesizing hormones were also emerging.[19] Moreover, Parke-Davis representatives regarded the steroid market as somewhat limited. During the early 1940s steroids were largely confined to medical treatments for cancer and gynaecological disorders. Only a few kilograms of progesterone appeared to be needed for this market each year. Merck, another pharmaceutical company, refused to finance Marker's venture for similar reasons.[20]

Frustrated, Marker decided to use his own money to manufacture progesterone. This meant working under very basic conditions. Marker collected 9 or 10 tons of the *Cabeza de negro* root with the help of a man with 'a little store in a small coffee-drying place' (see ill. 11).[21] The root was chopped into 'material like potato chips' and dried in the sun. Marker then took the chopped material to Mexico City to extract the chemical compounds. This he did with the aid of crude extractors. Having evaporated it down into a syrup, Marker returned with his material to the United States. There he borrowed laboratory facilities from a friend in exchange for a third of the profits to be gained from the processed progesterone.[22]

With 2 kilos of synthesized progesterone in his possession (worth $160,000 on the open market), Marker hunted for people in Mexico to help him exploit the new resource.[23] Expertise in organic chemistry, however, was scarce in Mexico during this period. Despite Mexico's long tradition of university education, it lacked graduates trained in this subject. Most Mexican chemists at this time were 'working in the petroleum or sugar industry, and at best, were trained as analytic chemists. The rest were educated to teach.'[24]

One of the few pharmaceutical laboratories then in existence in Mexico was Laboratorios Hormona. Established in Mexico City in 1933, Laboratorios Hormona was a small enterprise partly run by Emerik Somlo. Somlo had started off his career in Mexico in 1928 as a representative for the Hungarian company Gedeon Richter, which at that time was negotiating its agreement with Haberlandt in Europe to produce an oral contraceptive.[25] In Mexico Somlo had established a lucrative trade for Gedeon Richter due to the almost total absence of other drug houses. He soon realized he could push the business even further with the establishment of a laboratory within Mexico. Refused funding by Gedeon Richter to finance such a project, Somlo collaborated with a young German Jewish chemist, Frederico Lehmann, to set up the laboratory and their own company, Laboratorios Hormona, in 1933.[26] Much of the production of this firm was built up through the expertise of refugee European scientists recruited to the company in the 1930s. Fleeing the ravages of fascism, these scientists brought with them many of the advances in hormone knowledge and production in Europe in the interwar period.[27]

For Marker, Laboratorios Hormona was the perfect partner to help him mount the production of progesterone. In 1944 he persuaded Somlo and Lehmann to join him in establishing a new company called Syntex, which quickly became a leading international supplier of progesterone. Despite this success, Marker left the company within a year of its foundation because of a dispute over his shares and payment.[28] His departure was potentially disastrous for Syntex, because he took with him the asset that was most valuable to the company – expertise in steroid chemistry and the production of progesterone.[29]

In 1945 Somlo hired a Hungarian Jewish chemist, George Rosenkrantz, to replace Marker. Like many earlier employees of Laboratorios Hormona, Rosenkrantz was a refugee scientist with European credentials. Trained in technical sciences and chemical engineering at the Eidgenossische Technische Hochschule (Technical School of the Confederation) in Zurich in the 1930s, Rosenkrantz had worked alongside leading experts in the chemical synthesis of male hormones. His supervisor, Leopold Ruzicka, for instance, had received the Nobel Prize in 1939 as a result of his work on male hormones with Adolf Butenandt, one of the discoverers of oestrone. Migrating to Cuba in 1941, Rosenkrantz had subsequently become involved in the production of steroids from the sarsaparilla plant, Marker's original plant material.[30]

On joining Syntex, Rosenkrantz struggled to reconstruct Marker's work. In the beginning, he was handicapped by the fact that Marker had been incredibly secretive about his methods. For instance, he had never labelled his chemical ingredients properly. Most of Marker's workers had identified substances, such as solvents, by weight and smell. After some wasted time, Rosenkrantz began to devise his own techniques to produce progesterone and other steroid intermediaries.[31] Within five years, he had worked out the pathways for the synthetic production not only of progesterone but also of androgens, oestrogens and corticoids, using diosgenin, the same substance deployed by Marker.[32]

In 1948, Rosenkrantz was joined in these efforts by a young American (born in Vienna), the Jewish Carl Djerassi. Recruited together with a number of other scientists, some of whom had trained with Rosenkrantz in Zurich, Djerassi had a strong background in steroidal chemistry.[33] After leaving Europe in 1938, he had obtained a doctorate from the University of Wisconsin in 1945. His graduate work had focused on the chemical conversion of the male hormone, testosterone, into the female hormone, oestrogen. Djerassi subsequently worked for the American subsidiary of the Swiss company CIBA, which held the patent for cholesterol, whence he joined Syntex. Employed by Syntex as part of its drive to fulfil its industrial potential and expand its range of steroidal intermediaries, Djerassi not only brought with him industrial expertise and a knowledge of steroid chemistry, but also a desire to establish an academic and scientific reputation.[34]

For Djerassi, placement at Syntex represented a unique opportunity to investigate cortisone, an increasingly competitive research area which he had been unable to pursue while employed by CIBA.[35] Interest in cortisone had been awakened in part as a result of the research carried out around corticoids after 1942. These compounds were thought to have the strategic potential to reduce stress levels among Allied pilots fighting the Nazi air force.[36] The importance of corticoids did not diminish with the end of the Second World War, however. In 1949 corticoid research was reinforced by the discovery of cortisone as an effective anti-arthritic drug. Djerassi thus arrived at Syntex at a time when there was tremendous international pressure to find a means of synthesizing cortisone much more cheaply and on a large-scale.[37] Between 1949 and 1951 numerous companies, including 'a dozen of the largest American drug houses, several leading foreign pharmaceutical manufacturers, [and] three governments' were trying to find an easier and cheaper means of synthesizing cortisone. Indeed, the number of researchers working on cortisone in these years outweighed all the input that had been put into all other medical problems since the development of penicillin in the Second World War.[38]

By 1951 Djerassi and his team of workers had devised an easier technique for producing cortisone.[39] Unfortunately he was beaten to it by the American pharmaceutical company Upjohn, which had just developed a simpler and cheaper method of synthesizing cortisone using fermentation methods which rendered Syntex's techniques redundant. However, the fermentation process soon proved advantageous to Syntex for it was dependent on progesterone as the starting material. Armed with *Dioscorea*, Syntex was the only company at this time capable of providing a large enough supply of progesterone at affordable prices. Upjohn's new process for producing cortisone, therefore, catapulted Syntex and Mexico to the forefront of the international cortisone market.[40]

Nonetheless Syntex faced difficulties in meeting Upjohn's large demand for progesterone. One problem was to gather and conserve enough supply of the *Dioscorea* plant. Another was that the quantity of diosgenin and hormones that could be obtained from the plant was limited. Ironically this problem was partially solved by Marker, who had left Syntex to form his own company. In 1949 he had discovered that another Mexican yam plant, known as *Barbasco*, yielded three times as much diosgenin as *Cabeza de negro*. *Barbasco* also had a shorter life cycle than *Cabeza de negro* which made it quicker, and easier, to grow. Commonly used by the locals as fish poison and for alleviating rheumatic pain, the *Barbasco* came from the same Mexican yam family as *Cabeza de negro*.[41]

Taking advantage of Marker's discovery of *Barbasco*, Syntex scientists were able to increase their yield of diosgenin from the plant because new techniques for drying and processing *Barbasco* out in the field had been devised by one of Syntex's newly employed chemists, Alexander Zaffaroni. Up to this point agricultural workers had simply chopped up the *Barbasco* 'with machetes and left them to dry – and putrefy – in the sun'. Zaffaroni established a small laboratory and rudimentary processing plant on the edge of the tropical forest. Here he installed second-hand potato chopping and drying equipment to process the roots. By 1951, Zaffaroni's technique had proven successful in raising the amount of diosgenin obtained from *Barbasco*.[42]

Back in the laboratory, Syntex researchers were also exploring new techniques and equipment to boost production. Prior to the rush for cortisone, the final stages of synthesis had been done in 20-litre glass bottles. This limited the amount that could be produced. For a long time the yearly production of progesterone barely exceeded 20 kilograms.[43] With almost 'zero experience with chemical manufacturing on a sizeable industrial scale', Syntex thus had problems meeting Upjohn's order for 10 tons of progesterone at 48 cents per gram. The price at the time was $2 per gram. One of the ways Syntex resolved the problem was by joining forces with the larger American chemical manufacturing firm Pfizer. This helped Syntex to replace its old glass bottles with glass-lined reactors and other equipment necessary for large-scale production.[44] By the early 1950s Syntex possessed some of the most advanced equipment for steroid research in the world.[45]

In addition to Syntex, scientists employed in other Mexican laboratories were deploying other means to produce higher yields of progesterone derivatives. Alejandro Hernandez, for instance, who was a chemical engineer employed by Diosynth (one of Syntex's competitors, originally set up by Marker after his departure from Syntex), achieved greater yields of progesterone by modifying his equipment. Building a bigger vessel in which to effect chemical reactions, Hernandez discovered that by simply enlarging the container, he increased the yield of progesterone by more than 5 per cent. As Hernandez has pointed out, such modifications and improvements to equipment and processes are a standard part of chemical engineering practice in industry. Yet their contribution is often overlooked in standard histories of science, and is not cited in standard histories about the rise of the steroid industry in Mexico or the emergence of the pill.[46]

Synthesizing hormones for a contraceptive pill

At the same time that Syntex was reaping profits from the innovations in cortisone production, its scientists were developing another progesterone derivative that was to push the company's business success even further. On 15 October 1951 Djerassi, together with an undergraduate Mexican student, Luis Miramontes, synthesized a pure crystalline progesterone compound called norethisterone. Built on the foundation of earlier work carried out by Maximilian Ehrenstein, an American chemist at the University of Pennsylvania in 1944 and Arthur J. Birch, an Australian chemist at Oxford University in 1950, norethisterone was the first compound capable of being used as an oral contraceptive. It was produced in an effort to find new synthetic progesterone derivatives to treat problems such as menstrual disorders and recurrent miscarriage, and neither Djerassi nor Miramontes initially realized its potential contra-ceptive properties.[47]

Lacking biological laboratories to test the compound, Djerassi and Mira-montes sent norethisterone for tests elsewhere. One of the first to expound on its contraceptive value was Dr Roy Hertz. Based at the National Institute for Cancer in Bethesda, Maryland, Hertz had conducted experiments with various hormones since the 1930s. He had been involved in testing the progestational compounds synthesized by Maximilian Ehrenstein in the 1940s, which were being tested for the treatment of gynaecological disorders. Hertz had wide expertise in the physiology of reproduction and pharmacology. Together with other scientists based at the National Institute for Cancer in Maryland, Hertz was able to show that, when taken orally, norethisterone was five times more potent than pure progesterone, and four to eight times stronger than progesterone when given by injection. Moreover, norethisterone was five times greater in strength than the most orally potent progestogen of these years. From this research Hertz concluded that the compound could be an effective contraceptive.[48] In April 1952 Djerassi publicized these findings at a meeting of the American Chemical Society's Division of Medicinal Chemistry in Milwaukee.[49]

Syntex was not the only company that managed to synthesize a progestogen with contraceptive potential. With the rising interest in cortisone and the race to produce new synthetic progestogens, by the early 1950s many companies were eagerly manipulating steroidal structures. One such company was G. D. Searle, a small American pharmaceutical company based in Skokie, a suburb of Chicago. Searle began to invest heavily in steroid chemical research in 1951, with the objective of improving the steroid drugs then currently available, and creating new compounds to treat conditions for which there remained no medication.[50] More importantly, Searle had as one of its consultants Gregory Pincus. Pincus had just taken up Margaret Sanger's suggestion to develop a contraceptive pill. He was therefore on the look-out for any compound that had contraceptive potential. Searle was continually receiving requests from Pincus to provide him with potential contraceptive substances.[51]

Among those recruited to Searle's steroidal research programme was the young chemist Frank Colton. Joining Searle in 1951, Colton had completed a doctorate in organic chemistry at the University of Chicago in 1949. He had subsequently been based at the Mayo Clinic where the major innovations in cortisone had taken place. While there Colton had devised a better chemical method for synthesizing cortisone. Once at Searle, Colton began to explore the possibilities of producing simpler and cheaper steroidal compounds with the aim of improving the 'biological profile of cortisone or hydrocortisone'.[52] Within months of Syntex's success in synthesizing norethisterone, Colton had managed to produce norethynodrel, an equally active oral progestogen. Like Djerassi and Miramontes, Colton had taken the work of Ehrenstein and Birch as his inspiration. The actual measures he took to develop the compound nonetheless differed from those undertaken by the Syntex scientists. The process he used to devise norethynodrel was based on chemical steps he had learnt from his earlier search for an easier means of synthesizing cortisone and hydrocortisone.[53]

Although it was synthesized later, norethynodrel was patented in the United States earlier than norethisterone. This is slightly surprising given that Djerassi and Miramontes filed for their patent for norethisterone as early as 22 November 1951, nearly two years ahead of Colton, who filed his patent for norethynodrel on 31 August 1953. Norethynodrel was officially patented in November 1955, at least six months ahead of norethisterone, which was patented in May 1956.[54] There is no evidence to explain this delay, but it might have been nothing more than a question of negotiating red tape and bureaucracy. Belonging to an American company based in Chicago, officials at Searle were in a better position to tackle such bureaucracy than those at Syntex, who, because of their location in Mexico, had a less advantageous position and less experience with the American patenting process. Table 3.1 indicates the first nine patents issued for the principal progestogens used in oral contraceptives in the United States by 1973, and shows that it was not uncommon for patents to take time to be granted, especially to companies that were based abroad, such as British Drug Houses, Glaxo (based in the UK) and Schering AG (based in Germany), which had to wait between two and three years for their patents to be issued.

The critical decision

Norethynodrel was not only patented ahead of norethisterone, it was also the first compound adopted for use as a contraceptive pill. Djerassi has argued that Pincus favoured norethynodrel because he was a consultant for Searle.[55] In 1967, however, Pincus made it clear that in the early 1950s he had been willing to use any compounds submitted to him whatever their company origins.[56] In fact his decision to use norethynodrel was heavily

Table 3.1 US patents of principal progestogens used in oral contraceptives in 1973

Progestogen	Brand name	Patent number	Assignor(s)	Assigned to	Filing date	Issue date*	Date marketed USA
Norethynodrel	Enovid, Conovid	2,725,389	Colton, F. B.	G. D. Searle	Aug. 31 1953	29 Nov. 1955	June 1960
Norethisterone (Norethindrone)	Ortho-Novum, Norinyl	2,744,122	Djerassi, C., Miramontes, L., Rosenkrantz, G.	Syntex SA	Nov. 22 1951	1 May 1956	Jan. 1962
Megestrol acetate	Volidan, Nuvacon	2,891,079	Dodson, R. M., Sollman, P.	G. D. Searle	Jan. 23 1959	16 June 1959	–
Dimenthisterone	Oracon	2,927,119	Ellis, B., Petrow, V., Stansfield, M., Stuart-Webb, I.	British Drug Houses, Glaxo	May 15 1958	1 Mar. 1960	Apr. 1965
Norethindrone acetate	Norlestrin, Minovlar, Anovlar	2,964,537	Engelfried, O., Kaspar, E., Schenck, M., Popper, A.	Schering AG	June 11 1957	13 Dec. 1960	Mar. 1964
Quingestanol acetate	Riglovis, Unovis	3,159,620	Ercoli, A., Gardi, R., Brianza, C.	Vismara SpA	July 12 1963	1 Dec. 1964	–
Ethynodiol diacetate	Ovulen, Demulen	3,176,013	Klinstra, P.D.	G. D. Searle	July 25 1963	30 Mar. 1965	Mar. 1966
Norgestrienone	Planor, Miniplanor	3,257,278	Nomine, G., Bucarxt, R., Pierdelt, A.	Roussel	Sep. 3 1965	21 June 1966	–
Norgestrel	Ovral	Pending	Trademark authorized to Wyeth		1964		Apr. 1968

* US patents run 17 years from issue date.

Source: 'Oral contraceptives – 50 million users', *Population Reports*, Series A, no. 1 (1974), p. A-5, table 2.

influenced by the obstetrician John Rock, who at the time had no ties with Searle.[57] One of the other reasons that norethynodrel was favoured was because of its biological activity. On the surface the chemical structure of norethisterone and norethynodrel appear to be very similar, differing only slightly in the position of one double-bond (see figure 3.3 below). Yet this bond means they react very differently when metabolized. While both have progestational activity, norethisterone possesses minor androgenic (male hormone) properties, while norethynodrel has oestrogenic qualities.[58] In 1957 Pincus justified the decision to use Searle's compound as a contraceptive partly because it was devoid of the androgenic effects occasionally observed with Syntex's compound.[59]

Clinically norethynodrel also showed better results than norethisterone. Initial animal and small-scale human tests carried out by Pincus and his team showed both norethisterone and norethynodrel to be effective suppressors of ovulation. When Pincus and his colleagues launched their first large-scale human trials, however, they favoured norethynodrel as the testing drug. Rabbit studies had shown norethynodrel to be more active in

Figure 3.3 Diagram of the chemical structure of norethisterone and norethynodrel

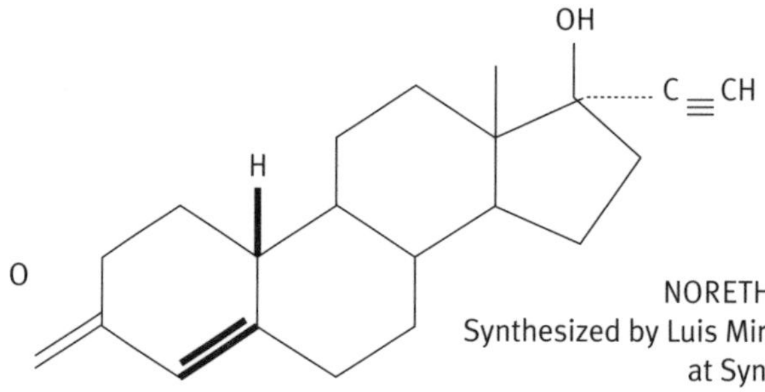

NORETHISTERONE
Synthesized by Luis Miramontes and Carl Djerassi
at Syntex, 1951

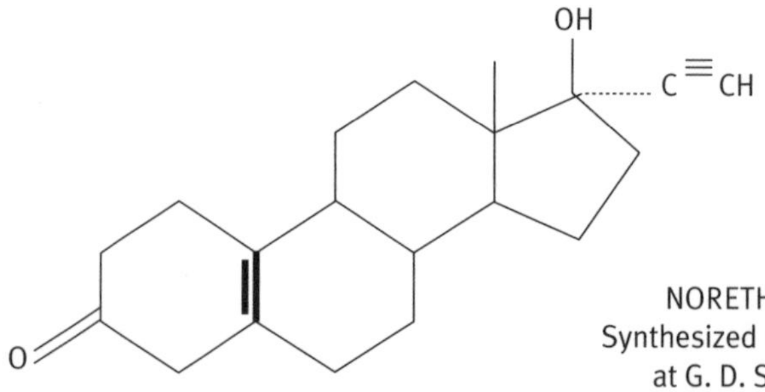

NORETHYNODREL
Synthesized by Frank Colton
at G. D. Searle, 1952

Source: C. Djerassi, The Pill, Pygmy Chimps, and Degas' Horse (New York, 1992), 57, 59, figs 5.14 and 5.15.

suppressing ovulation.[60] Large-scale human trials also indicated that because it had a small amount of oestrogen, norethynodrel was superior to norethisterone in controlling menstruation and preventing break-through bleeding.[61]

As early as 1956, Pincus and his colleagues had noticed that both norethynodrel and norethisterone appeared to have some oestrogenic contamination. When Searle was able to produce preparations of the compound which were free of oestrogen, Pincus and his colleagues discovered that the oestrogen component was crucial in preventing break-through bleeding. As a result of this discovery, Pincus and Searle decided against purifying norethynodrel and to standardize its oestrogen component instead. Moreover, they discovered that adjustments to the dose of oestrogen was crucial. While break-through bleeding occurred when the dose was too low, nausea and breast discomfort resulted when the dose was too high.[62]

Clinical trials carried out in Britain also indicated that when the oestrogen component was too low, pregnancy was not prevented. This discovery arose from a mislabelling by the manufacturer, as a result of which women had been given pills that contained a third of the originally intended oestrogen. While traumatic for the women on the trial who became pregnant, the error nonetheless provided valuable information for the investigators, because it showed the lowest dose to which oestrogen could be decreased before its preventive effect was diminished.[63] The accident also revealed the importance of the dose of oestrogen in the inhibition of ovulation.[64]

In 1957 Searle was able to market norethynodrel under the trade name Enovid for use as a treatment for gynaecological and menstrual disorders. Exactly the same formulation, which included oestrogen together with progestogen, was approved as an oral contraceptive for the US market in May 1960. The final 10-milligram Enovid tablet marketed in the United States contained 1.5 per cent mestranol (oestrogen).[65]

While norethisterone was also approved for gynaecological disorders in 1957 under the trade name Norlutin, it took much longer to materialize as a contraceptive pill. Norethisterone was Syntex's first commercial pharmaceutical speciality, but the company faced particular procedural difficulties in marketing it. In order to sell norethisterone, Syntex was forced to collaborate with a bigger pharmaceutical company, and its choice of Parke-Davis, which had strong historical links with Syntex but a very conservative marketing policy in the 1950s, turned out to be a mistake. After many delays on the part of Parke-Davis, Syntex was forced to turn to another company, Ortho Division of Johnson and Johnson, to market its compound as an oral contraceptive.[66] Norethisterone finally appeared in the form of a contraceptive pill in America in 1963. Called Ortho-Novin (or Ortho-Novum) this pill was a combination of norethisterone and oestrogen mestranol. This was different from Norlutin, which contained only norethisterone and no oestrogen.[67] Other pills approved in 1964, Norlestrin and Norinyl, also contained norethisterone with the oestrogen compounds ethinyloestradiol and mestranol.[68]

The competitors and successors of the first pill

The synthesis of norethisterone in 1951 and norethynodrel in 1952 were just the first of many compounds suitable for contraception. By 1954, Pincus was testing a number of compounds from pharmaceutical companies such as Merck, Upjohn, Frost, E. R. Squibb and Co. and Schering.[69] By the late 1950s a succession of compounds derived from norethisterone, including norethisterone acetate, ethynodiol diacetate and lynoestrenol were available for contraceptive trials as were progestogens derived from progesterone such as megestrol acetate, patented by Searle in 1959. Table 3.1 on p. 73 indicates the speed with which new compounds were being synthesized and patented in the United States in these years. In 1964 the pharmaceutical company Wyeth developed norgestrel, the first progestogen to be made from a total chemical synthesis. Subsequently licensed to Schering AG, norgesterol was used to develop levonorgestrel, another active progestogen later used for oral contraception. Today a third generation of progestogens is being used in oral contraceptives.

By the early 1960s, shortly after the original pill went on the market, new regimens were also being developed for the administration of the pill. These included sequential pills, which were different from earlier combined pills in that they were based on the inhibition of ovulation by the addition of extra oestrogen. Sequential pills worked by giving oestrogen on its own for the first ten or fifteen days before progestogen. By the mid-1960s progestogen-only oral contraceptives were also being introduced. These contained compounds such as the progestogen chlormadinone acetate, and were aimed at inhibiting conception by increasing the viscosity of cervical mucus and reducing the possibility of implantation of fertilized eggs.[70] Increasing variations in dosages, strength and packaging meant that by 1973 there were between 25 and 30 different kinds of oral contraceptive products on the market in many countries. In some cases the same product was being sold around the world under a dozen or more different proprietary names.[71] By 1992 there were at least 430 different brand names for oral contraceptives worldwide, manufactured by nine pharmaceutical companies.[72]

Table 3.2 Composition of a selection of oral contraceptives available on the British and US markets by 1969

Marketing date	Company	Product	Progestogen content	Oestrogen content
USA 1960	Searle (USA)	* Enovid	norethynodrel 10mg	mestranol 0.15mg
UK 1961 USA 1962	Searle (USA)	* (Enovid)/ Conovid	norethynodrel 5mg	mestranol 0.075mg
USA/UK 1962	Searle (USA)	* (Enovid-E)/ Conovid-E	norethynodrel 2.5mg	mestranol 0.1mg
UK 1962	Roussel (France)	* Prevision	norethyndorel 2.5mg	mestranol 0.1mg
UK 1962	Schering Chemicals (Germany)	Anovlar-21	norethisterone acetate 4mg	ethinyloestradiol 0.05mg
UK 1963	British Drug Houses (UK)	Volidan	megestrol acetate 4mg	ethinyloestradiol 0.05mg
USA/UK 1963	Ortho (USA)	* Ortho-Novin/ (Ortho-Novum) 2mg	norethisterone 2mg	mestranol 0.1mg
UK 1963 USA 1964	Parke-Davis (USA)	Norlestrin	norethisterone acetate 2.5mg	ethinyloestradiol 0.05mg
USA/UK 1964	Searle (USA)	* Ovulen	ethynodiol diacetate 1mg	mestranol 0.1mg
UK 1964	Schering Chemicals (Germany)	Gynovlar-21	norethisterone acetate 3mg	ethinyloestradiol 0.05mg
USA c.1964	Mead Johnson (USA)	Oracon	dimethisterone 25mg	ethinyloestradiol 0.1mg
USA c.1964	Upjohn (USA)	Provest	medroxyprogesterone acetate 2.5mg	ethinyloestradiol 0.05mg
USA c.1964	Eli Lilly (USA)	*† C-Quens	chlormadinone 2mg	mestranol 0.08mg
UK 1965	Organon (Netherlands)	* Lyndiol	lynoestrenol 5mg	mestranol 0.15mg
UK 1964	British Drug Houses (UK)	*† Serial 28	megestrol acetate 1mg	ethinyloestradiol 0.1mg

Table 3.2 Continued

Marketing date	Company	Product	Progestogen content	Oestrogen content
USA/UK 1964	Syntex (USA)	Norinyl	norethisterone acetate 1mg	mestranol 0.05mg
UK 1964	British Drug Houses (UK)	Volidan 21	megestrol acetate 4mg	ethinyloestradiol 0.05mg
UK 1966	Eli Lilly (USA)	*† Sequens	chlormadinone 0.2mg	mestranol 0.08mg
UK 1967	British Drug Houses (UK)	* Nuvacon	ethinyloestradiol 0.1mg	megestrol acetate 2mg
UK 1967	Ortho (USA)	* Ortho Novin SQ	norethisterone 2mg	mestranol 0.1mg
UK 1968	Eli Lilly (USA)	* C-Quens 21	chlormadinone acetate	mestranol 0.1mg
USA c.1964 UK 1968	Searle (USA)	* Demulen 0.5	ethynodiol diacetate 0.5mg	mestranol 0.1mg
UK 1968	London Rubber Industries (UK)	* Feminor	norethynodrel 2.5mg	mestranol 0.1mg
UK 1968	Syntex (USA)	* Norinyl-2	norethisterone 2mg	mestranol 0.1mg
UK 1968	W. J. Rendell[1]	* Norolen	norethynodrel 3mg	mestranol 0.075mg
UK 1968	Ortho (USA)	* Ortho-Novin 1/80	norethisterone 1mg	mestranol 0.08mg
UK 1968	Schering Chemicals (Germany)	Minovlar	norethisterone acetate 1mg	ethinyloestradiol 0.05mg
UK 1969	Ortho (USA)	Ortho-Novin 0.5	norethisterone 0.5mg	mestranol 0.1mg
UK 1969	Organon (Netherlands)	*† Ovanon	lynoestrenol 2.5mg	mestranol 0.075mg
UK 1969	Schering Chemicals (Germany)	Minovlar ED	norethisterone acetate 1mg	ethinyloestradiol 0.05mg
UK 1969	Parke-Davis (USA)	Orlest 28	norethisterone acetate 1mg	ethinyloestradiol 0.05mg

Bracketed drugs indicate trade name in the USA.

1 W. J. Rendell was one of the oldest contraceptive manufacturing firms in the UK, having made contraceptive pessaries since the 1880s. Their involvement with oral contraceptives indicates their strategy for diversifying.

* oral contraceptives not recommended for continued prescription by the British Committee on Safety of Drugs in 1969 due to high oestrogen component and its association with thrombosis.

† sequential preparations.

Sources: 'Safety of Drugs statement on oral contraceptives', *Pharmaceutical Journal*, 2 (20 Dec. 1969), 751; M. Roland, *Progestogen Therapy* (Springfield, Ill., 1965), ch. 4.

Table 3.2 indicates the composition of different oral contraceptives that were available on the British and American markets by 1969. From this it is clear that numerous companies in Europe and the United States were involved in the production of oral contraceptives. By 1973 twelve major pharmaceutical companies based in eight countries (excluding China) were producing and marketing oral contraceptives throughout most of the world. Table 3.3 lists these companies and the complex international networks that were necessary for obtaining the raw material and for processing the final product. The pill was clearly not only a product consumed worldwide, but was dependent on an intricate international network for its manufacture. Table 3.3 also shows the complex licensing and cross-licensing arrangements that existed for making and distributing the pill. Some drug firms even found themselves competing with their own licensees or selling two competitive products of their own. Indeed, marketing factors were to become as important in the distribution of the pill as were medical and pharmacological factors.[73]

Although Searle had beaten Syntex in the race to provide the first marketable contraceptive, Syntex later gained the upper hand in the contraceptive market. In 1961 almost half a million American women were taking Searle's first oral contraceptive.[74] Searle's market sales shot up from $37 million on the eve on the pill's launch in 1960, to $89 million just five years later. In 1964 Searle's net profits had 'rocketed beyond $24 million'.[75] By the mid-1960s, however, Searle was beginning to lose its lead in the market. Three of the first four brands of oral contraceptives launched in the United States, for instance, contained substances developed and produced by Syntex.[76] Moreover, by 1966 nearly 50 per cent of the world's oral contraceptives contained the compound norethisterone and were being manufactured either by Syntex or one of its four licensees.[77] Syntex's sales increased accordingly, rising from $7 million in 1960 to $60 in 1966. Between 1960 and 1966 Syntex's shares also increased from 3 cents to $2. During the 1960s the value of a share increased to $300. By 1993 each original share was valued at $8,000.[78]

Norethisterone and its relatives remain important components of oral contraceptives to this day.[79] This is partly because of the increasing reluctance dating from 1969 to prescribe high oestrogen pills because of their association with thrombosis (blood clots). Many of the pills which were dropped from prescription in Britain in 1969, for example, contained Searle's original compound norethynodrel. In this instance, norethynodrel was at a disadvantage compared to norethisterone because oestrogen was

Table 3.3 Major pharmaceutical firms manufacturing and marketing oral contraceptives, 1973

Parent company and country	Pharmaceutical division or subsidiary	Brand names commonly used for combination pills	Production			Marketing	
			Source of steroid (progestogen) intermediates	Country where intermediates converted to progestogen	No. of areas with tableting plants	No. of areas marketed	Estimated 1972 sales (millions)
Akzo NV (Netherlands)	Organon Diosynth[1]	Lyndiol, Minilyn	Mexico[2]	Netherlands	22	119	$30
American Home Products (USA)	Wyeth	Femenal, Anfertil, Ovral, Nordiol, Denoval, Stediril, Evanor	Total chemical synthesis: West Chester, Penn.		24	88	$67
Bristol-Myers Co. (USA)	Mead Johnson	Oracon, Femagest (sequential)	Purchased from Organon and Syntex (Licence from BDH)		7	13	$10
Ciba-Geigy (Switzerland)	CIBA	Anacyclin, Noracyclin, Yermonil	Mexico[2] licence from Organon	Switzerland	1	99	–
Gedeon Richter (Hungary)	Gedeon Richter	Infecundin, Bisecurin	Budapest		1	–	–
Glaxo-Holdings Ltd (UK)	BDH (British Drug Houses), Glaxo	Volidan, Voldys, Volplan, Ovucal			7	78	–

Johnson and Johnson (USA)	Ortho	Ortho-Novum, Ortho-Novin		Purchased on licence from Syntex (through May 1973)	13	73	–
Roussel UCLAF (France)	Roussel[1]	Planor, Miniplanor		Total chemical synthesis: Paris	6	31	–
Schering AG (Germany)	Schering[1]	Eugynon, Neogynon, Anovlar, Gynovlar, Minovlar, Microlut, Microgynon, Primovlar		Total chemical synthesis: Germany; Norgesterel licence from Wyeth	22	141	$53
G. D. Searle (USA)	Searle	Ovulen, Demulen, Enovid, Conovid	Mexico[2]	Caguas, Puerto Rico	(1)	111	$44
Syntex Corp. (Panama)	Syntex	Norinyl, Conlunett, Conlumin, Nor-SQ, Regovar, Conluten	Mexico[2]	Cuernavac, Mexico and Freeport, Grand Bahama Island	10	49	$30 (incl. bulk sales)
Warner-Lambert (USA)	Parke-Davis	Norlestrin, Loestrin		Licence from Schering and Syntex	21	86	$20
	Vister	Reglovis		Purchased from Milan	1	1	
	La Campana	Riglovis, Unovis		Syntex and Ono,	1	1	
	Apothekernes	Pilovtal		Japan	2	2	

Bracketed data are incomplete.

1 Bulk supplier of oral progestogens and oestrogens. 2 Member of Asociacion de Fabricantes de Esteroides (diosgenin producers from *Barbasco* root in Mexico).

Source: 'Oral contraceptives – 50 million users', *Population Reports*, Series A, no. 1 (Apr. 1974) p. A-4, table 1.

an intrinsic component of its compound.[80] Table 3.4 indicates the sharp drop in Searle's share of the British oral contraceptive market after 1968. Syntex's share of the British market is larger than appears in the table because the oral contraceptives marketed by Schering, Ortho, Parke-Davis and Lilly were all subject to licences granted by Syntex. Together these accounted for 50 per cent of the market in 1969.[81] Interestingly, the German and Dutch companies Schering and Organon have retained their lead in the British oral contraceptive market since the 1960s. Schering came out with its first pill shortly after the marketing of Enovid.[82] While these European companies had not taken the risk in developing the first pill, historically they were in a good position to take the lead in the subsequent manufacture of new oral contraceptives due to their investment in sex hormone production since the interwar years.

Table 3.4 Percentage market shares for oral contraceptives in Britain

Manufacturer	1964	1968	1974	1990	1994
British Drug Houses (BDH)	16	10	–	–	–
Duncan Flockhart	–	–	2	–	–
Gold Cross	–	–	–	2	1
Lilly	–	5	–	–	–
Organon	4	15	12	26	34
Ortho[1]	4	5	5	6	11
Parke-Davis	–	–	2.5	–	–
Schering	30	31	53	39	35
Searle	42	27	9.5	–	–
Syntex	–	c.4	8.5	1	1
Wyeth	–	–	8.5	20	16

[1] In the 1990s Ortho became known as Janssen-Cilag.

Sources: 'Oral contraceptives', *Pharmaceutical Journal*, 2 (1969), 181; Economist Intelligence Unit, 'Special report no.1: contraceptives', *Retail Business Market Surveys*, no. 138 (Aug. 1969), 19, table 5; Economist Intelligence Unit, 'The UK contraceptive market', *Retail Business Market Surveys*, no. 210, (Aug. 1975), 22, table 6; Economist Intelligence Unit, 'Market survey 4: contraceptives', *Retail Business Market Surveys*, no. 444, (Feb. 1995), 119, table 12.

Mexico and the pill

Despite its initial difficulties in marketing norethisterone, Syntex continued to influence the production and price of steroids, which were to affect the development of subsequent pills. By 1955 diosgenin made from Mexican *Barbasco* accounted for 80–90 per cent of the world's production of steroids. In addition to Syntex, six other companies, half of which were Mexican owned, were handling this production in 1954.[83] Up to the early 1950s however, Syntex had the business advantage over other companies in this area not only because of its lead in production but because it possessed access to and control over the raw material. As early as 1951 Syntex officials had managed to negotiate an official deal with the Mexican Ministry of Agriculture to regulate the commercialization of *Barbasco*. This had led to a presidential mandate which imposed a tax on the exportation of the *Barbasco* root and particular intermediates which were major precursors for hormonal contraceptive compounds.[84] Syntex's competitors were also denied the forest permits necessary to gather and transport *Barbasco*. These measures gave Syntex a significant lead over other companies in the area because at this time it was the only company with the technology and knowledge to produce the intermediates that could be exported without being taxed.[85] As a result of the legislation a number of Mexican subsidiaries of foreign companies such as the German company Schering went bankrupt.[86]

By 1954 some companies had caught up with Syntex and had adopted new synthesis processes which enabled them to produce compounds that were not subject to tax. Syntex tried to obtain further governmental protection, but failed because of pressure from three North American pharmaceutical companies which had complained to the US Senate about Mexico's earlier embargo, placing responsibility for the situation on Syntex. In response, Syntex renegotiated with the Mexican government and established a new policy. While this allowed foreign companies, along with Mexican companies, to collect and export *Barbasco*, foreign companies still faced more tax restrictions. As a result, six North American companies sent letters of protest to the American embassy in Mexico and to the Mexican Minister of the Economy, claiming that such limitations infringed the principles of free trade. The case was also presented to the US government, but it ruled in favour of the Mexican legislation.[87]

The case did not rest there. In July 1956 American drug manufacturers protested to the US Senate stating that Syntex had infringed the patent laws. Syntex had bought three patents which had originally been given to the American government by the German company Schering as part of the compensation settlement for the Second World War. Competitors perceived Syntex's action in buying the patents as monopolistic. Three months before the official Senate hearing was due on the matter, Syntex was sold to Ogden Corporation, a publicly owned US indust-rial holding company. At the same time, Syntex signed an agreement with the US Department of Justice, in which the company denied having restricted the activity of other companies in Mexico, but, interestingly, agreed at the same time never to restrict its competitors again. Syntex also asked the Mexican Ministry of Agriculture to rescind the policies.[88] Many aspects of these events were closely tied up with the power that the United States wielded overseas during these years, and the internal dynamics of Mexican politics.

From 1955, foreign pharmaceutical companies began to take over pre-existing Mexican laboratories and to set up their own subsidiaries within Mexico. These included G. D. Searle, Smith Kline and French Laboratories, Schering Corporation and the Wyeth Laboratories Division of the American Home Products Corporation. Each of these companies established *Barbasco* processing facilities.[89] This gave the companies control over the raw material and control over prices, thereby diminishing their dependence on others, such as Syntex, for their supplies.

In obtaining their supply of raw material, the companies were heavily dependent on the labour of local peasants. It was they who gathered the *Barbasco* root, which grew wild. For these peasants *Barbasco* represented a cash crop which provided a supplement to their subsistence farming, which to this day consists of maize, beans, fruit and occasionally coffee. Most of these peasants were based in the Mexican states of Veracruz, Oaxaca and Chiapas. Many lived in areas that were difficult to reach and inaccessible to pharmaceutical companies. The peasants were reliant on supplying *Barbasco* to an intermediary who sold it to the companies. The intermediaries, therefore, were able to take advantage of the peasants, insisting on their share of the profits from the *Barbasco*. Sometimes the peasants were only given their payment in the form of goods from stores which belonged to the intermediaries. Most intermediaries charged very high prices for goods purchased from these stores, thus reducing further the money the peasants earned from *Barbasco*.[90]

Overall, while vital in the peasant economy, the income provided by *Barbasco* was a pittance compared to the profits pharmaceutical companies were making from the hormonal products derived from the root. By the early 1970s, local peasants were being paid 0.50 Mexican pesos (2 US cents) per kilo of dried *Barbasco* root, while pharmaceutical companies were making 1000 pesos ($40) profit out of each gram of progesterone made from the *Barbasco*.[91] Approximately 250 kilos of *Barbasco* were needed to make 1 kilo of steroids.[92] The market price for 1 gm of progesterone was 11 US cents or 2.5 Mexican pesos. The very low wage paid to the peasants was one of the many factors which held down the cost of progesterone.[93]

During the 1970s the low wages paid to peasants for *Barbasco* became a major campaigning issue within Mexico. This was part of a more general protest about the poor living conditions of rural people. All of these issues led the Mexican government to re-evaluate its position on the *Barbasco* trade. In 1975, the Mexican president, Luis Echeverria, created Proquivemex (Productos Quimicos Vegetales Mexicanos), a regulatory body to protect Mexico's natural resources in order to improve the local economy and create new jobs. Proquivemex was established as part of a larger plan to develop a national Mexican pharmaceutical industry based on Mexican resources.[94]

The aim of Proquivemex was to control all the transactions involved in the gathering, processing and sale of *Barbasco*. It was to be more than just a commercial buyer and seller; it was to be a pharmaceutical company in its own right, intended eventually to compete with multinational companies abroad.[95] From this moment on, Proquivemex became the chief Mexican supplier of *Barbasco* to the pharmaceutical industry. This was achieved by buying up the entire stock from the intermediaries, and then buying the *Barbasco* directly from peasants through a network of a thousand locations in the south-west of Mexico. In accordance with this policy, peasants were now paid 2 pesos for each kilo of *Barbasco*, which was divided into 1.50 pesos for the root gatherer and 0.50 cents for the *ejido* (community)[96] to buy equipment or cattle.[97] Pharmaceutical companies were then charged 10 pesos per kilo of *Barbasco*, double the amount that intermediaries had previously charged.[98]

Despite its initial success in improving the wages for peasants, Proquivemex did not last long. In 1976 it attempted to triple the price of *Barbasco* per kilo, and began to demand that pharmaceutical companies allot up to 20 per cent of their manufacturing capacity to assembling some of Proquivemex's products. Many pharmaceutical companies began to resist, refusing to buy *Barbasco* from Proquivemex. With pressure from abroad, Lopez Portillo, the Mexican president from 1976 to 1982, ordered Proquivemex to reduce its prices. At the same time, Portillo removed Proquivemex's right to control the production of *Barbasco*.[99] Proquivemex's power was further diminished when the next Mexican president, Miguel de la Madrid, privatized the industry.[100]

The collapse of Proquivemex was also brought about by a more general trend away from the use of *Barbasco* for steroidal production. Long before

Barbasco had become a nationalized Mexican commodity, pharmaceutical companies had begun to look for alternative raw materials. By 1970, for example, only 50 per cent of the production of steroids was based on *Barbasco*, a fall of 30 per cent from 1958. This decrease can be partly attributed to the inadequacy of the Mexican-based companies in supplying steroids and failing to meet the deadline, quantity and supply requirements of the pharmaceutical companies abroad.[101]

More important, however, was the fact that *Barbasco* is difficult to cultivate on a commercial basis. The plant itself is slow growing. Yams with a good diosgenin content, for instance, can take more than 20 years to grow. Most suppliers were therefore dependent on gathering the plant in the wild. By the 1970s, however, many experts feared a depletion of the wild resource and the endangerment of the species. This led a number of pharmaceutical companies to explore alternative avenues. In addition to experiments with the planting of *Barbasco* outside Mexico, they had begun to look for other plants which could supply diosgenin. The Soviets, for instance, explored the possibility of two Australian Solanum species, known as 'Kangaroo apples' (*S.aviculare* and *S.laciniatum*). Selected mainly because of their wide availability, the fruit of these plants provided a raw material which could easily be converted into a useful intermediate for sex hormone synthesis. Companies based in other countries also organized botanical expeditions in Africa and other parts of the world to find new sources for steroids. Raw materials such as stigmasterol and cholesterol were to be increasingly exploited as substitutes.[102]

In addition to exploring the properties of new plants, better methods for synthesizing steroids began to be exploited. In 1974 the Mitsubishi Chemical Industries Company based in Japan disclosed a new means of manufacturing norethisterone for contraceptives using a microbiological conversion of cholesterol. The Mitsubishi method was greatly attractive because it not only offered an alternative source of contraceptive steroids but looked to make a sizeable reduction in manufacturing costs. Soon synthesis could be done independent of any natural steroid raw material, making the need for *Barbasco* obsolete.[103]

Conclusion

The appearance of norethisterone and norethynodrel marked a significant milestone in the search for a contraceptive pill. Scientists had finally found a way of making a hormone which was both active when ingested and had the desired effects on the reproductive system. These developments had been dependent on a range of discoveries in steroid chemistry. Scientists had come very close to finding a hormone and a mechanism for implementing hormonal contraception by the outbreak of the Second World War. They were severely handicapped, however, by an insufficient supply of cheap and effective hormones. This was partially resolved during the 1940s by Marker's breakthrough in steroid chemistry with the Mexican yam and the rush for easier and cheaper ways of manufacturing progesterone for the development of the anti-arthritic drug cortisone after the Second World War.

With Marker's discovery, steroid hormones became an increasingly profitable and competitive enterprise, paving the way for the development of new and cheap synthetic hormones. The abundance of these new synthetic hormones, however, did not rest on the efforts of Marker alone. Much of their development was linked to the increasing expertise then developing in the United States and Latin America with the arrival of European refugee scientists fleeing the ravages of fascism. Trained in European countries that had dominated the international sex hormone industry during the interwar years, these refugees provided the crucial skills needed to allow both the United States and Mexico to become international leaders in the sex hormone market. Their history, together with that of Marker, illustrates the ways in which individual entrepreneurs and scientists helped develop multinational businesses in the postwar years. This was to have a major impact on the international politics of pharmaceutical production and marketing.

By 1951 the sales of hormones in Britain were valued at £684,000. This was equivalent to 2.1 per cent of the market for drugs and pharmaceutical products.[104] Between 1951 and 1958 the growth of steroid hormones grew threefold. Much of this was based on the supply of the Mexican yam. By 1958 30 pharmaceutical companies around the world were seeking new and improved steroid hormones. That year the market in sex hormones was estimated at $25 million.[105] By 1958 steroid hormones ranked fourth among the big bestsellers in the USA, the first being antibiotics ($431 million), the second vitamins ($250 million), and the third tranquillizers ($175 million).[106] With this upsurge in production, hormones had also become less expensive. The price of progesterone, for instance, had fallen from $12 per gram in 1947 to just 15 cents per gram in 1957. Similarly, a gram of oestrone, a key intermediate compound for manufacturing oral contraceptives, declined from $100 in 1947 to $2.50 in 1957.[107]

Accompanying this rise in the steroid industry was a proliferation of different contraceptive pills. By the early 1960s oral contraceptives had become a profitable tool in the pharmaceutical industry. Within two years of launching Enovid, the first oral contraceptive, on to the American market, G. D. Searle had managed to increase the company's overall sales by 27 per cent to a record high of $56.6 million in 1962. Moreover, Enovid had been mainly responsible for doubling the total US sales of all types of medical contraceptives from approximately $20 million to about $40 million annually.[108] The financial importance of the pill in the pharmaceutical market can also be seen from the fact that in 1960 officials from a British pharmaceutical company, British Drug Houses, were able to prevent a takeover bid on the basis that it was about to launch an oral contraceptive.[109] This was launched as Volidan, the first British oral contraceptive, in 1964.[110] Moreover, in 1967 British Drug Houses was presented with a Queen's Award to Industry in recognition of its contraceptive.[111] Given for technological innovation, this award was significant in revealing not only the strides that had been made in chemistry but also the changes that had occurred in social attitudes to contraception. The profitable nature of the oral contraceptives can be seen from the list below, which estimates how fast the value of the British oral contraceptive market grew between 1964 and 1994:

1964	£1.5m
1966	£2.7m
1968	£3.6m
1970	£5.6m
1972	£7.4m
1974	£10.0m
1994	£59.5m[112]

Growth was also rapid in the USA: in 1992 drugstore purchases of oral contraceptives exceeded $1 billion.[113]

Oral contraceptives had become big business by the 1960s, yet few could have imagined this as a possibility only a decade before, when few scientists were working in the field and pharmaceutical companies were wary of undertaking any contraceptive research for fear of losing their reputation. Moreover, the hormones available in these years made such a project seem unrealistic. The development of norethisterone and norethynodrel and their successors provided the long-sought agents needed for oral contraception. Nobody, however, knew their contraceptive efficacy or their long-term safety. This could only be established through elaborate clinical testing over many years to come.

4
Human Guinea Pigs?

When Gregory Pincus decided to meet the challenge of finding a hormonal contraceptive he entered unknown territory. Although chemists had begun to synthesize a number of compounds which appeared to have contraceptive qualities from the early 1950s, no one knew what effects these chemicals might have on the human body and whether they would cause adverse reactions. The only way to find out was to test the pill on women themselves. This task was not going to be easy, however; it would require the aid not only of numerous scientists, but also of physicians, and the cooperation of hundreds of women volunteers. Challenging previous histories which have tended to champion individual male scientists in the making of the pill, this chapter highlights the multiple skills that were involved in its development and shows that they were not gender specific. It also reminds us that the expertise and knowledge involved in scientific work are not confined to the site of the laboratory and those who work there.

In addition to the team effort that went into the development and testing of the pill, it is important to remember the historical context in which the pill was tested. Much of the early testing of the pill took place at a time when there were few legislative regulations for testing drugs.[1] Safety guidelines were not an established feature of clinical trials until the 1960s, when the thalidomide scandal and the birth of children with deformed limbs prompted stricter protocols for the testing of drugs around the world.[2] Moreover, while scientists and medical practitioners had been troubled about the hazards of administering experimental drugs to humans since the nineteenth-century,[3] the oral contraceptive presented special problems. First, the monitoring and testing of the pill were more difficult than in the case of other drugs, because the pill was intended to be administered to healthy women out in the field and not, as was normally the case for other drugs, to sick patients under the close supervision of a hospital or out-patients' clinic. Intended to be given to healthy women of reproductive age for long periods of time, the pill also raised important questions not only about possible injurious effects to the women taking it, but also as to whether it might have an impact on their long-term fertility and on the health of their offspring. Fears that taking the pill might result in detrimental side-effects were heightened by the fact that contraceptive research was often considered socially immoral and medically question-able. Taking place in a number of different geographical locations and with different types of women, the early trials of the pill also raise ethical questions about drug research in the international setting and how this has changed over time.

Early animal testing

When Pincus began his search for a hormonal contraceptive he drew on the efforts of a number of bright and enthusiastic scientists and tech-nicians at the Worcester Foundation for Experimental Biology. One of the first people he approached was Min Chueh Chang (1908–91). Born in China, Chang was completing a doctorate at Cambridge when he was trapped in England by the Second World War. He arrived at the Worcester Foundation in 1945. Trained in pure basic science, Chang had a strong research interest in sperm. Today he is recognized as having provided the foundation for the development of *in vitro* fertilization. In the scientific community, Pincus depicted Chang as 'the sperm man' alongside himself as 'the egg man'.[4]

By the time Pincus started his contraceptive project, Chang had worked at the foundation for six years and had carried out a number of tasks assigned by Pincus, not all of his own choosing or liking. While he and Pincus had a warm relationship, it was not always an easy one. As the historian James Reed notes, Chang once 'joked that in his first years at the Worcester Foundation his contributions were so poorly understood by out-siders that a rumor circulated about a Chinaman who was being chained up in a cellar for experimental purposes'.[5] Some of the tension between the two scientists stemmed from Chang's dislike of undertaking scientific work for business and pharmaceutical companies, both of which were major sources of funding for the foundation.[6] For Chang the work on the pill represented a sideline to his real interests, which were artificial insemination and sperm capacitation.[7]

On 25 April 1951 Min Chueh Chang began the first animal experiments to develop an oral contraceptive. Drawing on work at the University of Pennsylvania by A. W. Makepeace, C. L. Weinstein and M. H. Friedman, who 18 years before had prevented ovulation in rabbits by injecting progesterone, Chang began to explore ways of deploying progesterone to suppress ovulation in women.[8] The progesterone he used was the standard kind of the time: the product Russell Marker had synthesized from the Mexican yam. The aim of Chang's work was to find the best method and appropriate dose for administering progesterone. Conducting tests with varying doses, he administered the substance in three different ways: by mouth, injection and vaginal suppository. On the basis of these tests, in January 1952 Pincus proclaimed that progesterone could effectively suppress ovulation and pregnancy without destroying fertility. The experiments indicated that progesterone worked most effectively and for long periods of time when given at high doses.[9] The research, however, also showed progesterone to be more effective when given by injection than when ingested. While today injected hormones have become a common contraceptive technique, Chang's results were troubling to Pincus and his collaborators in the 1950s because they believed that in the long run oral contraception would be more acceptable to women.[10]

Subsequent animal investigation was therefore directed towards finding a chemical substance which would be more active when taken orally.[11] Between 1952 and 1953 a large variety of compounds, including synthetic progestins, were tried out on animals. The explicit purpose of these tests was to find a compound suitable for human consumption.[12] This was not a quick process because the action of each compound was completely unknown until tested on animals. In each case a control group of animals initially had to be screened to determine the standard effect expected from different doses of pure hormones. The results were then matched against those produced in tests on synthetic compounds.[13]

Several types of animals were used for the experiments, but mostly rabbits and rats. Rabbits were used because they ovulate within ten hours of mating. They were thus easy subjects for monitoring the effects of the experimental substances. Rats were used because they exhibit a spontaneous ovulation in the course of their oestrous cycle which is comparable with the human female.[14] Work with each animal involved a great deal of preparation.[15] Animal experiments continued throughout the 1950s, the prime purpose being to screen different substances for their toxicity and success in inhibiting ovulation before they were administered to women.

While Pincus and Chang masterminded most of this experimentation, the day-to-day mechanics could not have been achieved without the expertise and knowledge of technicians. Yet their names are frequently missing from the official history of the pill. As is the case with many scientific and technological innovations, their role is often ignored because of their status as technicians. So entrenched is the status of Pincus and his fellow scientists in the history of the pill that the technicians themselves stress the importance of Pincus's work over their own.

One of the technicians who conducted the bulk of the animal tests and laboratory tests for humans was Anne Merrill. Pincus himself acknowledged that much of the animal experimentation for the pill could not have been achieved without her 'meticulous efforts'.[16] Merrill was assisted in this work by, among others, Mary Ellen Fitts Johnson. Their job demanded an intricate knowledge of the reproductive cycle of the experimental animals, as well as adept laboratory work and an ingenuity in working in locations with poor scientific facilities. Every stage had to be done by hand and was time-consuming.[17]

The work demanded an enormous amount of commitment from the technicians. Merrill and Fitts Johnson remembered having to do 'two hours here, and five hours here'. They often had to run into the laboratory 'at midnight to change something'.[18] For this they received minimal salaries. As they recalled, the Foundation was 'a non-profit place, and we were ladies, so we got minimum of everything!'[19] From their perspective they were willing to put in the hours for 'the dedication to science, and learning'.[20] They saw their work as helping women to have fewer children. They had no idea that the outcome of their efforts was going 'to turn the world upside down'.[21]

Human investigation begins

Since the 1930s medical practitioners had administered progesterone and oestrogen and their synthetic derivatives to women in substantial doses, primarily for gynaecological and reproductive disorders. When Pincus first began his research into developing a pill, both these hormones were being used for preventing threatened miscarriages. Much controversy remained, however, over how these hormones worked and their overall safety. While progesterone was favoured in Britain for the treatment of miscarriage, oestrogen was more popular in the United States.[22] Pincus, however, decided to focus on progesterone and its derivatives because he felt oestrogen and androgen substances had more side-effects.[23] Nonetheless, whether the progestational compounds could be used as an effective oral contraceptive in women remained a mystery.[24] In order to solve this Pincus enlisted the help of a variety of medical clinicians.

One of the most prominent physicians to take part in Pincus's testing was Dr John Rock, an eminent obstetrician and gynaecologist based at Harvard University and the Free Hospital for Women in Boston.[25] A devout Roman Catholic, Rock had long been interested in finding an easier means of detecting ovulation in order to improve the efficacy of the rhythm method. He also had a great deal of experience of using the hormones progesterone and oestrogen to treat female infertility. His aim in using these hormones was to stimulate a pseudo-pregnancy, which he felt would correct dysfunctioning wombs and fallopian tubes and thereby lead to fertility.

Both Pincus and Rock had known each other during the 1930s. Pincus had followed Rock's efforts to develop better methods for detecting ovulation, and had also placed several experimental compounds with Rock for clinical testing. They had lost contact during the 1940s, but renewed their connections when they met by chance at a scientific conference in 1952. At this conference Pincus revealed the contraceptive research he had been doing on animals and learnt of the work that Rock had been conducting on infertile women. Rock had tried using progesterone of between 50 mg and 300 mg on a number of women who had proved to be infertile for at least two years before joining the trial. Each of these women had also received a daily dose of oestrogen of between 5 mg and 30 mg. Receiving these hormones by injection for three to five months without a break, these women had experienced many symptoms commonly associated with pregnancy – tender and enlarged breasts, nausea and absence of menstruation. In many cases the women found it difficult to believe that they were not in fact pregnant and were bitterly disappointed to find that they were not. Four months after stopping the treatment, Rock discovered to his delight that an astonishingly high number of his patients had in fact become pregnant. Dubbing this effect the 'Rock rebound' phenomenon, because it seemed the women rebounded from being 'pseudo-pregnant' to the real thing, Rock remained uncertain whether the treatment had worked by maturing the women's reproductive system or by giving it a complete rest.[26]

On the basis of these tests it was clear to Rock that the hormone was an effective inhibitor of ovulation in women. It could therefore be used not only as a treatment for sterility, but also as a method of contraception. He himself had assured his patients that they could not become pregnant while taking the hormones because they prevented ovulation. For Pincus this research provided additional insights into the tests already conducted on animals at the Worcester Foundation. He was fascinated by the combination of progesterone and oestrogen deployed by Rock to achieve his results. The results Pincus had obtained using progesterone on its own, particularly because progesterone was known to be much safer than oestrogen, in turn intrigued Rock.[27]

As a result of a suggestion from Pincus, Rock decided to begin tests with the infertile women using only progesterone, and to limit the hormone to just 21 days of the menstrual cycle, as had been common practice in the treatment of menstrual abnormalities in the 1940s. It was thought that this regime, because it would encourage some menstrual bleeding at certain moments in the month, would also prevent raising false hopes and a belief in the women that they were pregnant when taking the hormones. Pincus might also have suggested this regime because he had been warned by Dr Frank Saunders, the chief chemist at G. D. Searle which was supplying the synthetic progesterone for Rock's trials, that the company would have nothing to do with a product that might tamper with menstruation and thereby interfere with nature.[28]

Within a short time of starting these tests, however, it became clear that the progesterone-only regime suggested by Pincus was not suppressing ovulation sufficiently. This was so even in the case of the highest doses given. Similarly the hormones appeared to be effective only when injected. Rock therefore argued that while such treatment might be used for cases of infertility, it would not do for contraception. For this reason Pincus began to search for compounds which might prove more successful. Between 1953 and 1954 dozens of new agents began to be tested on rabbits and rats at the Worcester Foundation, including norethisterone (from Syntex) and norethynodrel (from Searle).[29]

In conducting the human trials Rock had a number of assistants. One of these was Miriam Menkin. While not a medical practitioner, Menkin had a great deal of expertise in reproductive physiology.[30] Originally setting out to become an M.D., Menkin, like many other women at that time, had been thwarted in her ambition by the demands of a husband and family. This had not stopped her getting a bachelor's degree in science, specifically focusing on embryology and histology. She had also gained a master's degree in zoology, with an emphasis on genetics. Menkin had twice completed the requirements for a Ph.D at Harvard University but had been denied the degree because she was unable to pay the course fees.[31] During the early 1930s she had worked with Pincus on a project to understand how pituitary hormones regulate ovulation. She had later become pivotal to Rock's research into infertility, particularly in the development of *in vitro* fertilization. Menkin was no less important to Rock for his work on the pill in the 1950s. She not only carried out the necessary laboratory work for the clinical testing, but was also heavily involved in plotting the research and testing the strategies proposed. Menkin also supervised the daily running of the clinical trials with the patients. This involved interviewing patients and ensuring that they understood the instructions given by the doctors.[32]

In addition to Menkin, Rock had a number of physicians working with him. These included Herbert W. Horne, Angeliki Tsacona, Luigi Mastroianni and Celso Ramon Garcia.[33] Of these Garcia played a particularly influential role in the testing of the pill. A Spanish-American born in Manhattan Garcia was a gynaecologist and had originally met Pincus while based at the Puerto Rican School of Medicine.[34] Pincus had asked him to consider testing progesterone as a contraceptive for Puerto Rican patients suffering from cervical cancer, on the grounds that it might offer a cure. Although he refused to do the trial because he did not want to add to the patients' suffering, Garcia was instrumental in setting up a trial with American medical students at the Puerto Rican Medical School. This trial was decisive in determining the use of normal healthy women for subsequent testing.[35] Joining Rock in Boston in 1955, Garcia helped devise the protocols and procedures used in the physical examination of the women in trials, and monitoring side-effects. He also set up a meticulous data-keeping system for the trials.[36]

In mounting human trials, Pincus and his colleagues had few guidelines about the procedures they should follow. In the 1950s the United States, which was the first country to approve the oral contraceptive, had some of the strictest regulations concerning the approval of drugs through its regulatory agency the Food and Drug Administration (FDA). All drugs approved by the FDA had to be demonstrated to be safe for use as intended. Pharmaceutical companies were required to present data from animal and human trials, as well as the information to be provided to the consumer, before marketing a drug product. The emphasis of this regulation was to check for accuracy and to ensure that the statements made to the patient were in accord with the evidence presented and did not make any false therapeutic claims.[37] Yet these regulations did not dictate the terms of clinical trials. Distinctions between toxicity trials (known today as Phase I) and clinical efficacy trials (known today as Phase II) were in their infancy, and pharmaceutical companies largely designed their own trials. After 1962 the FDA acquired control over procedures for the testing of drugs, including those in the very early stages of experimentation. Moreover, it was not until after 1962 that doctors were required to inform patients of the experimental nature of a drug prescribed to them.[38] It is against this background that the pill trials have to be judged.

Small-scale human studies

Early in 1953 Pincus began to collaborate with a number of medical investigators around the world, including those in Israel and Japan, to undertake tests with individual women using different compounds. The aim of the tests was to work out the dose and the ways in which the compounds should be administered, as well as the length of time it would take for them to become effective.[39] In 1953 Rock and Pincus began to combine the trials on infertile women at the Free Hospital for Women in Boston with investigations into contraception with nurse volunteers at the Worcester State Hospital.[40] The initial object of the trials was to observe normal menstrual cycles (labelled 'control cycles') among the women. This was followed by observation of two subsequent cycles with the oral administration of progesterone (supplied by Syntex) between the fifth and the twenty-fifth day of each woman's cycle.

At each stage of the trials, women were expected to follow very complicated and time-consuming procedures. Some were required to take tablets every day (about one every six or eight hours). Others had to inject themselves or insert a vaginal suppository. Each woman had to take her own body temperature readings and vaginal smears on a daily basis. All this data had to be marked on a chart. She also had to collect urine over a 48-hour period on the seventh and eighth post-ovulatory days for hormone analysis. This was not an easy procedure for it required a woman to be within easy reach of a toilet, thus confining her to home. The smell of stored urine would also not have been pleasant. On top of this she had to have endometrial biopsies every month. These biopsies involved taking a few snips of tissue from the womb lining. This procedure is at best uncomfortable and at worst can be extremely painful. Two of the women were also given laparotomies (abdominal surgery) on the twenty-third day of their cycles. While cumbersome, all the procedures were designed to determine whether the compound suppressed ovulation, and therefore had contraceptive potential.[41]

By June 1954 60 women had participated in the trials in Massachusetts. The high degree of cooperation required meant, however, that only half managed to provide the accurate information necessary for proving the contraceptive potential of hormonal steroids.[42] Of the two groups, it had been the infertile women who had most faithfully stuck to the trial. The nurses found it difficult to continue because of summer vacations and job transfers.[43]

Difficulties in launching larger investigations

One of the advantages of the small-scale studies was that they were mainly conducted among middle-class women within a hospital or an institutional setting. If the pill was to be as acceptable and universal as the investigators intended, however, women from a wider range of educational, cultural, geographical and class backgrounds were needed as volunteers. Pincus and Rock also needed a much larger group of women if they were to prove to scientific and lay communities the safety and effectiveness of such an oral contraceptive. This was not going to be easy. Two issues faced the investigators: how to recruit women to the trials, and where to find patients who would be compliant with the procedures needed.

From the start it was clear that such large-scale trials could not be conducted in Massachusetts because contraceptive research was still illegal in that state. It was one thing to conduct trials under the guise of helping infertility, but quite another to conduct large-scale trials specifically to develop a contraceptive. As Rock was the medical practitioner in charge of the trials, this issue was much more pertinent to him than to Pincus, who could not test drugs directly. Rock realized that he could not undertake such trials at the Free Hospital or his private clinic without risking criminal prosecution. Those found breaking the law faced penalties of up to five years in prison and fines of up to $1,000 on each occasion that contraceptive advice and devices were provided. At the time of launching the large-scale trials, Rock was retiring from Harvard University and having to move his practice from the Free Hospital to the newly formed Rock Reproductive Study Center. Now working outside the protection of Harvard University, he had to be even more cautious about the legal implications of his work.[44]

Various possibilities were discussed about extending the studies to other places. These included New York, Puerto Rico, Japan, Hawaii, India and Mexico.[45] One of the major problems investigators faced was finding suitable research subjects who would be willing to follow complicated rules and undergo intense scrutiny, and sometimes even surgical investigation.[46] As Katharine McCormick admitted, the real problem was how to get a '"cage" of ovulating females to experiment with'.[47] She also noted:

> Human females are not easy to investigate as are rabbits in cages. The latter can be intensively *controlled all the time*, whereas the human females leave town at unexpected times and so cannot be examined at a certain period; and they also forget to take the medicine sometimes; – in which case the whole experiment has to begin over again, – for scientific accuracy must be maintained or the resulting data are worthless.[48]

Scientists were therefore reliant on the cooperation of women if they were to be successful in conducting the trials. A key question in launching larger-scale trials was whether women would continue to take the pills faithfully outside the clinical setting. McCormick writing to Sanger in 1954, outlined the problem:

> The *headache* of the tests is the co-operation necessary from the women patients. – There is so much of it and it must be accurate. I really do not know how it is obtained at all – for it *is* onerous – it really is – and requires intelligent attention, persistent attention for weeks. Rock says that he can get it only from women wishing to become fertile –: those who wish to be sterile are not ready to take so much trouble: I cannot see any way of overcoming this headache in the tests – unless one can furnish enough nurses to go around to their homes and see that the women patients do accomplish the tests regularly and correctly.[49]

The need for women to be able to monitor themselves was also particularly important in the context of understanding the effects of the drug. Self-monitoring was crucial, for instance, in seeing whether the women experienced any break-through bleeding, an important sign for seeing the impact of the drug on ovulation. Only women could detect this for themselves. This was undoubtedly very different from monitoring an animal in a cage. The doctors were therefore heavily reliant on the cooperation of the women involved in the trials.

Investigators wondered where it would be possible to find 'intelligent enough' women who could 'be relied upon to carry out' the procedures expected of them.[50] Infertile women participating in the trials were considered to be more highly motivated in adhering to the instructions than other women because they hoped their involvement would provide a cure for their infertility. Not all women, however, had such incentives, let alone the leisure or knowledge, to perform the intricate tests required. Women with families, for instance, could not be used in such trials as they did not have the time considered imperative for undertaking the elaborate tests on themselves. Making sure that the women performed the necessary tests was also time-consuming for the doctor.[51]

The problem of keeping women in the trials was most clearly illustrated in the case of a small-scale trial launched among American female medical students doing their internships at the School of Medicine at the University of Puerto Rico in San Juan in January 1955.[52] Investigators experienced great difficulties in retaining the students. Only 13 of the 23 women who started completed the trials. A number left despite being threatened with academic failure should they not comply with the procedures.[53] Some dropped out to take up internships in the United States. One was forced to leave the school because she failed her course. Even students who did complete the pilot study often did not adhere to the rules.[54] Pincus and his colleagues also regarded the study as limited because the number of women included in the trial was too small to make the results conclusive. Medically trained, these women were also regarded as too sophisticated for demonstrating how well women with less education could deal with the contraceptive.[55]

Investigations were undertaken to see if the trial in Puerto Rico could be extended to student nurses from the San Juan City Hospital and female prisoners from the Women's Correctional Institute at Vega Baja, but these proved fruitless. Resentment on the part of the female prisoners towards the project proved enough to disrupt the discipline of the prison.[56] Clearly these women would not comply with the procedures necessary for the success of the project. In January 1956 investigators at the medical school decided not to pursue any further work with the pill because of the difficulty of recruiting suitable subjects, as well as the opposition they faced from Catholics higher up in the university's hierarchy.[57]

More success was achieved with 15 psychotic women studied at the Worcester State Hospital in 1956. Overseen by the Commonwealth of Massachusetts, this hospital had long-standing ties with the Worcester Foundation and had received funding from Katherine McCormick in 1927 to establish a Neuroscience Research Foundation. For the hospital's director, a trial of the pill on the hospital's patients provided an attractive source of income at a time when money for state mental care was very hard to obtain. As a result of the trial, the hospital received funds from McCormick to paint and refurbish the wards used for the trial. Pincus and his colleagues considered the psychiatric patients ideal for the trial, because they were confined within a hospital setting and therefore easy to monitor and control. Unlike the previous trials, the doctors were therefore less dependent on the women remembering to perform their own temperature readings, vaginal smears and other tests necessary for the project. All the women chosen for the project were between the ages of 18 and 43 and were classified as psychotic, suffering from serious conditions such as schizophrenia or manic depression. In addition, 16 men were included in the trial to see what impact the drug might have on their fertility and whether it would help to reduce their psychotic behaviour.[58]

The trials soon proved to have a major disadvantage for the investigators in that none of the women were having sexual intercourse. This made it impossible to ascertain the contraceptive effects of the administered hormones. It was similarly difficult to establish whether the compounds had any impact on ovulation because menstrual cycles are frequently disturbed by psychiatric problems. In the case of the men it proved impossible to obtain specimens of their semen to check the effect of the drug on their potency. One man, however, appeared to have smaller testicles after having taken the pill for five and a half months.[59]

In extending the trials the investigators had the difficulty not only of finding suitable research subjects but also of ensuring a uniform scientific standard. Checking vaginal smears, performing endometrial biopsies and analysing urine required special expertise, and allowed great potential for error and faulty diagnosis.[60] Similarly, finding cooperative and suitably trained personnel abroad was not easy. One of the problems in setting up a trial in Japan, for instance, was the overall 'jealousy and resentment of American doctors' in the country, which investigators feared would jeopardize the accuracy of any investigation.[61]

Puerto Rico was favoured because many of its medical practitioners were American trained and thought to 'have the American approach'.[62] In addition, the island was near enough to the United States to allow close supervision. Pincus and his team could visit the site easily and collect the vaginal smear slides and urine samples to analyse at the Worcester Foundation's laboratories.[63] It was also regarded as an ideal setting because it had no laws prohibiting contraception. Moreover, it had an active family planning movement and a well-established network of birth control clinics. The island was also important because of its growing population and poverty. Many women were keen for contraception and most were semiliterate or fully illiterate, and had large families. They were therefore considered perfect models for testing whether the pill could be used for women around the world, particularly in places where population problems were thought to be at their worst.[64] Finally Puerto Rico was an island and therefore had a relatively stationary population that could be easily monitored.[65]

Large-scale trials

Launched in 1956, the first large-scale Puerto Rican trial was conducted under the medical supervision of Dr Edris Rice-Wray. Rice-Wray was an ideal ally for Pincus and his colleagues because she had an American training and approach to medical care that guaranteed the collection of accurate data.[66] It was vital to have a person who could accurately assess the reproductive and menstrual patterns of patients and was skilled at taking vaginal smears.[67] She was a member of the faculty at the Puerto Rico Medical School and director of the Public Health Department's Field Training Center for nurses. Rice-Wray was also medical director of the Puerto Rican Family Planning Association and ran a contraceptive clinic where she trained medical students in contraceptive work. She had also conducted a number of trials with conventional barrier methods.[68] Rice-Wray not only had experience in the organization of family planning programmes, but the necessary contacts for gaining access to possible test locations for the pill.[69] For her the pill project provided a financial opportunity to boost the poorly funded Planned Parenthood Federation in San Juan.[70]

It was Rice-Wray's networks that decided the location of the first large-scale human trials. She proposed conducting the trial in Rio Piedras, a suburb of San Juan, where a new housing project had been set up as part of a slum clearance campaign. Many families there prized their new accommodation highly and were therefore unlikely to move away during the course of the trial. This would make them easy to monitor. While Pincus and Rock were responsible for the overall research design of the Rio Piedras trial, Rice-Wray was in charge of the fieldwork. She was expected to recruit subjects, distribute the pill, monitor the reactions and collect the necessary data.[71] The Puerto-Rican Secretary of Agriculture and the Director of Social Relations granted permission for the project.[72]

Many of the women participating in this trial had previously taken part in short-term contraceptive trials (using conventional barrier methods) and were known to be keen for an alternative means of contraception. Several had to cope with large families on a very small income and with little support from their husbands. As the American technician Anne Merrill observed, many were struggling to survive:

> I would see these young women with many, many children, although I wouldn't know they were young women until I'd looked at their records. Some of them looked like what I would think of as a great-grandmotherly type ... All wizened up and gaunt to the point where you wanted to do something for them. I'd think it was due to old age, but then I'd look at the records and the women would be thirty-four ... with ten children.[73]

The desperation of some of these families is summed up by the sad story of one husband who hung himself in 1956 on account of the poverty he and his family were facing.[74]

All those included in the study had to be under 40 years old and already to have borne children to show they were fertile. They also had to be prepared to have another child if oral contraception failed. All the women had to guarantee long-term residence in the same area so as to remain on the trial for a year.[75] The women were divided into two groups: those who were testing the pill; and those who formed a control group, who were expected to use conventional contraceptive devices.[76] Those in the pill group were told they were participating in a birth control trial, while those in the control group were informed they were part of a survey on the size of the families residing in the housing project. In each case they were told that the trial was run by the Family Planning Association of Puerto Rico which was a private agency with objectives of family planning and no governmental links.[77] While the ways in which these women were informed about the trial would not meet the ethical standards of today, they were not unusual for this time.

Soon after the Rio Piedras trial, another trial was established in Puerto Rico under the supervision of the American-born and trained Dr Adaline Satterthwaite in April 1957.[78] Undertaking obstetric and gynaecological work on patients attending a small mission hospital and a separate family planning clinic in Humacao, Satterthwaite was in an ideal position to launch trials. Humacao was a municipal district in a predominantly rural area in the eastern part of Puerto Rico, where much of the population worked cutting sugar cane. The women taking part in the trials were therefore good subjects to compare with the more urban subjects based in Rio Piedras.[79] Supervised by Pincus, Satterthwaite received her funding for the project from the philanthropist Clarence Gamble.[80] Overall, the cases from Humacao accounted for 30 per cent of the cases Pincus used as data for gaining official approval for the contraceptive pill in 1959.[81]

The women in Humacao were in a generally worse state of health than those in Rio Piedras. Most were anaemic and suffered greatly from intestinal parasites as well as malnutrition. Many of them walked miles, sometimes taking days, in order to reach the hospital. For Satterthwaite the pill project represented a major step forward. She had frequently encountered women who had been sterilized and who then wanted to have more children. Sterilization was widespread in Puerto Rico. The experiences of sterilized women who had changed husbands or lost a baby and could not have another convinced her of the need for a reversible contraceptive method.[82]

Trials were also established elsewhere. By 1960, when the first pill, Enovid, was approved, clinical trials were being conducted in various parts of the United States, including in the mountains of Tennessee, in Seattle, Chicago and Los Angeles, as well as in other parts of the world such as Haiti, Mexico City, Hong Kong, Australia, Ceylon, Japan and Britain.[83] These trials not only tested Enovid but a range of pills from different pharmaceutical companies. Many of the procedures used for testing the pill in subsequent trials were formulated during the first trial in Puerto Rico.

While the women participating in the Puerto Rican trials were not expected to follow so complicated a set of procedures as those who had taken part in the Massachusetts trial, each woman had to undergo a preliminary medical examination and was required to take a pill for a set number of days.[84] Adherence to the instructions was ensured by the regular visit of a social worker to each woman at the end of her month's supply of pills. The social worker checked whether the right number of pills had been consumed at the appropriate time and asked detailed questions concerning side-effects such as break-through bleeding, length of menstrual cycle and frequency of intercourse.[85] Such observation, however, was not always foolproof. Social workers, for instance, did not always find the women at home when they called, and sometimes were unable to make the visits when there had been very heavy rain. Where too much time lapsed between visits, women found it hard to recall crucial personal medical details.[86]

Problems also occurred in monitoring the consumption of the pills. Initially women were given a bottle with only one month's supply of pills in order to make it easier for them to know when to stop taking the medication. The pills were replaced by the social worker at the end of each month. This arrangement soon proved impractical, however, because many women were absent when the social worker called. It thus became necessary to provide two bottles to ensure continuation of the regime. This system did not always work. Some women, for instance, took all the pills without stopping for the required five days in between cycles to allow for menstrual bleeding. Others became agitated when their pills ran out, fearing that any gap in taking the medication would result in an immediate pregnancy. In order to combat such confusion, simple printed instructions were given out on the assumption that most women would be able to read or have a schoolchild read the instructions for them.[87]

Those conducting subsequent trials faced similar problems in ensuring that women adhered to the regime. In Haiti, for instance, over 20 per cent of the women on the trial forgot to take the pill and some stopped the medication whenever their husband went away.[88] Many of them were illiterate and innumerate, which made instructions difficult to follow. Even when supplied with a calendar as a reminder device, many could not remember when to take the pills. Some women were given rosary beads that they were to move individually each day on taking a pill. This, however, was not foolproof. A number of the women wore the beads in the belief that they alone provided protection against pregnancy and that there was no need to take the pill. Others ignored the instructions altogether and presumed that they had to take all of the pills in one go.[89] Such difficulties, however, were not universal. In Humacao and Mexico City, for instance, even very poor and illiterate women took the pill correctly.[90] Clearly much depended on individual motivation, as well as the skill of the instructor.

A major problem for all the trials was the unpleasant side-effects caused by the pill, such as nausea, dizziness, headaches and vomiting. This resulted in many women leaving the trials prematurely.[91] Rice-Wray calculated that in the first few months 17 per cent of the subjects in the Rio Piedras trial had these reactions. Initially she feared this would threaten the long-term viability of the pill.[92] Women also dropped out of the trials in Haiti, Humacao and Mexico City, averaging between 10 and 30 per cent of the total cases recruited. In Los Angeles, where trials were set up in 1956, the drop-out rate was particularly high (66 per cent), with at least 37 per cent leaving because of side-effects.[93]

Initially Pincus and his colleagues presumed leading questions by social workers had resulted in psychosomatic symptoms rather than real reactions.[94] This was somewhat ironic, for initially many of the questions were posed because women were shy of reporting any unpleasant reactions for fear of displeasing the investigators.[95] The undesirable reactions, however, lessened the longer a woman stayed on the medication and decreased as the dose of the pill was lowered. Distributing antacid tablets also relieved some of the symptoms.[96] The number of subjects who left the trials also diminished over time, so that those participating for lengthy periods increased the longer a trial was conducted.[97]

Side-effects were not the only problem. Some women were forced to abandon the Rio Piedras trial because of objections from their husbands, or because they moved to another area. Others stopped because they wanted either to become pregnant or to be sterilized.[98] Finding replacements was easy, however. Women were continually begging to join the trials. As the social worker Iris Rodriguez wrote of the Rio Piedras trial: 'we have more cases than what we can take for our study. Continuously they are ringing this office asking for the pill, going to see Dr Rice-Wray and calling on me when I make the visits.'[99] In many trials elsewhere, a waiting list had to be drawn up to cope with the demand. During the early years the only way many women could gain access to the contraceptive was by volunteering to be on a trial.[100]

More serious than the drop-out of women was the hostility the investigators encountered to such trials. Within the first month of the Rio Piedras trial, for instance, 30 women dropped out when a local newspaper claimed the trial to be a 'neomalthusian campaign' to sterilize and harm women.[101] Similar problems occurred in Humacao, where women not only faced negative reporting from local newspapers but opposition from local priests.[102] In the end Rice-Wray and Satterthwaite faced so much hostility from their colleagues that they were forced to resign their positions and abandon their trial work in Puerto Rico.[103] Such opposition was not unique to Puerto Rico. Rice-Wray, for instance, had to tread very carefully in setting up subsequent trials in Haiti and Mexico.[104]

Part of the difficulty was the taboo nature of contraception. In Mexico, for example, Rice-Wray could not even mention the word for fear of opposition not only from the Roman Catholic church but also from the government.[105] Mexican government officials were more interested in promoting population growth, which they saw as key to industrialization, than in curbing the birth rate.[106] Working conditions were thus not easy and the survival of the trials was constantly threatened.[107] Rice-Wray's difficulties were compounded by the fact that she was from the United States. As she wrote to a British representative for Searle in the early 1970s:

> There is such a prejudice against Americans here in Mexico that in order for our clinic to collaborate with government in their family planning program, we had to get rid of the American image – meaning me – our clinic had been called Dr Rice-Wray's clinic for too long. So I am out – retired – I remain as chief technical advisor. But the truth is that the less my American face is seen in the clinic, the better.[108]

During the early 1960s she battled to keep the Mexican trials going when the government forced the temporary closure of her clinic and some of her staff began to siphon off money from the project for their own purposes.[109]

Ethical and safety considerations

The testing of the pill on psychiatric women in the United States and then on poverty-stricken women in Puerto Rico, Haiti and Mexico has raised many questions retrospectively about the ethical nature of the early pill trials. In the late 1950s and 1960s Puerto Rican newspapers insinuated that 'Nordic white' American drug companies were using non-white women as 'guinea pigs'.[110] In Mexico doctors were accused of putting 'poison into the veins of … patients'.[111] Neither was it simply a question of perceived racial abuse. American white women, when protesting about the side-effects of the pill and the lack of warning about its health implications in the 1970s, accused scientists and medical practitioners of treating them just like guinea pigs.[112] Subsequent feminist literature on the history of the pill has also tended to reassert these accusations.[113]

To see the testing of the pill on women in impoverished areas such as Puerto Rico merely as a question of easy access to human guinea pigs and the exploitation of women, however, misses the range of social, political and economic considerations, outlined above, that influenced the setting up of these trials. Moreover, from the start the original developers of the pill were very concerned about its safety.[114] Early on, Rock confessed to McCormick that he had reservations about using synthetic progestins, because they might (1) lead to permanent sterility by diminishing ova production; and (2) cause long-term damage to the lining of the uterus.[115] In addition some feared that the pill might cause congenital or androgenous defects in future children. The early investigators were thus greatly relieved when women began to produce healthy babies once they came off the pill. Equally troubling was whether the oral contraceptive would have long-term side-effects such as cancer. As early as the 1930s oestrogens had seemed to be implicated in carcinogenic growths in animals.[116]

A major criticism levelled at the investigators is that they neglected to attach any importance to the fact that one woman died from congestive heart failure and another developed pulmonary tuberculosis while in the Puerto Rican trial.[117] In the light of what we know today about the connections between thrombotic complications and the pill, the failure to comment on such cases would indeed appear to be negligent. In retrospect, however, there was very little to alert suspicion about the connection between the pill and thrombotic problems in the late 1950s.[118] When the pill was first approved chronic disease epidemiology was also still in its infancy.[119]

In all the trials women were expected to have a complete medical examination to check that they were in good health before participating, and this included gathering information on their menstrual and pregnancy patterns. The patients were also followed up during the trials. This included investigations for liver function, cervical smears and tests for blood clotting. The tests became increasingly elaborate as time went on and scientists learnt more about which side-effects they should look for.[120] Regular medical check-ups were installed as part of the trials in Puerto Rico and Haiti.[121] Investigators also spent a great deal of time chasing up women who failed to return to the clinic. Special attention was paid to those who got pregnant, and the babies were carefully monitored.[122] For those conducting the trials, these tests were not only important for the information they provided on the drugs tested, but because many of the women had little access to good health-care services, particularly in places such as Puerto Rico and Haiti. Those conducting the trials pointed out that even in places such as Los Angeles and Britain, women participating in the trials were often receiving better health-care attention than they would have done if they had merely been prescribed the pill by a private physician.[123]

What is interesting about these tests is that not everyone agreed they should be performed. Celso Ramon Garcia recalled that during the early small-scale trials conducted at San Juan Medical School, he fought with the professor of preventive medicine who was unconcerned about the possibility of hazardous effects and saw such tests as pointless. The professor's attitude reflected a more general attitude for the period. Tight codes for testing drugs were not an established feature of clinical trials until the 1960s when the thalidomide disaster prompted stricter protocols for the testing of drugs across the world.[124]

Undertaking regular medical check-ups and investigative examinations of the women, however, was not always an easy operation. In the Caribbean the tests took place at certain prearranged times of the year when the technicians and medical practitioners flew out from Massachusetts. In many cases the tests were performed in a central place and women frequently found it difficult to get there. In Haiti, for instance, some had to walk all night in order to be tested, and then had to wait for several hours before being seen. Women also did not know what to expect and took a lot of persuading to come in for the tests.[125] Even basic gynaecological tests were often unfamiliar as they were unaccustomed to seeing a doctor except when giving birth. Only a small number of those in the Caribbean trials, in fact, underwent all of the rigorous physical examinations expected of them.[126] In his 1958 publication on the Rio Piedras trial, Pincus admitted that they had only been able to collect blood samples from 39 women, and urine samples from 42. Endometrial biopsies had proved even harder to obtain.[127] The difficulty of getting women to undergo these tests underlines the fact that many of them were unpleasant and even painful. Moreover, women were active subjects who could choose whether or not to undergo these tests.

Not only was it difficult in places like Puerto Rico and Haiti to encourage women to attend the check-ups, there were also technical obstacles to overcome. The technicians undertaking the bulk of the work for such investigative tests pointed out that they lacked even the very basic facilities for undertaking such work. It was not uncommon for equipment to be lost on the way. This was a major problem as the provisions could not be replaced once they were in Puerto Rico or Haiti. In addition to this, none of the equipment was disposable, which meant that everything (needles, syringes and glass slides) had to be washed in order to be reused. Even this was not straightforward because distilled water was unavailable. Because of the difficulties of conducting the tests out in the field, only the most basic of tests were performed there. Blood and other samples were preserved so that more elaborate tests could be done once back in Worcester. This in itself was problematic because of the difficulty of storing specimens collected.[128]

One of the most troubling features of the early trials of the pill in places like Puerto Rico was that women were not asked to sign forms of consent. As Satterthwaite has pointed out, however, this was not a common procedure at the time.[129] Dr Luigi Mastroianni, a colleague of John Rock, also recalled in the 1980s:

> The concept of informed consent that is so talked about now, and is a legal requirement of any research project involving human volunteers, didn't exist then. But Rock practiced it [informed consent] before it was ever defined. There were always long and large discussions of the risk factors. It didn't matter that Rock had no formal guidelines, he set his own and they were high standards indeed.[130]

Later trials in Britain included provisions for patients to sign consent forms. Women were expected to sign these forms with their husbands because family planning was then believed to be a joint decision. Yet, as was the case with many drugs, the amount of information they could expect to be given about the pill was limited, thus making the value of the consent forms questionable.[131] Few knew what the long-term effects of the oral contraceptive would be.

Women in the trials sometimes exercised their power to change its terms. Satterthwaite remembered that in the case of a study conducted in Humacao to study the carcinogenic effects of the pill in the early 1960s, women refused to take part when they were assigned to the control group using contraception other than the pill. Women taking the pill in this instance were to be decided blind on the basis of a piece of paper in an envelope. Satterthwaite quickly dropped the study because she found that she could not deny the pill to those women wanting it. As she stated, the blind procedure used to decide which contraception a woman took 'just wasn't acceptable to my patients'. These women usually argued with the doctor or quit if they did not get their way.[132]

Of all the trials conducted on the pill, those which were probably the least ethical by today's standards was the one carried out on the psychiatric patients at the Worcester State Hospital.[133] While the investigators sought the consent of each patient's family, the psychiatric patients themselves were far from having any choice over whether or not to participate in the trial. Historically, such trials with psychiatric patients were not unusual. Sex hormones were being widely tested in the 1950s as tranquillizers on psychiatric patients. Homosexuality, for instance, then believed to be a mental illness, was also commonly treated with sex hormones.[134] It is noticeable that Pincus and his colleagues not only tried the pill on male schizophrenic patients at the Worcester State Hospital, but also on some male prisoners in Oregon in 1958, some of whom were homosexual. One of the aims of these trials was to see whether the pill had a calming effect on the patients, as well as an impact on sperm production.[135]

Evidence in the approval of the pill

Many of the allegations made by critical journalists and feminists since the 1970s about women being used as guinea pigs assume not only that the women were used badly in the clinical trial process, but that the product was launched too soon. They have argued that insufficient evidence was collected prior to the first pill's approval and that too few women had been tested for too short a time to prove the drug's safety.[136] Demonstrating the safety of any drug is never a clear-cut issue, however. In the United States, for instance, numerous drugs were approved and left on the market by the Food and Drug Administration even though they caused significant, and occasionally rare and fatal, side-effects.

In the case of the pill it is difficult to establish the precise number of women on which its approval was based. In the United States the first pill, Enovid (10 mg), was put forward by Searle for FDA approval as an oral contraceptive on the basis of 897 women on trial, 132 of whom had taken the pill for over a year. Additional data from Searle suggests that the total number of women who had received Enovid was 1,200. An extra 995 women had taken a lower dose of Enovid at 5 mg.[137] These figures should be considered alongside the women who began to take Enovid when it was first released on to the American market to treat gynaecological disorders in 1957. Between 1957 and 1959, 500,000 American women took Enovid for therapeutic purposes.[138] With hindsight, and by comparison with today's standards, the numbers of women who took Enovid 10 mg on trial for contraceptive purposes may appear quite small. By 1965, the FDA required that new formulations of the pill be tested on no fewer than 1,000 women before approval be sought.[139] It is important to remember that protocols for appropriate sample sizes in clinical trials continued to be contentious even after the tightening of drug testing in the wake of the thalidomide affair.

Whether the pill was sufficiently tested before it went on the market should be considered in the context of other pharmaceutical investigations of the time. This can be done by comparing the pill with Librium Hydrochloride, a drug aimed at 'removing "emotional overlays" complicating the treatment of organic disease'.[140] Approved within months of each other, both Librium and the pill (though not in the same formulation as Enovid) are still on the market and widely prescribed today. Librium and the pill are unusual in that – in aiming to prevent stress and prevent pregnancy, respectively – they are intended to act on conditions not widely regarded as diseases. Librium, like Enovid, came to be hailed as a revolutionary drug, primarily helpful in treating psychiatric disorders.[141]

Unlike the pill, which was designed as a contraceptive, the value of Librium was unknown before its clinical testing. Librium was thus tested on a much wider range of conditions than the pill. It could be prescribed by any medical practitioner for any patient of any age and gender. In total Librium was tested on 1,163 patients. On the surface this seems larger than the 897 included in the clinical data originally put forward for the approval of the pill. When broken down by specialty prescribers, however, the totals for Librium were much smaller. In some conditions, such as epilepsy, Librium was tried on as few as three patients. Psychiatric patients formed the largest trial group, totalling 570. In addition, the evidence collected for Librium did not make clear for how long each patient had taken the drug.[142]

What many have found most interesting about the evidence of safety presented on oral contraceptives is the fact that women were represented as 'menstrual cycles' or 'woman years'. In justifying the FDA's approval of Enovid, for instance, the FDA's commissioner, George Larrick, stated: 'Altogether in the entire clinical cases, 897 women representing 801.6 women-years and 10,427 cycles have been studied.'[143] Nelly Oudshoorn, a sociologist, argues that this method of presentation:

resulted in a major increase of scale: the grand totals of the trials now included much more impressive numbers than a focus on the individual subject might have achieved. The trials were thus presented as having met their purpose: the testing of progestins on large numbers of women over longer periods, as a prerequisite for its approval as a safe and reliable contraceptive.[144]

This representation of women in terms of woman years undoubtedly did mask some of the experiences of individual women and might have created a false impression of the number of women who had taken the pill continuously. It certainly did not reveal the number of women who dropped out in the process of the trial. Nonetheless, it would be a mistake to see this statistical device as a deliberate distortion on the part of the investigators. Rather, they were using a shared and well-established methodological framework that had evolved since the 1930s.[145]

For the investigators and regulators the key issue was whether the drug was an effective and safe contraceptive. In their eyes the crucial evidence did not rest on the numbers of individual women tested, but on whether the pill was effective in suppressing ovulation without affecting future fertility. From their perspective, animal testing and early clinical trials showed Enovid to be physiologically effective, as did the physical examinations of women.[146] The prevention of pregnancy, plus the birth of babies among women who had taken the pill at other times, also made it clear that Enovid had the desired physiological effect.[147]

Regulators were most concerned about Enovid's ability to prevent pregnancy. If it were ineffective, or even less effective than the mechanical contraceptives already available (condom and diaphragm), then they would need more convincing about its safety.[148] Such an evaluation was not easy for it was dependent on variables such as formal education, socioeconomic background, and motivation to control fertility.[149] The trials, however, indicated that the pill was much more use-effective than any other contraceptive or contraceptive method then available.[150] Final approval of Enovid by the American FDA was partly justified on the basis of the drug's extraordinary use-effectiveness. The FDA reported that investigations led by Pincus with Enovid 10 mg had resulted in 2.7 pregnancies per 100 woman-years, and the failures had been attributable to 'irregular tablet taking'.[151] Pregnancies were more likely to occur the more frequently a woman forgot to take the drug. As with other contraceptives, Enovid was effective only when used 100 per cent of the time.[152]

One of the accusations levelled against Enovid and other pill formula-tions was that the initial dose was too high. Investigators worldwide soon learned that a much lower dose of hormones would suppress ovulation just as effectively as the higher dose. Moreover, the lower doses produced fewer side-effects and were cheaper to produce. Studies carried out in Puerto Rico and Japan had already demonstrated that the original 10 mg of the chemical progestogen compound could be successfully reduced to 2.5 mg.[153] Searle originally asked the FDA to consider simultaneously an application for three dosages of Enovid: 10 mg, 5 mg and 2.5 mg. The company was particularly interested in promoting the lower dosage forms of Enovid because the chief criticism of the pill up to that point had related to an economic rather than a medical problem. Partly developed in response to concerns about world overpopulation, it was clear that the present oral contraceptives would prove far too expensive for women in poorer countries. G. D. Searle, therefore, had a great incentive to prove the safety and efficacy of its lower dosage pills. As far as Searle officials were concerned, the lower dose of Enovid was merely an alternative dose of the same drug.

The FDA, however, viewed the dosage question differently. Any reduction in the dosage could theoretically have allowed ovulation and thereby destroyed Enovid's effectiveness as a contraceptive, rendering it unsuitable for approval. The FDA was therefore very cautious in consider-ing any alteration in the original dose formulation of the pill.[154] The agency required that Searle gain approval for the 10 mg dosage first, and then file a new application for the lower dosage forms. This decision initially operated in Searle's favour because the evidence demonstrating the safety and effectiveness of the 10 mg dosage of Enovid was solid. Problems, however, had already been observed with the lower dosages. The most important one was an increased incidence of break-through bleeding. A disturbing side-effect for women, it also concerned researchers who feared that the break-through bleeding was an indication that ovulation was not being effectively suppressed in the lower dosages. Had Searle insisted on having all three dosages approved simultaneously, the approval would have been much delayed.[155] As it was, approval for Searle to market 5 mg Enovid tablets did not come until two years after the original approval of Enovid 10 mg.[156]

Britain, in contrast to the United States, had a very different perspective on the lower dosage pills. Unlike the United States Britain released the lower dose formulation (5 mg) first. The 10 mg Enovid, approved for gynaecological purposes in 1957 and still available on prescription in 1961 in the USA, was never prescribed for contraceptive purposes in Britain.[157] Part of this can be explained by the fact that British rules governing the establishment of the dosage of drugs were fairly relaxed during this period. In the United States experimental trials were more regimented. FDA regulators required the establishment of a test dosage at a very early stage, and were thereby committed to the 10 mg dosage of Enovid as a standard dose long after it had become clear that the 5 mg dose worked and caused fewer side-effects.[158]

Another major criticism of the approval of the first pill by journalists in the late 1960s and the 1970s was that it had been tested for too short a time before its release. Officials in Britain and the United States, however, recommended strict limits on the length of time the pill could be prescribed for an individual woman.[159] This fact has been virtually ignored in all discussions of the subject.[160] When approved for gynaecological treatments in the United States, for instance, Enovid was restricted to between three to four months' consumption, with a maximum of ten months in the case of endometriosis.[161] Officials were well aware that approving the safety of the drug for use over a short period of time for menstrual disorders was very different from allowing it to be taken on an indefinite basis as a contraceptive. Initial FDA guidelines for Enovid as a contraceptive recommended, for instance, that individual prescriptions be limited to two years.[162] This two-year restriction continued well into the 1960s until enough evidence had been collected to show that the drug could be used safely by most women who chose to do so for longer periods of time.[163] Nonetheless, physicians were always free to exceed the recommendations.

Conclusion

Considered in their historical context and by comparison with others who released drugs on the market at the same time, the original developers of the pill have been unfairly accused of experimenting on women as though they were guinea pigs. The very trial process could not have worked without the full cooperation of women. Unlike animals, women could not be caged and watched constantly once given certain compounds. Women were free agents whose cooperation had to be constantly sought and won. Their agreement was vital if they were to swallow the pill regularly and submit to the investigative tests needed to check its action. Physicians working in

Britain realized that it was the women who were the most successful monitors of the effects of the pill. As Dr Margaret Jackson pointed out in 1960, 'Greatly to my interest, I find that one of my best assessors of dose are the patients themselves. They settle their doses very often, and they settle them very well.'[164] The active cooperation of women in the investigative process thus throws into question the idea that they were guinea pigs. It would also be wrong to see the clinical trials as directed at the most vulnerable and impoverished groups of women of the third world. As we have seen, trials were conducted on women from a variety of locations and class backgrounds.

Any analysis of the pill has to take into consideration the historical context in which it was developed. If the pill is compared with other pharmaceutical products also coming on to the market at the time, those conducting the trials cannot be accused of negligence and supplying a questionable drug. The standards of the time required only very basic and simple toxicity tests in running the trial which Pincus and his team undertook before launching large-scale trials in Puerto Rico. Indeed, it could be argued that Pincus and his team, in carrying out large-scale field studies in Puerto Rico and elsewhere, did their utmost to monitor and test the pill with strict scrutiny.[165] In doing this, however, they not only had the difficulty of monitoring the population in the trial, they were also unaware of exactly what to look for and had only very basic equipment at their disposal to do the tests. At the end of the day the regulatory bodies considered the pill to be a safe and effective contraceptive.

5
Doctors and the Pill

Shortly after the first oral contraceptive was officially marketed in Britain in 1961, a general practitioner, practising in a remote rural part of Norfolk, had his lunchtime drink interrupted by medical colleagues. They had come to protest about his prescription of oral contraceptives. Outraged, they saw his action as 'totally unethical' and 'undermining the reputation of the medical practice in the neighbourhood as well as the morals of the public at large'.[1] Their complaint was not an isolated event. Indeed, many doctors in the early 1960s were opposed to prescribing the pill. One British doctor, Dr J. W. Dignan, summed up the attitude of many when he stated in 1962 that 'the provision of contraceptives is not the function of a doctor'.[2] A similar argument was made by Dr A. Hill in the same year when he argued that 'medicine's calling is to guard against illness ... and to treat established diseases through appropriate remedies'. From his point of view the prescription of oral contraceptives was thus a 'debasement' of the medical vocation, 'a misapplication' of medical 'knowledge and totally unworthy of a great profession'.[3] Such views were not confined to Britain. In the United States a former president of the Academy of General Practice reflected a common feeling in the 1960s when he stated: 'Physicians have one job and one job only – healing the sick.'[4]

Over the next decade, however, most British and American doctors changed their attitude towards contraception in general,[5] and part of this can be attributed to the appearance of the pill. It radicalized the medical profession's view of contraception. Prior to oral contraceptives doctors had mainly issued the diaphragm, but many disliked this device because it needed careful fitting which was regarded as an 'improper' medical pursuit.[6] By comparison hormonal contraception relied on a pharmaceutical drug which required medical prescription. Because of its physiological effect, the pill had potentially dangerous medical consequences if not administered correctly. Necessitating greater medical supervision than previous birth control devices, oral contraceptives thus turned contraception into a legitimate medical activity.

The pill not only increased physicians' contact with contraception, it also promoted a new form of preventive medicine. Unlike other forms of pharmaceutical drugs, which were prescribed to cure an illness, oral contraceptives were intended for the prevention of pregnancy in healthy women. It was therefore important that the women were constantly checked. Physicians were expected to conduct a full medical examination of the women prior to issuing the pill, as well as to undertake regular breast examinations and cervical smears thereafter. Such procedures coincided with an increasing emphasis on preventive medicine and the ascendance of cancer-screening programmes generally. While physicians varied in the degree to which they examined their patients, the rising number of women who were coming into a doctor's surgery for oral contraceptives made such screening easier. In addition to encouraging more regular examinations, the pill generated widespread medical investigation into its side-effects. Large epidemiological studies to detect the long-term effects of the pill were established early on, making it one of the most intensively studied medicines in history.[7] The pill thus brought an unprecedented number of healthy women under the scrutiny of the medical profession.

It would be a mistake, however, to see the pill as the sole reason for the growth of medical interest in contraception. To some extent the pill accelerated a process that had begun before it. A number of physicians, for instance, had begun to see themselves as pivotal to the provision of contraception long before the pill was developed. The medical response to oral contraceptives was part of the wider phenomenon of increasing medical intervention in areas of women's reproductive health, such as pregnancy and childbirth, since the early twentieth century.[8] As with all previous medical interventions, physicians varied in their response to the pill. This chapter focuses on the medical profession's reactions in the United States and Britain, which were among the first countries to market it.

Medical profession and the provision of contraception

When considering the medical response to the pill it is important to under-stand the historical context in which contraception had been distributed prior to its development. For much of the early twentieth century, family planning clinics, set up by birth control campaigners, were the chief providers of contraceptives in Britain and the United States. Many within the medical establishment were disdainful of the work done in these clinics. Part of this stemmed from the fact that they were controlled by lay committees rather than medical practitioners. The medical establishment also associated much of the work undertaken at such clinics with unortho-dox practice and quackery.[9] Those working in family planning clinics were considered to be committing 'professional suicide'. Significantly, the majority of physicians staffing these clinics were part-timers volunteering on humanitarian or eugenic grounds. A large proportion of the doctors working in these clinics were also women or immigrant doctors who struggled to get medical positions elsewhere. Working in such clinics was particularly attractive for women because it could be combined with the demands of a family.[10]

Nonetheless, family planning clinics were an important source of contraception for many women in both the United States and Britain. Voluntary birth control clinics had been set up in the United States as early as 1916, and in Britain in 1921. In the United States the clinics came under the umbrella of the Planned Parenthood Federation of America (PPFA) and in Britain under the Family Planning Association (FPA). The prime aim of the clinics was to help women who could not afford to buy contra-ception through a physician or from other sources.[11] Overall the British clinics were more numerous and served a greater proportion of women than those in the United States. Indeed the FPA had become an accepted auxiliary medical service, albeit financed on a voluntary basis or by local authorities.[12]

One of the reasons for the larger number of women visiting birth control clinics in Britain was the absence of other contraceptive providers until the 1960s. As early as 1930 the British government permitted local authorities to establish maternal welfare clinics funded by rates. They were designed to give contraceptive advice to women suffering from medical problems contra-indicating further pregnancies but their function was restricted to advice and did not extend to supplies. In addition, few authorities provided such services. In 1948, with the establishment of the National Health Service, grants began to be given for the provision of contraception to those suffering from problems that were not necessarily medical.[13] Despite such funding, only about a quarter of all local health authorities in 1954 were making use of the government money provided. Few authorities saw contraception as necessary for conditions other than medical ones and feared political problems if they were to make such provision.[14]

The reluctance of local authorities to provide contraceptives mirrored that of the medical establishment. The British Medical Association, for instance, was unwilling to have any association with the subject.[15] Medical students also received little training in the area. In 1950 the British Medical Women's Federation published a survey which showed that only 5 of 27 medical schools provided special lectures on contraception to their students. A survey carried out in 1957 indicated that fewer than half of medical graduates had received instruction on contraception and sexual relations. Teaching on these subjects continued to be poor until the 1970s. Up to the late 1960s the FPA was the main agency which taught medical professionals about contraception, and until 1969 it received no central funding for such training.[16]

Not all British medical practitioners, however, were opposed to contraception. Neither was teaching on the subject totally absent. Young doctors who were trained in the years after the Second World War were more favourably disposed towards contraception. Some received training in the subject while working on obstetric wards. Dr I. Loudon, for instance, who worked as an obstetric houseman in 1950 in a large maternity ward in a hospital in Oxford, remembered being taught how to fit diaphragms as a regular part of postnatal care. Contraceptive advice, moreover, was not confined to postnatal care. When Dr Loudon went into general practice in the early 1950s he and many of his peers were routinely fitting diaphragms and offering contraceptive advice. Overall, however, Dr Loudon and his young colleagues were a minority within the medical profession. Many of the older prewar generation of general practitioners had little interest in contraception, like the medical establishment in general.[17] In 1963 less than 50 per cent of a sample of 157 British general practitioners thought that contraception should be within the jurisdiction of general practice.[18]

The aversion of many British medical practitioners to contraception stood in marked contrast to the attitudes of doctors in the United States.[19] In spite of the greater formal restrictions imposed by legislation, American medical practitioners started issuing contraceptives much earlier than in Britain. By the 1940s many American physicians were beginning to support birth control and were routinely providing information on demand to their wealthy private patients, even in states where the Comstock laws were strongly enforced and contraceptive provision was severely restricted.[20] In 1947 a national survey indicated that more than half of America's physicians in private practice were prescribing contraception to any married woman who wanted it.[21] To some extent the difference in medical attitudes towards contraception between the United States and Britain reflected the wider structure of the medical marketplace. While American physicians were able to deal with their patients directly and charge for their services, those in Britain were increasingly reliant on public funding and constrained by attitudes about what was deemed appropriate to cover through public expenditure.

The growing number of physicians in the United States providing contraception by the 1940s partly reflected changes that had accompanied the *United States v. One Package* case in 1936. This had 'explicitly ruled that the medical prescription of contraception for the purpose of saving life or promoting the patient's well-being was not a "condemned purpose" under the Comstock law'. The pronouncement 'effectively legalized birth control because it did not require the presence of disease to legitimate contraceptive prescription'.[22] In 1937 the American Medical Association reluctantly agreed to reverse its previous condemnation of contraception and accept it as a legitimate medical practice.[23] Medical schools also began to include contraception in the curriculum. In 1940 60 per cent of approved medical colleges provided some instruction in contraceptive techniques. Two years later the American Medical Association recommended that medical students be 'taught the clinical considerations and therapeutic application of contraceptive methods'.[24]

The increasing involvement of the American medical profession in contraception was accompanied by a shift in ideas about when it was appropriate to issue contraception. For much of the early twentieth century the established medical profession had argued against the prescription of contraception requested for reasons other than medical and were hostile to family planning clinics that contravened this principle.[25] By the 1940s, however, many doctors were issuing contraception to women on grounds that were not entirely medical. In 1958 the American Public Health Association captured the widening definition being applied to contraception when it declared family planning to be a proper and legitimate aspect of public health.

Reflecting this change between 1953 and 1958 the PPFA found that the number of medical professionals who were willing to join its executive committee had more than doubled. Many of those joining the committee were distinguished medical professionals from a variety of disciplines. They ranged from obstetrics and gynaecology to public health, internal medicine and psychiatry.[26] The increasing enthusiasm of the medical profession continued into the 1960s. In 1964 the American Medical Association and the American Gynecological Society recognized for the first time that the provision of contraception need not be confined to those with medical problems. As the American Gynecological Society resolution stated, 'The proper prescription of child-spacing measures is an essential aspect of preventive medicine. It should be available to all who desire it, whether they obtain their medical care through private physicians or tax-supported health services.'[27]

In some ways the American physicians' acceptance of contraception was merely an extension of their increasing involvement in other areas of reproductive health. This was most noticeable in the field of childbirth, where obstetricians had replaced midwives by the mid-twentieth century. Childbirth had not only come to be dominated by obstetricians, but was increasingly taking place in hospitals. By 1950 98 per cent of American urban births were taking place in hospitals. (In Britain only 50 per cent of such births occurred in hospital.[28]) Many American obstetricians and gynaecologists regarded contraception as another avenue for gaining clientele. This was reinforced by the appearance of the oral contraceptive.

Pharmaceutical companies were quick to point out the advantage the pill brought to the doctor. Emphasizing the newly augmented role of physicians in family planning, one advertisement for the oral contraceptive Norinyl also pointed out in 1964 that the drug not only allowed the physician to 'offer a dependable and physiologic approach to fertility timing that is under his control', but that the 'opportunity to further his patient's happiness and to promote family harmony is greatly increased'.[29] Many of the pharmaceutical advertisements appearing in medical journals in the United States indicated the potential expansion of patients and earnings physicians could gain by providing oral contraceptives. Moreover it potentially allowed doctors more regular contact with their female patients.[30]

Many gynaecologists had initially become familiar with the first pill, Enovid, when it was released for the treatment of gynaecological disorders in 1957. As soon as Enovid had been released as a gynaecological drug, Searle had sent out letters to leading obstetricians, gynaecologists and general practitioners indicating that 'there is adequate evidence to indicate that the drug will inhibit ovulation when the physician so chooses and that it is safe for this purpose in short-term medication', and went on to describe how the drug might be used to achieve this effect.[31] Thus, while the drug was not being explicitly distributed as a contraceptive, physicians quickly learnt of its contraceptive potential. It is difficult to know how many physicians used it in this way until it was approved as a contraceptive in 1960. Nonetheless, within five years of Enovid's appearance as a contraceptive in 1960, 95 per cent of American obstetricians and gynaecologists were prescribing it.

Part of this speed of take-up reflected the vigorous campaign by the pharmaceutical companies to promote the drug. Many physicians first learnt about the contraceptive through the promotional literature from the pharmaceutical companies. The strength of this promotion campaign cannot be underestimated. With approximately fifteen thousand pharmaceutical sales representatives in the United States, it was hard for doctors to miss the message.[32] By the 1970s private physicians delivered at least 50 per cent of domestic contraceptive services. Obstetricians and gynaecologists dominated the field, partly reflecting their overall command of reproductive health. By 1976, 61 per cent of the American physicians providing contraception were obstetricians and gynaecologists, while 28 per cent were general practitioners.[33]

To some extent the appearance of the pill in the United States merely accelerated doctors' interest in contraception. In Britain, however, the pill had a more dramatic effect on the medical profession, most notably the general practitioner. This is particularly striking given that general practitioners traditionally had little experience with contraception and were not expected to provide it automatically under the National Health Service. Nonetheless, by the mid-1960s general practitioners had begun to usurp the FPA clinics as the main providers of contraception. Many of these doctors had first learnt about the pill from medical journals, and the prescribers' book sent to all medical practitioners by the Ministry of Health.[34] By the 1990s general practitioners were writing at least 90 per cent of all prescriptions for the pill in Britain.[35]

Government and general practitioners in Britain were drawn into increasing involvement with contraception because oral contraceptives had to be prescribed. Initially, guidelines were unclear about how far such prescriptions would be paid for under the National Health Service, and whether women could expect to have them free or pay a standard charge. In December 1961 the Minister of Health indicated that the National Health Service would only cover oral contraceptives prescribed for medical conditions, as had been laid down by legislation governing contraceptives in the 1930s. From 1964 doctors within the National Health Service were allowed to give private prescriptions for oral contraceptives not issued on medical grounds. From 1967 the British government agreed to pay general practitioners a special fee for prescribing private prescriptions for the pill, and for fitting contraceptive appliances and intrauterine devices when given on non-medical grounds.[36] While the British Medical Association frowned on doctors selling oral contraceptives for profit, for the first time general practitioners now had a financial incentive to provide contraception.[37] The sum they could earn from such a service was not unsubstantial. In 1988, for instance, general practitioners earned on average an extra £1,540 per annum for contraceptive services, the second largest contribution to their income from item-of-service payments after maternity services.[38] Not surprisingly the number of general practitioners providing contraceptive advice was to rise over the decades following 1967. Much of this reflected the fact that prescribing the pill was a much more cost-effective use of doctors' time than fitting the cap.

Part of the increase in contraceptive services provided by doctors came about in response to a greater demand from patients for contraceptive devices of all sorts.[39] In many cases doctors found themselves being asked for the pill by patients.[40] This was slightly unusual in the history of medicine because, prior to the pill, drugs were usually prescribed by the doctor with little prompting from patients.[41] A national survey conducted between 1967 and 1970 among parents from 12 areas in England and Wales revealed that four-fifths of general practitioners who had been in practice for five years or more were spending more time discussing birth control than five years previously. It also revealed that they had become the main sources of information about contraception.[42] A different study of 1,989 doctors in England and Wales in the 1960s indicated that most doctors, while concerned about the social problems of their families, were more likely to raise the subject of family planning where there were clear clinical indications.[43]

General practitioners were known to recommend the pill more frequently than other forms of contraception. Of the mothers interviewed for the British study of parents in 1967–70, nine-tenths of those who had taken the pill indicated that it had been a general practitioner who had first offered and prescribed them the drug. This investigation also followed up 527 general practitioners and found that 95 per cent of them prescribed the pill. The preference of the general practitioners for oral contraceptives in the 1960s contrasted with family planning clinics, where the diaphragm remained the dominant type of contraception recommended. Many of the women chose general practitioners over family planning clinics not only because they issued the pill, but because they were more familiar to them and easily accessible.[44] By 1970, 700,000 (14 per cent) of the 5 million married women aged 16–40 were obtaining contraceptives from general practitioners, the majority being prescribed the pill.[45] This was a trend which was to increase in coming years. A national survey conducted in 1985 indicated that 55 per cent of women preferred to consult a general practitioner for their contraceptive provision, compared to 33 per cent who preferred a clinic. The remaining 12 per cent showed no particular preference. Women tended to favour the general practitioners not only on the grounds of familiarity, but also because they were more likely to have daily office hours and provide greater continuity of care. Moreover, the purpose of a visit to the general practitioner could be more easily disguised to friends and neighbours.[46]

General practitioners were not uniform in their prescription of the pill. In Britain, for instance, younger general practitioners working in the late 1960s prescribed oral contraceptives more frequently than their older colleagues. A survey of 525 British general practitioners in 1967 indicated that younger doctors also tended to be more aware of the risks associated with the pill than the older generation. It also showed that doctors with larger surgeries (over 3,500 patients) were more likely to see their work as including the provision of contraception. Overall male doctors were more prepared to prescribe the drug than female doctors. Part of this stemmed from the fact that women physicians were much more concerned about the risks associated with the pill. For this reason they were more likely to offer the cap or the IUD. When giving out oral contraceptives women doctors also restricted their prescription of the drug to six months or less.[47]

Medical care of women taking the pill

From the time of the pill's experimental introduction through to the time of its marketing, physicians were expected to undertake rigorous medical examinations of the women to whom they prescribed pills. The FPA's

Clinic Handbook specified that doctors should take a full medical history and examine the woman's breasts, abdomen and cervix. Where possible women were also to have cervical smears and their blood pressure and weight taken.[48] A report by the World Health Organization in 1966 also recommended these procedures, with regular check-ups every six months.[49] In many ways the doctors' prescription of oral contraception afforded them the opportunity of carrying out preventive check-ups they could not otherwise have done because of women's reluctance to come forward for such tests. As one British medical textbook published in 1969 stressed, 'The family doctor may be the only physician that the woman sees with any regularity and a cervical smear and questions on lumps in the breast can be life-saving.'[50] The provision of contraception could thus be used as a convenient reason for recalling women for routine measures in preventive medicine.[51]

Many of the examinations recommended for patients taking the pill were not new. Cervical smears, for instance, had begun to be used by the medical profession in the United States as early as the 1940s, and started being used on a small scale in screening programmes in the 1950s. By contrast, in Britain the routine use of cervical smears in medical practice began in the late 1950s and became part of the National Health Service in 1967.[52] What is noticeable about Britain is that cervical screening increased at the very time the pill appeared, so it can be argued that the pill was influential in promoting cervical smears in Britain. The rise of patients coming forward for oral contraceptives certainly made it easier to target patients for screening.

Wherever they were based, doctors varied in the level of care they gave to their patients.[53] Physicians working in family planning clinics in both the United States and Britain paid much greater attention to their patients. In the United States, for instance, the obstetrician-gynaecologist Edward Tyler, who carried out some of the early clinical trials of the pill in Los Angeles, insisted his daughter obtain the pill from a family planning clinic rather than a private physician because the clinic offered better medical supervision.[54] In the early years British family planning clinics gave greater attention to pill patients than did general practitioners.[55] General practitioners said they were handicapped by the pressures of time and on occasion were known to prescribe pills without seeing their patients at all.[56] The 1967–70 British investigation of parents revealed that only 36 per cent of women who first received oral contraceptives from a general practitioner had been given a medical examination at the time. This was a much lower percentage than women receiving their pill from a family planning clinic, where the proportion was 97 per cent.[57] The same survey indicated that despite an increase in publicity about thrombotic risks between 1969 and 1970, the proportion of general practitioners who undertook a medical examination of their patients taking the pill went down rather than up in 1970.[58] A questionnaire posted by the pharmaceutical company Syntex in 1968 to 1,240 specialists and completed by 356 respondents revealed that most consultants saw their patients on an annual basis.[59] The disparity in medical care offered to women taking the pill between general practitioners and clinics continued on into the 1980s. A British survey of 1988 also indicated that general practitioners overall provided their patients with a less balanced discussion of the risks and benefits of the pill than did practitioners in clinics.[60]

Liberation from pregnancy and childbirth

Much of the care doctors took of their patients depended on their attitude towards the safety of oral contraceptives. Reflecting the greater emphasis on surgical and medical intervention within the American medical world than in Britain, American physicians tended to dismiss the dangers of the pill more quickly than their British counterparts. National differences, however, were not rigid.[61] Doctors in the United States could be just as cautious about the drug as those in Britain and vice versa.[62] Much depended on a physician's particular medical speciality and who employed them. Physicians involved in the pill's initial trials and promotion, or those who had stronger ties with the pharmaceutical industry, tended to stress the benefits of the pill. Those involved in state committees to assess the safety of drugs, or in research exploring the possible side-effects of the pill, were more critical in their approach.

One of the medical justifications for prescribing the pill was that it protected women against dangers associated with pregnancy and childbirth. As one American doctor arguing in favour of the pill put it, pregnancy could not be regarded as completely 'benign'.[63] Many saw the risk of dying as a result of pregnancy as greater than the potential risks of the pill.[64] Much of the argument was based on the notion that many pregnancies, particularly those that were unwanted, resulted in maternal deaths, either because of ill-performed abortions or inadequate access to good obstetric care. The high incidence of maternal mortality, especially among underprivileged women, gave strong credence to this assertion. A powerful proponent of this view was Dr Joseph Goldzieher.[65] He showed that in America underprivileged women faced a risk of dying in childbirth from complications during delivery that was five times greater than that of economically privileged women. The maternal mortality rate among underprivileged women was 250 per million. In developing countries the rate was often much higher. In Ceylon, for instance, the death-rate was between 6,000 and 7,000 per million pregnant women.[66]

Goldzieher and other medical professionals argued that all women of childbearing age were potentially at risk, even if they were taking contraceptive precautions other than the pill. This they justified on the grounds that other forms of contraception were far less effective than the pill in guarding women against pregnancy and possible death. If side-effects, such as thrombosis, were taken into account, the number of women dying as a result of taking oral contraceptives would be between 15 and 40 per million. By comparison, the number of deaths per million among women exposed to the failure rate of other methods of contraception varied between three and 300.[67]

In this context pregnancy and childbirth were viewed as pathological and requiring medical intervention, rather than as natural processes. Such ideas were not new. During the interwar years a number of physicians, driven by concern about rising rates of maternal mortality, had advocated greater medical intervention, such as prophylactic episiotomies and the use of instruments in deliveries, to shield women from the fatal consequences of childbirth.[68] Some physicians saw such intervention as necessary because they believed that women's bodies had been weakened by the process of civilization and could no longer withstand the difficulties of labour.[69] Other medical practitioners were not quite so confident. As one British doctor asked in 1961:

> Are none of my colleagues as apprehensive as I am about the threatened advent of oral contraceptive therapy? The prime function of the human race was to reproduce itself, and we are threatening to strike a blow at the very heart of the process which is responsible for the miracle of life itself. Will Nature let this indignity go unchallenged? Will she allow the creatures to whom she has given the privilege of existence to interfere with the process that gave them the existence?

To prevent contraception by mechanical barriers is a different thing altogether – this is merely controlling the end product of a natural process, not interfering with the process itself. If Nature decides that science has invaded the very heart of her domain, what terrible penalties may she inflict upon the female of the species. Sterility? Ovarian atrophy? Malignant disease?[70]

Other doctors agreed with this reasoning. One American obstetrician and gynaecologist, Dr Hugh Davis (director of a contraceptive clinic and assistant professor of obstetrics and gynaecology at Johns Hopkins Medical School), contended that the difference was that while the pill might be more effective than other contraceptives, it produced systemic changes in the body which other contraceptives did not.[71] Similar arguments were made in the British journal the *Lancet* which, in listing 50 metabolic side-effects of the pill, stated:

These changes are unnecessary for contraception and their ultimate effect on the health of the user is unknown. But clearly they cannot be ignored, since they raise the possibility of irreversible structural changes, such as arteriosclerosis, after 10 or 20 years. In view of these doubts, the wisdom of administering such compounds to healthy women for many years must be seriously questioned.[72]

British doctors involved in cancer research also called for caution in using the pill, arguing that it should be used only for medical and not social reasons.[73]

Dr William Inman, who undertook pioneering research in Britain on the thromboembolic effects of the pill for the Committee on Safety of Drugs (later renamed Committee on Safety of Medicines) in the 1960s and 1970s, also contested the arguments used by Goldzieher and others. As he pointed out in 1970:

Many comparisons with the risks of pregnancy have ignored the obvious fact that a woman has to become pregnant before she can run any risk of dying as a result of this pregnancy. If, for example, mechanical methods of contraception had a failure rate of 10% per annum, as against nil for oral contraception, the mortality due to the latter should be compared with one-tenth of the mortality associated with one pregnancy.[74]

Similarly, he warned that any evaluation of the risks of the pill against maternal mortality should take into account the fact that many of the women who died in childbirth had not died as a result of their pregnancy. A report from the Department of Health and Social Security in the early 1960s showed that, with the exception of abortion, at least 30 per cent of the women dying during pregnancy, delivery or the puerperium, died of underlying medical or surgical complications they had suffered before becoming pregnant.[75] This indicated the fallacy of regarding all pregnancies as pathological and posing a greater risk than the pill.

What was at stake in the debate was whether unwanted pregnancies constituted a 'pre-existing pathological state'. As Dr Roy Hertz, associate medical director of the biomedical division at the Population Council in America,[76] put it in 1970:

The view we have to take, I think ... is that we are now seeing the emergence of a new preventive public health practice; namely the prevention of births. We have not yet socially agreed to what extremes we have to go in order to protect ourselves in terms of survival.[77]

For these reasons the degree of risk involved in averting an unwanted pregnancy remains a tremendously undefined term, both in social as well as medical terms.[78]

For some doctors the risks associated with oral contraceptives were minimal compared with those associated with routine activities such as travelling by air, by car or by motorbike, rock climbing, smoking, domestic accidents or playing soccer. As a medical textbook on contraception pointed out in 1969:

There are a large number of recreational activities which are more dangerous than taking the Pill. In the USA there are over 5,000 boating and swimming fatalities a year and there is ten times the likelihood of a death in the family if father buys an outboard motor boat than if mother uses oral contraceptives. It is probable that the amateur cricketer or footballer (activities which caused twenty-seven deaths in the UK, 1955–8) is more likely to die playing sports at the weekend than his wife is to die from using oral contraceptives.

This comment is particularly interesting for understanding the ways in which questions of gender informed the debate about the risks of the pill. What is most noteworthy is that it was primarily recreational pursuits that were used as the comparative tool for assessing the risks women faced when taking the pill. Clearly the authors of the textbook viewed the use of oral contraceptives as merely a matter of recreation. The choice made by a man to sail a boat, swim or play football or cricket was equated with that made by a woman when engaging in sexual intercourse and presenting herself with the possibility of pregnancy. The same medical textbook went on to point out:

Almost without exception the consequences of contraception are beneficial and contribute significantly to the health and well-being of the community. In contrast, many societies permit drugs and other practices which are of questionable value or are demonstrably harmful. The ill-effects of alcohol and tobacco, which are tolerated for no better reason than that they provide comfort and pleasure, add appreciably to the mortality and morbidity rates of many societies, but they are inadequately regulated by civil law and social custom and do not fall within the sphere of medical prescription at all.[79]

Many went further to argue that oral contraceptives brought 'an inestimable benefit to mankind'.[80] In this statement, the choice of an individual woman and her health fades from view and is pushed to one side in favour of the good of society as a whole.

The pill as 'normal hormone'

In many cases doctors justified the prescription of the pill on the grounds that it induced a 'natural state' for women, merely mimicking the natural hormones of a menstrual cycle or pregnancy. Such thinking can partly be attributed to the original developers of the pill. As the obstetrician-gynaecologist John Rock put it, the pill merely provided 'a natural means of fertility control such as nature uses after ovulation and during pregnancy'.[81] Explanations given to doctors and patients replicated this model in explaining how the pill worked and its side-effects.[82] Thus symptoms such nausea, breast changes, fluid retention, headaches, depression, abdominal cramp, weight increase and glucose intolerance were initially dismissed on the grounds that they also occurred during the menstrual cycle and pregnancy.[83]

Comparable arguments were also made in relation to the possible long-term effects of the pill. In 1963, for instance, Dr A. S. Parkes, a British scientist closely involved in the initiation of the first clinical trials of the pill in Britain, argued that the contraceptive would not have a detrimental effect on the anterior pituitary gland. He declared:

> In fairness it should be pointed out that the ovulation-producing activity of the human pituitary gland is inhibited for a year or more during pregnancy and lactation; so in this respect the continued use of the pill may be likened to a rapid succession of pregnancies. However undesirable in other ways, a succession of pregnancies is not usually regarded as carcinogenic or endocrinologically catastrophic.[84]

Not everyone was happy with such thinking. Many, for example, feared that interference with the pituitary gland might cause cancer. Dr Hilton Salhanick, professor of obstetrics and gynaecology at Harvard University, stressed that contraceptive steroids were not equal to natural hormones. They differed substantially both in their chemical structure and in their biological function.[85] This was a view also promoted by Dr Hugh Davis, who argued that to think of oral contraceptives 'as natural is comforting but quite false'. He went on to warn: 'In using these agents, we are in fact embarking on a massive endocrinologic experiment with millions of healthy women.' Dr Victor Wynn, who helped to expose the negative metabolic effects of anabolic steroids in the 1950s, revealed in the early 1960s that oral contraceptives had abnormal metabolic side-effects on women's bodies such as increasing their weight.[86]

'Normalization of women'

One of the most controversial debates about the pill centred on its psychological effects. Many pharmaceutical advertisements for oral contraceptives emphasized not only the drug's prevention of pregnancy but also the emotional distress women might experience during their normal menstrual cycle. Capturing this view in 1964, an advertisement for Envoid claimed:

> *Unfettered.* From the beginning woman has been a vassal to the temporal demands – and frequently the aberrations – of the cyclic mechanism of her reproductive system. Now to a degree heretofore unknown, she is permitted normalization, enhancement or suspension of cyclic function and procreative potential. This new method [of] control is symbolized in an illustration borrowed from ancient Greek mythology – Andromeda freed from her chains.[87]

In alluding to Andromeda the advertisement drew on the story of a woman saved from death by Perseus. Rescuing her from a rock where she had been chained naked by her parents in a sacrificial bid to assuage the anger of the god Poseidon, Perseus won Andromeda's hand in marriage.[88] Now Enovid was being offered to save women from the age-old torment of their reproductive functions.

The Andromeda advertisement shows that the debate on the pill represented more than just a question of freedom from pregnancy. Indeed, it would seem that the pill symbolized the possibility of the 'normalization' of women's cycles. Such claims also appeared in the literature put out by other pharmaceutical companies for different formulations of the pill.[89] Yet what was meant by 'normalization' is unclear and raises interesting questions about the ways in which women's bodies were perceived. In America and to a lesser, but still significant, extent in Britain, women's reproductive organs have often been regarded by some of the medical profession not as natural but as something of a nuisance and in need of control. This can be most clearly seen from the justifications used in America for undertaking hysterectomies. As one American obstetrician/gynaeologist, Dr Ralph C. Wright, put it in 1970: 'After the last planned pregnancy, the uterus becomes a useless, bleeding, symptom-producing, potentially cancer-bearing organ and therefore should be removed. If, in addition, both ovaries are removed, further benefits accrue.' A similar attitude appeared in 1975 in the widely used American *Novak's Textbook of Gynecology*, which declared, 'Menstruation is a nuisance to most women, and if this can be abolished without impairing ovarian function, it would probably be a blessing not only to the woman but to her husband. ...

Thus one can make a rather convincing case for the value of elective hyseterectomy.'[90]

Such attitudes to women's bodies and their reproductive organs can be traced back to well before the twentieth century. Indeed, it had many parallels with earlier medical interventions to control women's suscepti-bility to 'hysteria' in the nineteenth century. Within this context medicine was seen as saving women from the emotional instability caused by their reproductive organs. Some of these beliefs can be linked to earlier medical understandings, which as late as the mid-nineteenth century still depicted the woman's body and her reproductive organs in accordance with a model of the male body.[91] Like hysterectomies, the pill could be viewed as nor-malizing women's bodies, bringing their reproductive organs under control and making them function in the way that men in general imag-ined women would like their bodies to behave. Yet the changes that the pill could induce were more subtle and complex than the more overt and instrumental procedures obstetricians and gynaecologists had used in the past to treat women.[92]

Some of the major benefits promoters promised the pill would confer was relief for those suffering from pre-menstrual tension, dysmenorrhoea, migraine, breast discomfort, nervousness, irritability, excessive menstrual loss, irregular menses, acne, spots, greasy hair, lack of libido and sleep-lessness.[93] For many women oral contraceptives did indeed offer an enormous advantage in alleviating such problems. However, in some cases such promises were also used to dismiss the negative effects of the pill. Much of the debate centred on the perceived emotional vulnerability women experienced as a result of their hormonal changes during the menstrual cycle. Clinicians involved in the early trials of the oral contra-ceptive, for instance, were slow to recognize the pill's side-effects on the grounds that they were 'subjective symptoms influenced by many emotional factors', and that they were 'often present in normal women'.[94] Reactions such as vomiting, nausea, dizziness, headache and 'gastralgia' were all labelled 'psychogenic'.[95] Some doctors attributed the side-effects to apprehension that women experienced when first taking the pill. Once on the pill many women showed fewer nervous symptoms and fewer reactions than those who were completely new to the drug.[96] The importance of women's psychological state was also seen as vital in determining who should be prescribed the contraceptive. Those considered to be anxious and worried were thought liable to exaggerate anything that was slightly wrong and were therefore not recommended to be prescribed the pill.[97]

One of the difficulties was to separate these reactions from coincidental symptoms women experienced in their everyday life. As one study put it, the difference between these conditions and the pill was that 'usually there is no one around to ask them about the way they feel'.[98] Doctors were initially particularly dismissive of depression as a reaction because women often experienced this as a result of normal hormonal changes in menstruation, pregnancy and menopause. The extent to which depression was seen as a natural part of women's lives can be seen from the reactions of women themselves. Many did not associate such symptoms with the pill because they regarded depression and mood swings as a normal part of their lives. Others who recognized feeling more tired, depressed and irritable as a result of the drug continued to take it because they felt its contraceptive benefits outweighed its disadvantages.[99]

Mood fluctuations as a result of the pill were therefore difficult to distinguish from what was perceived as 'normal'.[100] In some cases doctors did not dissuade depressed women from using the pill precisely because such mood swings were regarded as quite normal.[101] Others argued that the pseudo-pregnant state that the pill induced in women could result in their becoming more depressed if taken off it, resulting in a similar depression to postpartum psychosis. One American physician argued that patients who had a history of psychiatric illness and who had no alternative contraceptive options but to take the pill should be prescribed anti-depressants alongside the pill. In doing this he stressed the need to inform women of the implications of this measure and to leave taking the pill to their discretion.[102] Significantly, rather than recommending a withdrawal of the pill altogether, he argued instead that women should take extra drugs. This view may have reflected a general tendency among medical practitioners towards pharmacological solutions, as had been witnessed during the early 1950s with the widespread prescription of Valium to housebound mothers with small children.

Another area under dispute was whether the pill caused loss of libido. In 1964 discussions held between British doctors conducting oral contraceptive clinical trials highlighted the fact that many of their patients complained of a decrease of libido. Further investigation into the problem, however, was rejected because it was seen as 'such an indeterminate symptom ... that it would be impossible to measure'.[103] Interestingly, by contrast, initial tests to develop the male oral contraceptive had been abandoned because of its effect on the male libido.[104] To some extent initial reluctance to recognize the problem reflected the denial of female sexuality that had dominated social and medical debates well before the twentieth century.[105] Nonetheless, one of the explicit arguments medical professionals and the pharmaceutical industry used in promoting the pill was that it would enable women to enjoy sex; they stressed the enhancement women experienced in their libido as a result of taking the pill.[106] Only in 1970 was serious attention beginning to be paid to the effect the pill had on the female libido.[107]

Conclusion

Ever since the 1920s Margaret Sanger, the American birth control activist, had been looking for a way to encourage the medical profession to take an interest in contraception.[108] To some extent it can be argued that the appearance of the pill and the concurrent rise in the medical provision of contraception indicated that her dream had finally been realized. This was most noticeable in Britain, where doctors had remained reluctant to be involved in anything to do with birth control until the marketing of oral contraceptives. By the end of the 1960s, however, general practitioners had replaced voluntarily funded family planning clinics as the main providers of contraceptives. This was reinforced by the reorganization of the National Health Service in 1974, which resulted in the disappearance of many family planning clinics. The need for a prescription for the pill, together with the establishment of a special payment to doctors by the National Health Service, created a new revenue stream from contraception. In the United States, the pill was less dramatic in its impact on the medical profession. Here obstetricians and gynaecologists had already begun to prescribe contraceptives on a growing scale from the 1940s as part of their increasing control of the reproductive field. In this country, therefore, the pill thus merely accelerated a process that had already begun.

The most striking difference oral contraceptives made to the medical profession in both the United States and Britain was in the number of women it brought into doctor's surgeries. This not only made contraception a lucrative avenue for medical practitioners but increased the potential for more preventive healthcare among women, such as cervical smear tests. To some extent such scrutiny coincided with a rise in such medical procedures anyway. In many instances, however, women would not have come forward for such testing had it not been for their strong desire for the pill. Equally the potential side-effects of the pill made women and doctors more conscious of the need for regular check-ups.

While many medical practitioners were quick to embrace the pill because it was a pharmaceutical drug that required legitimate medical supervision, many of their arguments for its use were rooted in medical ideas about women and their bodies that stretched back to the nineteenth century. In praising the virtue of the contraceptive in protecting women against the hazards of pregnancy and childbirth, medical professionals reflected the earlier arguments used to justify invasive medical intervention to combat maternal mortality. Similarly the drug's promise of control over women's menstrual cycles and reproductive functions might be seen as a new twist in an old debate about women's propensity to hysteria because of their aberrant reproductive organs, and the implied necessity of ovariectomies.

While this can be regarded as one more example of primarily male medicine and attempts by the pharmaceutical industry to control women, such an interpretation distorts the much more complex history of the medical profession's response to the pill. The drug generated many contradictory and contrasting debates about women and their bodies within the medical profession. This in part reflected the diversity of backgrounds and affiliations of the medical professionals involved in work on the pill. Moreover, such a black and white picture hides the very real fears and anxieties initially expressed by the doctors themselves and the drug industries about prescribing the pill and the long-term implications this might have for women's health.

Much of the debate over the use of oral contraceptives and their safety hinged on whether they could be considered natural. While decrying the hazards of childbirth, many within the medical profession, particularly those involved in the pharmaceutical industry or running the initial clinical trials, saw the side-effects women experienced on taking the drug as reflecting the pseudo-pregnant state it caused. Thus the pill was regarded as a natural extension of the hormones in women's bodies. This was used to explain symptoms such as nausea, breast tenderness, depression or the more major disease of thrombosis that women experienced on taking the pill. Other doctors, however, particularly those monitoring the adverse reactions to drugs, were less happy with this conclusion, seeing the pill as a synthetic compound that had systemic effects throughout the body beyond controlling women's fertility. They pointed out the difficulties of equating the pill with a normal pregnancy, arguing that other forms of contraception were more localized in their impact on women's bodies and therefore posed less risk to their health.

The medical profession's response to the pill therefore varied. While many accepted the efficacy of the method, many continued to fear its safety. After the 1960s, fears about the hazards of the pill did not abate. The death of women from thrombotic complications in the 1960s reinforced the anxieties of many in the field, as did the lack of hard evidence about the effect of the pill in relation to cancer. Whether or not the pill was linked to these diseases continued to puzzle medical practitioners long after its first appearance.

6
Handling Health Concerns of the Pill: Thrombosis

In November 1961 a British family doctor from Suffolk wrote to the *Lancet* of a disturbing case he had seen of a woman who had developed thrombotic (blood-clot) complications after taking the first marketed oral contraceptive pill. Prescribed the pill for recurrent endometriosis, the woman had experienced nausea and intense vomiting. Three days after she stopped taking the drug the woman appeared to return to normal health, but ten days later she developed a blood clot in her lungs (pulmonary embolism).[1] She returned to normal health after three months, but was the first of many such cases to be reported in the British medical press in the months that followed. They included women suffering from a variety of thrombotic disorders, some with fatal consequences. Such disclosures were not confined to Britain. In December 1961, the Food and Drug Administration (FDA), the American drug regulatory agency, began to receive reports of women who had died from the oral contraceptive. By August 1962 the FDA had received reports of 26 women who had suffered from blood clots in their veins (thrombophlebitis), six of whom had died.[2] Such complications were not only alarming but were totally unexpected. Up to this point the major concern about the pill had focused on its potential carcinogenic effects.

News of the possible links between the contraceptive pill and thrombotic disease were especially worrying in the light of the thalidomide tragedy that was hitting the headlines in the early 1960s. The concern was particularly acute in Europe where the impact of thalidomide had been most catastrophic. One of the most drastic reactions to the negative reports about the pill occurred in Norway. Here, in August 1962, the Norwegian Directorate of Health temporarily stopped the sale of the pill 'pending investigation of the possible association between the pills and thrombosis'. The drug was only let back on to the Norwegian market in 1964. Other countries were less radical in their action. Governments in Britain and the United States, for instance, did not withdraw the pill from circulation. Instead they sent warnings to doctors, and provided government funding for investigating the problem.[3]

The varying responses of the United States and European countries in 1962 demonstrates the problems that confronted governments and medical experts in handling the question of the pill and thrombotic disease. What was at stake was not only the possibility of women dying from the drug, but also questions about banning what was becoming a very popular form of contraception. In addition to its popularity, the pill was championed by political figures and policy-makers as the key weapon for solving the highly politicized issue of population growth.

Focusing on Britain and the United States between the years of 1960 and 1970, this chapter explores the diverse reactions of medical experts and political figures to the issue of thrombosis and the pill. While medical practitioners and scientists were keen to unravel the connection between oral contraceptives and thrombotic disease, they were not always united in their interpretation and acceptance of the evidence presented. Indeed, there was some debate to and fro across the Atlantic between medical experts and scientists over what constituted the most appropriate procedure and valid evidence for answering the question and determining whether action should be taken. The acceptance and implementation of the findings of the scientific and medical community also varied between the two countries, reflecting their different legal, medical, social and political traditions.

The most distinctive difference between the United States and Britain lay in their policy moves after 1969. In December 1969, Britain restricted the prescribing powers of doctors, confining them to prescribing oral contraceptives with less than 50 micrograms of oestrogen, a dose shown to carry less risk of cardiovascular complications. Up to 1969 higher dosage pills represented about 50 per cent of the total sales. By 1970, however, pills containing more than 5 mg of oestrogen had almost completely disappeared from the market.[4] Indeed, many British medical practitioners had changed their prescribing habits by the early 1970s.

By contrast, American doctors continued to prescribe on a large scale pills that were restricted in Britain.[5] As late as 1978, 40 per cent of all women taking the contraceptive in the United States were prescribed pills containing 100 micrograms of oestrogen. Between 1970 and 1986 the American use of oral contraceptives containing more than 50 micrograms of oestrogen decreased from 65 per cent of the market to 3.4 per cent. While this meant the number of women taking the higher doses dropped from 7.5 million in 1970 to 400,000 in 1986, this still represented a significant number.[6] What was most disturbing was that women aged 35 to 39, that is, the group most at risk of developing thrombotic complications when taking oral contraceptives, were twice as likely to be recipients of high dose oestrogen pills than younger women. Moreover, more than 400,000 women were taking oral contraceptives containing between 80 and 100 micrograms of oestrogen. Only in 1988 did the FDA finally persuade the last three pharmaceutical companies who were manufacturing high dose oestrogen pills (over 50 micrograms) to withdraw them from the market.[7]

One of the reasons for the slow withdrawal of high oestrogen pills in the United States was the government's emphasis on providing better package inserts to alert women to the thrombotic dangers of the pill. This contrasted with Britain, where measures were targeted at directing doctors' prescribing habits. Many of the differences in the approach taken by the two countries can be attributed to the distinct values they attached to the legal and social status of the medical profession and the autonomy of the patient–consumer. Equally important were the nature of each country's regulatory philosophy and how much power pharmaceutical companies could exert over governmental decisions. The medical research orientation of each country was also a crucial determinant in defining the scope of the problem. British researchers, for instance, demonstrated what is now seen as the first conclusive link between high dose oestrogen pills and thrombosis. This partly reflected the strong British epidemiological tradition and the researchers' ability to draw on data from a centralized health-care system.[8]

Thrombotic disease and its links with the pill

When the first reports on thrombotic disease and the pill began to appear, it was clear that the blood clots varied in their severity. The intensity of the problem was partly determined by whether a clot had formed in the arteries or in the veins. Where a clot or 'thrombus' forms in a vein, most often in the thigh or lower leg, the condition is called thrombophlebitis.

Such problems can occur either following a minor injury to the leg, such as after a surgical operation or childbirth, or spontaneously, for example, when a person is immobile for too long on aeroplane or car journeys. In some instances these clots are minor and disappear of their own accord without becoming life-threatening. Where clotting occurs in one of the deep veins, a person can experience a large swelling in the leg. Moreover there is also a risk that part of the clot will break loose from the vein, where it originally developed, and form what is known as an embolus. The clot can then travel through the great veins to the heart and then to the lungs, where it can interfere with lung circulation (pulmonary embolism). The great majority of pulmonary embolisms are not fatal, but when the embolism is massive, death is very sudden.[9]

Clots that form in the arteries can occur anywhere in the body. Those that affect the heart, known as coronary thrombosis, can result in what is called myocardial infarction, which involves either the destruction or scarring of some of the heart muscle. Clots that affect the brain, cerebral thrombosis, one type of stroke, can lead to permanent brain damage, loss of speech or paralysis. In both instances a number of patients die soon after the event. Occasionally arterial thrombosis can occur in unusual sites such as the limbs, resulting in gangrene, or in the retina, leading to blindness.[10]

While reports in the 1960s indicated that some of these conditions occurred in women who were taking the pill, medical experts could not be sure whether the pill was the only cause, for many seemingly healthy people suffer such disorders without ever taking oral contraception. Pregnancy and operations, for instance, can lead to complications such as deep vein thrombosis. People who are obese, diabetic or smoke also have a greater propensity to suffer arterial thrombosis.[11] Such factors confused the medical community when trying to establish whether the pill alone could cause thrombosis.

The problem was made greater by the absence of reliable statistics concerning the natural occurrence of thrombotic complications in the general female population at various ages. In the early 1960s many patients who were hospitalized for thromboembolic morbidity were not officially reported. This was compounded by the fact that diagnosis was difficult and often inaccurate, and autopsies were not always carried out in the case of death. Moreover, prior to August 1962, very few doctors were aware of the possible connection between thrombotic disease and oral contraceptives, and thus failed to ask patients presenting with such disorders whether they were using the pill. This made it difficult to assess how the numbers of deaths which were considered to be associated with oral con-traceptives compared with the natural incidence of the disease in women of reproductive age.[12]

Drug monitoring and the structure of health care

Each country's framework for monitoring drugs determined the ways in which evidence was collected. When the first reports began to appear on thrombosis and the pill, the United States had a much longer and stronger legal tradition for monitoring the manufacture and safety of drugs than Britain. By the 1960s the FDA was a well-established institution. Set up to assess and monitor the safety of drugs, the powers of the FDA were extended in 1962 to allow for the withdrawal of a drug from the market where it had proved dangerous to public health. From 1962 onwards all advertising of prescription drugs in the United States was also expected to carry information on side-effects.

By comparison Britain had a much weaker tradition of regulating and monitoring drugs, only founding the Committee on Safety of Drugs (CSD) in 1964 in the wake of the thalidomide disaster.[13] However, by the mid-1960s Britain had established a better mechanism than the United States for the long-term surveillance of drugs once they were released on to the market.[14] Much of this was funded by the Medical Research Council (MRC), a body set up under government auspices. Part of the strength of the British system can be traced to the structure of the CSD, as well the National Health Service (NHS), which provided more centralized health care, with better monitoring of patients and tracing of reactions to drugs than was available in the United States.[15] One of the weaknesses of the American system was that all statistics were kept at the level of individual states. In the 1960s no US state had an exposed population of a size to compare with that of the whole of England and Wales for undertaking any epidemiological investigation.[16]

The pill posed special problems for those gathering evidence on its side-effects. While given on prescription, the pill was different from other medicines because it was a contraceptive and as such had its own patterns of distribution. Oral contraceptive prescriptions were available to women in both countries through a variety of medical practitioners, which made monitoring adverse reactions difficult. In the United States, the problem was exacerbated by the fact that no individual doctor was responsible for the overall care of a particular woman, and coordination between hospitals and individual practitioners was weak. Women could thus go from one doctor to another without automatically being monitored in any way. Coordination between family planning services and other health-care facilities was also poor.[17] Networks between different medical specialties were also sometimes weak. Thus, while some specialists, such as ophthalmologists and neurologists, were seeing women with complaints that seemed to stem from taking the pill, such information was not always channelled back to other specialists, such as gynaecologists or general practitioners, who were the ones responsible for the initial oral contraceptive prescription.[18] In addition to this, many American doctors prescribing the pill were hesitant to report adverse reactions for fear of litigation.[19] The transmission of data was also hindered by the diversity of health-care agencies across different states and the absence of a centralized recording system for patient records and prescriptions.[20]

Collecting evidence from pharmaceutical companies was also inadequate in the United States. Many pharmaceutical companies did not have a uniform policy for gathering reports on deaths notified to them by individual doctors, and the FDA did not provide clear guidelines to manufacturers over the type of investigational evidence that was required. The FDA tried to tighten the reporting system for deaths on the part of the pharmaceutical industry in 1966, but such improvements took time to materialize.[21] The situation was not helped by the absence of a consistent method for recording and following up patients. Important information was thus often duplicated or difficult to retrieve.[22]

While Britain also experienced an under-reporting of adverse reactions,[23] British doctors were less frightened of litigation than their American counterparts, and were thus probably more likely to report side-effects. Britain also had a better infrastructure for monitoring the effects of the pill than the United States. In Britain, general practitioners were primarily the first point of call for patients within the NHS, and they were the main coordinators of treatment. Under this system, general practitioners ideally kept running files on each patient's prescription history and other case notes. Thus general practitioners could keep track of whether a woman was receiving a prescription for an oral contraceptive, even when they had not issued it.[24] Initially British family planning clinics also made a special point of informing general practitioners when putting one of their patients on an oral contraceptive. General practitioners were called on to inform the clinics of any medical contra-indications which indicated that the pill should not be prescribed, and to report any adverse reactions once a woman was taking the pill.[25] Aimed at maintaining good relations with general practitioners, this policy meant that coordination between the clinics and general practitioners was generally good. This ideal was not always achieved, however. Family planning doctors, for instance, had to respect the confidentiality of their patients when asked not to inform the general practitioner that they were taking the pill.[26]

British family planning clinics not only had more effective coordination with other medical practitioners than their counterparts in the United States, but were also alerted to the thrombotic problem earlier. This stemmed partly from the fact that very early in its clinical trials, the British Family Planning Association (FPA) witnessed three women who developed thrombophlebitis within six weeks of each other. Clustering within such a short time, and from a sample of only 300 to 350 patients on trial, these cases made the FPA particularly watchful. As early as 1961 the FPA was careful not to admit patients to clinical trials who had suffered thrombotic complications during pregnancy, although some did slip through the net.[27]

Studying the problem

Much of the problem in determining whether the pill was a risk in thrombotic disease was bound up with questions of what constituted affirmative evidence. Medical practitioners differed in their opinions on this. Much depended on their specialty and the type of contact they had with women taking the pill, as well as whether they had any attachment to a drug regulatory agency or to a pharmaceutical company.[28]

Among the difficulties confronted by investigators was the fact that the effects of the pill could not be treated in the same way as diseases such as malaria or other infectious diseases, for it did not involve the presence of a micro-organism which could be easily isolated and studied. Moreover, it was difficult to separate the pill from the many factors known to cause thrombotic disease. While epidemiologists were dissatisfied with methods which did not seem to progress 'beyond the clinical impression phase' and stressed the need for good statistically designed studies, other medical experts felt that epidemiological studies provided an unsatisfactory and inconsistent picture and were 'too blunt a tool for the detection of small risks'. For these doctors only basic clinical medical research could provide the answer.[29]

Even where investigators agreed that epidemiological studies were the way forward, it was unclear which technique would yield the best results. One of the major difficulties confronting epidemiologists was finding a large enough sample of women to work with. This was particularly important given the infrequency of thrombotic illness, which necessitated very large samples in order to detect the disease.[30] One of the problems in the early 1960s was that the number of women taking the pill was still relatively small and it was hard to find institutions with adequate concentrations of women for conducting a study. By contrast, in later years, once oral contraceptives had become universally available and widely consumed, it became harder to find women who had not taken the pill for any period who could act as controls. The problem was not made any easier by the fact that women did not necessarily stick to one method of contraception, often switching between oral contraception and mechanical methods.[31] Women also varied in the length of time they remained on the pill. The problem was made even more complicated by the ever-increasing diversity of oral contraceptives on the market, which consisted of differing types and doses of hormones and involved different daily regimes for consumption. Under these circumstances, and with women often changing their medication or even dropping it, it was difficult to isolate which pill, and what component of that pill, was linked to thrombotic disease.[32]

Studies undertaken

A variety of methods was deployed in various developed countries during the 1960s to investigate the possible thrombotic hazards of the pill, with differing conclusions.[33] One of the earliest investigations in the United States was undertaken by an ad hoc committee for the FDA in 1963. This committee concluded that the incidence of deaths among Enovid users was 12.1 per million users, while it was 8.4 per million in the general population.[34] While these rates were regarded as not statistically significant, the investigators argued for more work in the area.[35] Two years later the FDA issued another report which again found no direct link between oral contraceptives and thrombotic disease.[36] It was to take another three years before US-based investigations showed any direct association between the pill and cardiovascular problems. Evidence collected from a number of hospitals between 1963 and 1969 showed that oral contraceptive users faced 4.4 times the risk of thromboembolism compared with non-users, and that the risk was even higher for those taking 100 microgram oestrogen pills and sequential pills.[37]

British investigators concluded much earlier that thrombotic disease was linked to oral contraceptives. One of the first studies to suggest a connection between the pill and vascular complications stemmed from the research prompted by the receipt of a number of notifications of complications from the pill by the CSD soon after its establishment in 1964.[38] By August 1965, evidence collected by the CSD revealed that thromboembolic death was much higher among oral contraceptive users than among the general female population, and that pulmonary episodes were particularly high among pill users.[39] Further investigation by the CSD medical officer, William Inman, revealed a link between the types of pills taken and the number and types of death that had occurred. A significant excess of thrombosis seemed to be associated with pills containing the synthetic oestrogen mestranol.[40]

The CSD findings did not tally with other studies published in 1966. Based on national mortality rates and death reports in Britain and the United States, these investigations indicated that there was no direct link between oral contraceptives and thromboembolic disease.[41] In order to probe the issue further, Inman and the CSD looked to other researchers to launch other studies that could deploy different methods from their own.[42] The first, conducted by the Royal College of General Practitioners (RCGP), called on 60 general practitioners to monitor any cases of thrombosis in their practices. The second study, launched by the MRC's Statistical Research Unit, involved an investigation of patients admitted to various hospitals with thrombosis. In May 1967 the evidence collected from the two studies, together with the research from the CSD, had advanced far enough for the MRC to publish an article in the *British Medical Journal* announcing, 'there can be no reasonable doubt that some types of thromboembolic disorder are associated with the use of oral contraceptives.'[43] Venous thrombosis (superficial and deep), pulmonary embolism and myocardial infarction were found to be the most common types of thromboembolic disease women experienced when taking the pill, and rates were found to be three times greater among them than among those who did not use oral contraceptives.[44]

These preliminary findings were substantiated by later studies. As early as 1970 evidence collected in Sweden and Denmark as well as Britain confirmed the earlier British conclusions. In addition, it was found that women over the age of 35 had a greater risk of developing thrombo-embolism if taking the pill. The risk of developing thromboembolic problems also appeared to be less among those women taking pills with lower doses of oestrogen.[45] In 1970 Inman and others calculated that the relative risk of death was 2.8 per million for women taking pills with 150 micrograms of oestrogen (mestranol), while the risk was only 1.3 and 0.50 respectively for pills containing 100 and 50 micrograms.[46]

Throughout the 1970s other investigations reinforced such conclusions, adding smoking as a factor that increased a woman's risk of experiencing thrombotic complications while on the pill. By 1978 enough evidence had been collected in the United States, Britain and elsewhere to show that a woman's risk of developing thrombotic complications increased between five and tenfold when taking an oral contraceptive.[47] During the 1970s and 1980s further studies indicated that fewer thrombotic complications were associated with oral contraceptives with lower doses of oestrogen. Moreover, evidence from Sweden suggested that thromboembolic morbidity and mortality reduced significantly with the withdrawal of high dose oral contraceptives.[48]

Overall, however, the risk of thrombotic complications was regarded as modest. In 1968 a British study showed that the risk was much smaller compared to the risks women faced during pregnancy and childbirth, and also other dangers in life (table 6.1). Summing up the risk the authors of this study argued:

On balance, it seems reasonable to conclude that the risk of death from pulmonary embolism during one year's treatment with oral contraceptives is of the same order as the comparable risk of bearing one child. In assessing the risks, however, it is important to remember that women in the United Kingdom give birth, on average, to only two or three children in their lifetime, that other methods of contraception are reasonably effective, and that birth control may be practised during most of a woman's child-bearing years.[49]

Moreover, women taking oral contraceptives also ran a greater risk of developing cardiovascular problems than women using other forms of contraception.[50]

Table 6.1 Estimates of risk of death from pulmonary embolism or cerebral thrombosis in users and non-users of oral contraceptives compared with risk of death from certain other causes, 1968

	Age 20–34	Age 35–44
Estimated death-rate per 100,000 healthy, married, non-pregnant women from pulmonary cerebral thromboembolism		
Users of oral contraceptives	1.5	3.9
Non-users of oral contraceptives	0.2	0.5
Annual death-rate per 100,000 total female population from:		
Cancer	13.7	70.1
Motor accidents	4.9	3.9
All causes	60.1	170.5
Death-rate per 100,000 maternities from:		
Complications of pregnancy	7.5	13.8
Abortion	5.6	10.4
Complications of delivery	7.1	26.5
Complications of the puerperium:		
phlebitis, thrombosis and embolism	1.3	2.3
other complications	1.3	4.6
All risks of pregnancy, delivery and puerperium	22.8	57.6

Source: W. H. Inman and M. P. Vessey, 'Investigations of deaths from pulmonary, coronary, and cerebral thrombosis and embolism in women of child-bearing age', *British Medical Journal*, 2 (Apr. 1968), 196, table 7.

External pressures on policy

While medical evidence increasingly showed a positive link between the pill and thrombotic disease, by the late 1960s external pressures were mounting from other quarters, such as in the media and among politicians, for stronger action to be taken in curbing thrombotic deaths from the pill. This had a powerful effect on government policy.

The safety of the pill had been the subject of parliamentary and congressional hearings in Britain and the United States from the early 1960s. In Britain, for instance, from 1962 onwards Baroness Summerskill made vehement appeals in Parliament for the withdrawal of the pill until adequate investigations resolved the issue.[51] Similarly, in the United States the pill was the object of much debate in hearings concerning government regulation of pharmaceutical drug monitoring and testing and safety.[52] Over the years the national media in both countries also kept the issue alive, with newspapers and television reporting cases of women who had died from thrombotic complications while taking the pill.[53]

Publicity over the pill's medical complications reached a crescendo in Britain in late 1969. That August the *British Medical Journal* published an article which challenged the medical profession for its complacency regarding the pill and its side-effects.[54] Between October and November a stream of articles also began to appear in non-medical newspapers highlighting the possibility of death associated with the pill, and calling on medical practitioners to do more to educate women on the risks they faced.[55] On 29 November the popular British tabloid newspaper the *Sun* announced that Professor Victor Wynn, an endocrinologist and an expert on the metabolic effects of the pill, was about to publish his own book on the side-effects of the pill; it requested that he disclose his findings without delay and called on the CSD to provide more information.[56] Six days later, on 5 December, Victor Wynn appeared on a television programme hosted by David Frost, during which he divulged to large numbers of British viewers the various risks of the pill, including thrombosis, depression and the possibility of cancer. Wynn appeared on a total of three David Frost programmes that month, one of which was broadcast to an American audience, and his testimony caused public and parliamentary uproar.[57]

Prior to Wynn's appearance, the CSD had been facing increasing pressure to make a public announcement. Calls from the press and from Richard Crossman, the Secretary of State for Social Services, added to the urgency. As a result, in November Inman prepared a preliminary draft report for the CSD on the links between thrombotic disease and the different doses of the pill. The report was to be finalized in early January. In the draft report he argued against making his work public because of the haste with which it had been prepared and the fact that the data were still incomplete. One area that still needed exploring was whether progestogens were as important as oestrogens in causing thrombotic complications.[58] Nonetheless, despite Inman's words of caution, on 11 December 1969 the CSD made an official statement through national media networks recommending that doctors prescribe certain low dose oestrogen pills (under 5 mg), which effectively excluded two-thirds of the pills on the British market (17 out of 21 types of pill).[59]

Inman attributes this radical measure not only to the mounting pressure of the media, but also to the political priorities and ambitions of certain civil servants and Crossman, all of whom were unwilling to listen to his advice. Crossman had been very ill, and was losing the political will to continue in office. He was also part of a government that was losing popularity and he himself had recently been subject to public criticism.[60] The CSD had also just experienced a change in personnel, and the new members were less experienced than their predecessors. All these factors, together with the David Frost programmes, and an unintended press leak to the *Daily Express* about the impending report from the CSD which warned of the dangers of high dose oestrogen pills, meant that the CSD was forced to take swifter action than originally intended. This led to the announcement that doctors should only prescribe lower dose pills. Within days there was chaos as desperately worried women phoned doctors who were unprepared and had received no official letter warning them of the CSD's recommendations.[61]

Meanwhile, similar concern over the pill's safety was mounting in the United States. Part of this stemmed from the publication of a book, *The Doctor's Case against the Pill*. Written by the journalist Barbara Seaman, and published in October 1969, the book exposed the suffering many women had experienced on taking the pill, including thrombotic disease, and aired criticisms from medical practitioners over the safety of the oral contraceptive.[62] While others, such as Morton Mintz (a journalist from the *Washington Post*), had written similar books exposing the negative medical effects of the pill, Seaman's book was the first written by a woman and to focus on women's own experiences.[63] Passed on to the Wisconsin Senator Gaylord Nelson, Seaman's book galvanized congressional hearings on the safety of the pill, with Seaman playing a crucial role in choosing who was to testify.[64] Commencing on 14 January 1970, and completed in March, the Nelson hearings were made even more urgent by the action taken by the British government the previous month. The Nelson hearings formed part of a general series of congressional hearings which had been running since 1967, the aim of which was to investigate the pharmaceutical industry and the monopoly of businesses.[65] Rather than seeking to restrict the pill on the market as the British had done, the overall aim of the hearings was to provide better information for patients on its adverse effects, on the understanding that it was silence which killed women. The hearings contributed to the FDA decision to formulate a patient package insert to warn women about the side-effects of the pill.[66]

The Nelson hearings alerted the public to the hazards of the oral contraceptive. Between January and March 18 per cent of American women taking the pill discontinued to do so as a result of the publicity from the hearings and 23 per cent seriously considered quitting.[67] In the months after the hearings the issue continued to provoke much interest. This stemmed partly from the very active campaigns mounted in the wake of the hearings by women, who were infuriated by the lack of representation of women during the hearings, and the opposition from the American Medical Association (AMA) to creating a patient package insert. They vehemently canvassed the FDA in the following months and years to take better measures to ensure the safety of the pill and that women were better informed of the complications it could cause.[68]

What is most interesting about the congressional hearings was their focus on providing the consumer with information, rather than changing the prescribing habits of doctors, as had been the case in Britain. While measures to provide patient package inserts had been considered in Parliament in Britain in 1967, these had been dismissed on the grounds that the doctor had the professional responsibility of advising the patient and providing any warnings, and that women themselves would either not read the package inserts or would become unnecessarily panicked by such information.[69]

Similar concerns were also articulated in the United States. In June 1970 the AMA passed a resolution opposing the insert 'on the grounds that it would "confuse and alarm many patients"'. What was at issue was the medical profession's fear that its authority over the patient would be undermined by such an insertion. Eventually a compromise was reached 'wherein a modified version was mailed to physicians to hand out with every Pill prescription'. Effectively this policy defeated the original purpose of the insert, which had been to inform women directly of the ill-effects of the pill. Between 1970 and 1975, for instance, it was estimated that the AMA only distributed 4 million copies of the inserts to the 10 million women who were taking the pill each year.[70]

Nonetheless, the opposition from the American medical profession never fully blocked the moves to establish a patient package insert. Partly this stemmed from the power of the consumer culture in the United States. It can also be attributed to the strength of the women's health movement, which was beginning to blossom in the late 1960s. This movement saw patient package inserts as an empowering device that would enable women to take more informed decisions on their own without being totally dependent on doctors.[71] It was only in the late 1970s, however, that mounting pressure from consumer groups finally overcame opposition from the medical profession and the pharmaceutical industry. In the late 1970s the FDA changed its policy to permit the distribution of the inserts in pill packets sold through pharmacists. Moves were also made to make the leaflet insert more comprehensible; up to 1980 it remained almost unintelligible to the lay reader.[72]

Drug regulations and the pharmaceutical industry

The differing drug regulations in the two countries determined the continuance of high dose oestrogen pills in the United States and the faster introduction of low dose pills in Britain. This difference was marked from the time of the introduction of the pill. In the United States, for instance, the first oral contraceptive approved for the market contained 10 mg of oestrogen. This dose was deliberately high because it was seen to be more effective, and neither the original developers nor FDA officials wanted to have the risk of a pregnancy on their hands.[73] This was particularly important given that abortion was still illegal and contraception remained taboo in many states at the time of the first approval of the pill. It was therefore imperative to have a foolproof product. Partly reflecting this concern, the FDA was very cautious in considering any alteration to the original dose formulation of the pill, only approving the 5 mg pill in 1962.[74] By contrast in Britain the first oral contraceptive that was marketed contained 5 mg of oestrogen. This partly stemmed from the fact that the research leading to the approval of the pill was undertaken by the FPA, which had been involved in trials specifically designed to test for the effectiveness of lower dose pills.[75]

Britain also had fewer hurdles than the United States in the reformulation of pharmaceutical drugs.[76] Lengthy and costly trials, for instance, were not required for the reduction of doses of drugs which had already passed the initial clinical tests necessary for their first approval for the British market. Britain also did not require evidence of efficacy in the same way as the United States did.[77] Interestingly, within days of the CSD statement in December 1969 that only lower dose pills should be prescribed, the pharmaceutical company G. D. Searle replaced its higher oestrogen oral contraceptive Ovulen in Britain with the lower dose pill Ovulen-50, indicating that drug companies had anticipated such action and had been attentive to the reports coming out in previous years.[78] It also demonstrates the speed with which a pharmaceutical company could lower the dose of a drug and put it on the market in Britain.

By contrast, prior to 1970 every pharmaceutical product in the United States, even if it merely consisted of a lower dose version that was reformulated from an old product, was expected to undergo rigorous testing from scratch prior to getting approval. This not only involved more expense for the pharmaceutical industry, but also more time.[79] Nonetheless, attempts were made to get round this problem in 1970. Soon after news broke about the policy changes in Britain, Dr Edwards, an FDA commissioner, after consulting British medical experts who had linked thrombosis with the pill, indicated to several US manufacturers of oral contraceptives that he would expedite any reformulations they had of old oral contraceptives which involved lowering the oestrogen dose. Part of this was to prevent a shortage in supply of low dose oestrogen pills, as had happend in Britain as a result of the CSD statement. One of the pills that was approved on this basis was Searle's pill Demulen, an American version of the British Ovulen.[80] In 1970 regulations were formally introduced which required less clinical data and a shorter testing period for a lower-dose product that had already been shown to be safe in a higher dose.[81]

What was probably more important in determining the American policy relating to the high oestrogen pills, however, was the strength of the pharmaceutical companies and both their fears and those of the medical profession about litigation. Minutes from FDA meetings in the 1970s and 1980s reveal that medical representatives from pharmaceutical companies frequently argued against the restriction of high dose oestrogen pills on the grounds that each woman had individual needs and that high-dose pills were the only products that were effective for some women. The major concern was that women experienced greater break-through bleeding and were more liable to pregnancy on lower dose pills. FDA officials and pharmaceutical representatives were also worried about the possibility of litigation should they decide to phase out the higher dose pill.[82]

Conclusion

In May 1969 in the United States, the husband of a woman who had died from a pulmonary embolism while taking the pill tried to sue a pharmaceutical company for the death of his wife. Although he lost his case, his testimony touched the hearts of many who had been present in court, and many others who had read the newspaper reports from the trial. His last comment on leaving the court, to be repeated later by many relatives of many others who had lost wives and friends in similar circumstances, was that his wife was not just 'a statistic', but 'a real person'. His statement is a poignant reminder that the women who died or were disabled by thrombotic complications while taking the pill were not simply a matter of statistics. What was at stake were the health and lives of real women, whose suffering would affect not only themselves but also those around them.[83]

For medical professionals and government officials, the numbers of women who were affected by thrombotic complications from taking the pill were also not merely a matter of statistics. At the heart of their agenda was what constituted a 'correct' statistic, that is, what constituted conclusive evidence in determining the link of the pill to the disease. For many medical professionals the risk of dying from thrombotic disease was equivalent to the risk women faced when pregnant or giving birth. Oral contraceptive users, for instance had a 1.5 risk of dying from a pulmonary embolism or cerebral thrombosis, while those who suffered complications in pregnancy and childbirth ran a risk of about 7. The effectiveness of the pill in preventing pregnancy compared to other forms of contraception made it a product for which the risk was worth taking. The ways in which such statistics were translated and used as evidence depended on the type of specialism and the medical orientation of the medical expert.

Even after conclusive evidence was finally collected linking the pill to thrombotic disease, such statistics were still open to debate in the formulation of policy. Much of this was determined by the tradition of litigation and the consumer culture of each country. Equally important was the power of the state and its relationship to the medical profession and the pharmaceutical industry. Britain, with its highly centralized health-care structure and better mechanisms for tracing side-effects of pharmaceutical drugs, seems to have made a quicker and more radical response than the United States, limiting the prescription of high dose oestrogen pills in December 1969. By contrast, America, which had a less centralized health-care system and poor systems for monitoring the side-effects of drugs once they were on the market, waited till 1988 to take such action. Fears of litigation, together with the power of a consumer culture, meant that the United States initially opted to provide information to the patient through package inserts, making the issue one of individual rather than collective responsibility.

The ways in which evidence was collected were highly circumscribed by the health-care structures and procedures for monitoring drug reactions that existed in the United States and Britain. One of the major problems in tracking the thrombotic effects of the pill was finding an adequate means of testing the risk. Pre-marketing testing in the late 1950s was on far too small a scale for the detection of the problem and researchers were not necessarily alert to it.[84] Even today FDA requirements of preclinical testing (about 600 women years of exposure) provide too little information about the long-term risk of lethal cardiovascular or carcinogenic disease.[85]

Whatever the difficulties of studying the connection between the pill and thrombotic disease, the policy to limit the potency of oestrogen in pills has been tightened over the years. Part of this can be linked to the continuing affirmation of the link between oestrogen dose and thrombosis. In 1989 a British study, for instance, indicated that the rate of venous thrombosis and thrombotic stroke was 12 per 10,000 women in those who had taken oral contraceptives containing over 5 mg of oestrogen, while it was only 3.5 per 10,000 for those who took under 5 mg.[86] Another investigation conducted among Michigan Medicaid women aged 15 to 44, published by the FDA in the early 1990s, also suggested a relationship between oestrogen potency and venous thromboembolism, confirming that oral contraceptives containing less than 5 mg of oestrogen were safer than the higher doses. In 1993 an American inquiry indicated that the risk of cerebral thrombo-embolism was reduced by a third for those taking oral contraceptives containing 3–4 mgs of oestrogen by comparison with those using preparations with 5 mg of oestrogen. Moreover, it was on the basis of this and other evidence that the FDA extended its policy of 1988, which had led pharmaceutical companies to phase out all pills containing more than 5 mgs of oestrogen, to include pills that contained 5 mg.[87]

The reduction in the dose of oestrogen, however, has not stopped the controversy over the safety of the pill. In October 1995 the pill once again hit the headlines in Britain. Preliminary research conducted in numerous countries together with the World Health Organization indicated that seven brands of low dose pills, containing the progestogens gestodene or desogestrel, could cause thrombosis. This was particularly disturbing given that these pills, developed in the 1980s, had originally held the promise of cutting the risk of thrombosis. Instead the pills were thought to have twice the risk of other brands on the market.[88]

While many governments, including that of the USA, decided not to take any action until the research was fully concluded, the British government swiftly requested doctors to switch their patients away from the brands considered more hazardous for thrombosis.[89] As had been the case in December 1969 the British government's action in 1995 was prompted by a press leak and came at a time when it was rapidly losing popularity. The decision, however, created uproar among the medical community, which regarded the government's deed as premature and incompetent. Many pharmaceutical companies also speculated that the alert was part of the government's ploy to save National Health Service money on expensive third generation contraceptives.[90]

With 1.5 million British women (50 per cent of all oral contraceptive users)[91] taking the new lower dose tablets, chaos threatened as patients flocked to their doctors' surgeries for information or simply stopped taking their pills. In the aftermath of the news the percentage of British women taking third generation oral contraceptives fell dramatically from 55 to 12 per cent of total use. At the same time the percentage taking second generation pills rose from 30 to 62 per cent of total use.[92] A similar decline in the uptake of third generation pills occurred elsewhere, even in countries where governments had issued no warnings, and rates of abortion and pregnancy increased because many women stopped their oral contraceptives mid-cycle.[93]

What doctors resented most was that the government had given inadequate warning of its action prior to media publicity and that its decision was based on inconclusive evidence.[94] Observers at the time were aware of the parallels with 1969.[95] A few months after the British government's action in 1995 further evidence confirmed the greater risk of thrombosis caused by third generation pills.[96] Within a couple of years, however, researchers believed that the risk was in fact less than had been specified and that it had been blown up out of proportion.[97] Nonetheless the affair indicated that controversy continued as to what constituted affirmative evidence in understanding the effect of the pill on thrombosis. Moreover, governments around the world were not united in their response to the news. Clearly the matter had not been closed in the 1960s.

In 1994 it was established that a mutant gene – called factor V Leiden – puts some women at increased risk of venous thrombosis. With the recent commercial availability of genetic screening for this gene, women now have the option of being screened before they take the pill.[98] Controversies, however, remain about the effectiveness of the test.[99] Moreover, given the small proportion of women affected by the gene, it is disputable how cost effective the test would be if implemented as a mass screening procedure.[100]

7
The Pill and the Riddle of Cancer

While few suspected the pill's potential to cause thrombotic complications, from the time of its development many had feared it might promote cancer.[1] Investigators running the early clinical trials of the drug were themselves concerned about the problem of conducting regular vaginal and cervical smears, as well as endometrial biopsies and breast examinations. The level of anxiety about the relationship between hormones and cancer can also be seen from the fact that, just before approving the pill, the American Food and Drug Administration had stopped feeding chickens with oestrogens to fatten them because of the potential carcinogenic effects.[2] While such fears did not prevent the marketing of the pill in either the United States or Britain, apprehension nonetheless remained.

One of the main anxieties troubling both medical practitioners and government officials was that the carcinogenic repercussions of the pill would not become apparent for many years. As one cancer expert advising those running British clinical trials stated in 1960, 'The induction period of all cancers in man is long (15–25 years) and therefore the effects of these compounds in cancer induction will not be seen for many years to come.'[3] For this reason women taking the pill were recommended to have regular examinations to check for cancer. From 1963 the American Food and Drug Administration and the British Family Planning Association were also cautioning against the prescription of oral contraceptives to women who had a history of cervical or breast cancer.[4] Such measures, however, did not do enough to prevent public alarm.

The earliest public alarms about cancer and oral contraceptives occurred in 1964 when a team of researchers at the University of Oregon demonstrated that certain hormones, such as the progestogen and oestrogen contained in Enovid, promoted the growth of cancers in animals such as rats. While the American Medical Association advised women that the pill nevertheless carried no risk, the news resulted in the immediate plummeting of G. D. Searle's shares on the stock market.[5] Fears continued to be heightened during the late 1960s and 1970s with news that female dogs had developed breast cancer when tested with certain oral contraceptives, and reports began to show links between oral contraceptives and non-malignant tumours of the liver, an extremely rare condition that can prove fatal should the tumour rupture and cause internal bleeding.[6] In 1975 sequential pills were also withdrawn from the American market when the FDA indicated that they suspected the drugs of increasing the risk of endometrial cancer.[7]

During this period suspicion about the pill was reinforced by the news that stilboestrol, a steroid drug containing high oestrogen, had caused vaginal cancer (an extremely rare disease) in the daughters of women who, from the 1940s, had taken the drug to prevent miscarriage. The same drug was then being explored for its properties as a morning-after contraceptive.[8] By 1984, some women who had been given stilboestrol 20 years earlier were discovered to have breast cancer.[9] With the possible links between stilboestrol and cancer having taken years to emerge, many people wondered how long it would take to prove the oral contraceptive pill unsafe.[10]

Not all the information about the pill was so troubling. As early as 1961, just months before news broke about the association of thrombotic deaths with the pill, Gregory Pincus announced that Enovid could potentially prevent breast and cervical cancer. His declaration offered an important glimmer of hope for American women, some 15,000 of whom were dying from cervical cancer in these years.[11] During the late 1970s, a number of epidemiological studies began to show that some of Pincus's predictions about the anti-cancer effects of the pill might in fact be correct. Evidence that the pill offered some protection against ovarian and endometrial cancer in particular seemed to be accumulating.

In 1983 the tenuous confidence that had begun to be built around the pill's protective effects against ovarian and endometrial cancer was shattered when a number investigators revealed that oral contraceptives might in fact increase the risk of breast and cervical cancer among women in later life. Those most at danger were young women who had taken the pill for many years before the age of 25. Such news was particularly disquieting given the rising incidence of breast cancer in many countries in the developed world, and the increasing mortality from cervical cancer in the developing world since the 1950s.

What was most disturbing in 1983 was that the progestogen compounds seemed to be associated with the cancer. This was particularly worrying because many women had switched to pills containing high doses of progestogen in the wake of the thrombotic scare and the phasing out of high oestrogen pills. Now it seemed that not only was oestrogen a problem, but progestogens might also be. This did not leave many pills from which to choose.

Despite the fears generated by the studies in 1983, many within the medical profession felt the evidence was still inconclusive; this provoked bitter debates about what methodological tool was most appropriate and led to fierce rivalry among epidemiologists. Many feared that breast cancer was the one risk, apart from cardiovascular complications, which might outweigh all the contraceptive benefits of the pill.[12] Yet, it was to take many more years and arguments before the riddle of the pill and cancer could be unravelled. Examining the twists and turns in the debate about the oral contraceptive and cancer, this chapter explores the ways in which the drug shifted from being a contraceptive tool with potential carcinogenic effects to becoming a major weapon in the fight against cancer.

The context of the debate

One of the difficulties throughout the debate on the pill and cancer was that nobody could be sure of the effects of the drug without a long passage of time. The carcinogenic effects of the pill differed from those of thrombosis in that they could not be detected immediately. The delay in time for a cancer to develop (known as the latent period) made it difficult to ascribe the resulting disease definitively to the pill. This was not made any easier by the fact that those patients who develop cancer experience few symptoms during the latency period. It also soon became clear that oral contraceptives were not universal in their effect on female reproductive organs and other parts of the body such as the liver. Moreover it was difficult to know whether the carcinogenic influence of the pill was dependent on when in her life a woman was exposed to an oral contraceptive. Was there, for instance, a difference in the effect if the drug was taken earlier rather than later in a woman's reproductive life? Any overall assessment of the risks and benefits of the pill was therefore complex. This was further complicated because there are multiple causes of cancer: genetic, viral, cultural, geographic, dietary and environmental.

Discovering the connections between the pill and cancer was not made any easier by the fact that both breast and cervical cancers were increasing. As figure 7.1 on p. 162 shows there was a considerable rise in mortality from breast cancer in Britain, the Netherlands, the United States and Australia, all countries where oral contraceptives were consumed on a large scale. As early as 1969 breast cancer was calculated to be the leading cause of all early deaths from cancer among women in Britain and America. The number of women dying annually from breast cancer in 1969 in these countries was 10,000 and 29,000 respectively. During the 1970s at least 1 in 17 British women and 1 in 14 American women developed the disease. By 1987 the lifetime risk of breast cancer had increased in both countries, reaching 1 in 13 in Britain and 1 in 10 in the United States. Overall, between 1955 and 1985 the crude death-rate from breast cancer shot up in Britain from 36 to 52 per 100,000 population. Most of this rise was among older women. In the United States during the 1980s breast cancer was the most common of all causes of death among women aged 40 to 44. By this decade at least 37,000 American women were dying annually from the disease. Breast cancer had also risen in other parts of Europe.[13]

While rates of breast cancer seemed significantly lower in the less developed regions of the world, these areas were experiencing an increasing mortality from cervical cancer. By the 1990s cervical cancer had become the leading cause of death from cancer among women in developing countries. Of the approximately 370,000 new cases of cervical cancer identified worldwide each year, 80 per cent occur in developing countries: 184,000 in Asia, 60,000 in Latin America and the Caribbean, and 48,000 in Africa. This is all the more serious because of the fact that the peak age of women during which the disease strikes in the developing world is between 30 and 40 years old. This contrasts with the case in many Western countries, where cervical cancer tends to peak in the age group of 50–60 years old. Moreover, many developed countries have experienced a significant reduction in mortality from cervical cancer since the 1950s (figure 7.2, p. 162).

One of the most dramatic falls in mortality was seen in the United States, where cervical cancer among white women decreased from 32 to 8.3 cases per 100,000 between the 1940s and the 1980s. This contrasts with the rates for developing countries. Mexico, for example, experienced a

Figure 7.1 Mortality rates from breast cancer in selected countries, 1950–1997

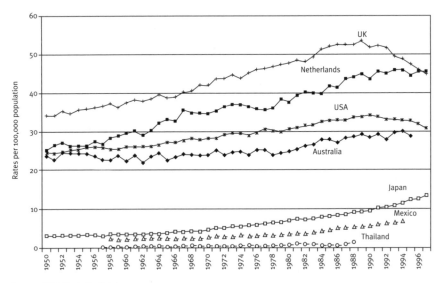

Source: WHO Mortality Database.

Figure 7.2 Mortality rates from cervical cancer in selected countries, 1950–1997

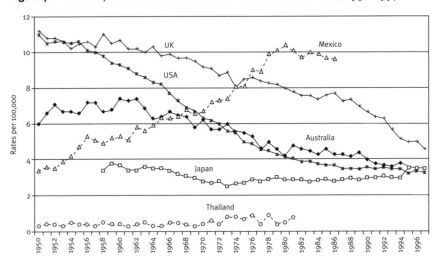

Source: WHO Mortality Database.

significant rise in mortality from cervical cancer dating from the 1950s (see figure 7.2). It has been argued that the decline in many developed nations is attributable to the establishment of intensive cervical screening programmes in such places, although some would dispute the efficacy of such screening. Nonetheless, while cervical cancer may have declined in some parts of the world, it continues to be one of the most significant reproductive health problems for women, with approximately 200,000 women dying from the disease each year worldwide. Indeed, overall it is the third most common cancer. During the 1980s and 1990s cervical cancer accounted for at least 3 to 5 per cent of all adult female deaths in many parts of the world.[14]

Debates about cancer and the pill in the 1960s

In April 1956, the month that the first large-scale trials were mounted for Enovid in Puerto Rico, Gregory Pincus was appointed chairman of the endocrinology panel of the Center for Cancer Chemotherapy of the US Public Health Service. Reflecting a general rise of research into endocrine carcinogenesis which had started before the Second World War, the aim of this panel was to test steroids as chemotherapeutic agents for the treatment of cancer. Interest in the relationship between hormones and cancer had first been sparked in the early 1930s when experiments with oestrogen, one of the hormones of early oral contraceptives, implicated the hormone in the growth of uterine and breast tumours in certain animals such as mice.[15]

While disturbing, it was uncertain how such research related to humans. Experiments with primates, for instance, showed hormones to have no carcinogenic effects. It was also unclear what the time threshold was for humans. A cancer that develops in a mouse in five months may take years to manifest itself in humans, if at all. Nonetheless, by the interwar years a number of investigators had begun to discover that some hormones, rather than being detrimental, could actually ameliorate certain symptoms of cancer. This included stilboestrol, which by the late 1930s had been shown to be highly effective in the treatment of prostate cancer. The excitement this generated cannot be underestimated, for this was the first time that a synthetic drug had induced an unquestionable improvement in malignant disease.[16] By the early 1950s, medical experts were carrying out experiments to see whether some oestrogenic substances could relieve the symptoms of inoperable breast cancer in women.[17] Others were looking into whether the hormone progesterone would help in the treatment of cervical cancer. Pincus himself had looked into the possibility of trying Enovid as a treatment for Puerto Rican patients suffering from cervical cancer as part of his initial contraceptive experiments in the early 1950s.[18]

In the end Pincus never tested Enovid on patients with cervical cancer. Nonetheless, he retained an interest in the area, and gained extra impetus to explore the matter when he and his co-workers found a surprisingly low incidence of early stages of cervical cancer among the pap smears taken from Puerto Rican women participating in the contraceptive trials. On the basis of data collected from 800 women over a four-year period, Pincus hypothesized that Enovid could help protect against cervical cancer. In 1961 he received some funding from the American Cancer Society to launch trials in the United States, Sri Lanka, Japan and Haiti to see whether Enovid was truly an inhibitor of cancer.[19] By 1965 Pincus and other investigators had collected enough evidence to announce that women taking oral contraceptives had a lower incidence of cervical problems than non-users. While Pincus acknowledged that the data from his own study was 'too scant to afford statistically significant figures', he nonetheless interpreted his findings as suggesting oral contraceptives could prevent cancer of the cervix.[20]

Not everyone, however, was convinced by Pincus's evidence. Indeed, by the early 1960s a number of medical practitioners were becoming increasingly uneasy about the potential carcinogenic effects of the pill.[21] One of the prominent figures to sound a note of caution was Dr Roy Hertz, who had been the first to point out the contraceptive potential of Syntex's compound in 1951. Based at the National Institute for Cancer in Bethesda, Maryland, Hertz was a trained obstetrician and gynaecologist who had wide experience with hormonal steroids and cancer. One of the reasons he had tested Syntex's compound stemmed from his interest in whether progesterone could alleviate cervical cancer. On the FDA's Advisory Committee on Obstetrics and Gynecology from the mid-1960s, Hertz played a key role in cautioning against the mass use of oral contraceptives before their carcinogenic risks had been assessed.

In late 1961 Hertz expressed his first public doubts about the long-term safety of the pill to a committee of the Planned Parenthood Federation of America. He was concerned that women who used the pill for long periods of time might develop abnormal endometrial growths, which could be a prelude to cancer. Moreover he felt it important to alert the public about the possible risks of the long-term use of Enovid.[22] Three years later Hertz submitted a paper, jointly written with J. C. Bailar, to Pincus and a number of the other investigators involved in the clinical trials of oral contraceptives as well as to members of the FDA and the Cancer Institute and National Institutes of Health. Written on the eve of the FDA's approval of the use of oral contraceptives for up to four years, the aim of the paper was to examine some unresolved problems with the contraceptive.[23]

Hertz's particular concern was to assess the potential hazards of the drug for the breast, endometrium (lining of the uterus), cervix and ovaries. Not only did his joint paper challenge some of the assumptions made by previous investigators regarding the state of knowledge of the effects of hormones on the human body, but it also argued that the carcinogenic effects of the pill might possibly not be known for many years. The authors pointed out that while hormones such as oestrogen had been clinically used over the previous 25 years, they had primarily been used in older women and only for short periods. Knowledge was therefore limited as to what effect such hormones would have if given to younger women over a long period. Arguing that existing data was insufficient to draw any conclusions about the safety of the pill in relation to cancer, Hertz and his co-writer argued that further study was necessary and that patients be informed about the drug's carcinogenic potential.[24]

The paper provoked an immediate critical response from Pincus and others. Pincus not only disagreed with Hertz's methodology, but argued that the paper seemed to be 'an attempt to substantiate a biased rather than a completely objective assessment of the available facts'. Pincus added, 'I have such a great respect for your scientific conscience that I hope to see a much better job than the one which is now on my desk.'[25] Others were equally harsh in their criticism.[26] Having received these communications Hertz decided not to publish the paper officially at this stage.[27]

Nonetheless, a few months later, in July 1964, Hertz once again publicized his concerns and the urgent need for more research to a National Advisory Cancer Council subcommittee that had been convened to consider the question of carcinogenesis and prevention in relation to oral contraceptives. The meeting took place within months of widespread media publicity over the possible links between cancer and the pill, and the collapse of Searle's shares on the stock market, in the wake of the Oregon research on rats.[28] The aim of the meeting was to design studies for assessing the potential risks of drugs taken over extensive periods of time. The meeting had a wide range of investigators from the scientific and medical community, including Roy Hertz, Gregory Pincus, FDA staff, and representatives from the pharmaceutical companies.

Throughout the proceedings it was clear that no one had a clear vision of how to examine the links between the pill and cancer. One of the main problems was that cancer, like thrombosis, was not a reportable disease in the United States at this time. Thus, while pharmaceutical representatives might forward any report of malignancy appearing in women participating in their oral contraceptive trials, the many physicians routinely prescribing the drug were not mandated to report cases to any business or government organization.[29] In addition to this difficulty, investigators were unsure about the direction future studies should take. One of the tensions that surfaced at the meeting, for instance, was whether animal experiments were relevant. While some felt that data collected from animal studies could not be extrapolated to humans, others felt the opposite.[30] The major problem was that while scientists remained unsure of the significance of animal data, there was no adequate 'scientific means for assessing the impact in man'.[31]

Confusion also emerged over the ways in which the research should be conducted with women. As with thrombosis, any study of the pill and cancer required careful selection of the types of women chosen for study, and was complicated by the differing doses of pills on the market, as well as by the different lengths of time over which women were taking the drugs. Investigators also differed in their estimates of the number of women needed to study the risk, depending on the type of cancer to be studied. Numbers ranged from 3,000 to 80,000 women studied over ten years. Given the uncertainty of how long it would take for any carcinogenic effects of the pill to be ascertained, investigators were also doubtful as to the exact amount of time to be allowed for significant results to be obtained. Some felt a study of five years would be sufficient for examining the problem, while others felt that a ten-year investigation would be more apposite. Yet many were concerned that a longer study would increase the costs.

Another dilemma was how a control group might be established given that oral contraceptives were so widely used, and what type of investigation should be set up. Among those thought to be appropriate for comparison with takers of oral contraceptives were young healthy women who had been sterilized by tubal ligation. Various research approaches were discussed. These included (1) an evaluation of the various internal hormone excretions that could affect cancer incidence; (2) the monitoring of an administered exogenous (non-bodily) agent; (3) an investigation of oestrogens alone; and (4) an examination of oral contraceptives within the overall context of cancer.[32] The interesting feature of these suggested studies was that they were primarily individual case-control studies, which was very different from the epidemiological population-based investigations adopted later on.

In 1966 the FDA followed up the meeting of the National Cancer Council with its own assessment of the carcinogenic safety of oral contraceptives. This was done alongside the examination of other side-effects of the pill such as thrombosis. Once again Hertz was an active player. Not only were his concerns included in a major appendix at the end of the FDA report, but they were also reprinted, almost verbatim, in two medical journals in 1966 and 1968.[33] In discussing the pill in relation to oestrogen and breast cancer, Hertz pointed out: 'Our inadequate knowledge concerning the relationship of estrogens to cancer in women is comparable with what was known about the association between lung cancer and cigarette smoking before extensive epidemiological studies delineated this overwhelming significant statistical relationship.'[34] Alongside expressing his concern about the carcinogenic potential of oestrogen, Hertz also made it clear that he was wary of the safety of progesterone.

Hertz did not call for a ban on oral contraceptives, however. Instead he reiterated the need for more long-term clinical trials and for physicians to be cautious in their prescription of the drug.[35] In line with this thinking, the FDA cautioned physicians and decided to support a number of investigations to look into the issue, ordering the mandatory testing of 'all currently licensed and investigational hormonal contraceptives on monkeys throughout their lifetimes and on dogs for 7 years'.[36] By 1969, when the FDA issued a second report on the safety of oral contraceptives, two oral contraceptives had been withdrawn because they had caused mammary tumours in beagles and were considered to offer 'no clear therapeutic advantage over previously available hormonal contraceptives'.[37]

One of the interesting features of the FDA reports was the evidence they contained contradicting Pincus's earlier assertion that the pill might prevent cervical cancer. The report in 1969 included research into the incidence of cervical carcinoma in 34,000 women attending Planned Parenthood Federation clinics in New York City. Started in 1965 this research had shown the incidence of cervical abnormalities to be twice as high among women using oral contraceptives than among those using the diaphragm.[38]

As one of the largest studies carried out on the pill and cervical cancer to date, this research attracted a great deal of attention from both FDA officials and the external medical community. The study itself was subsequently found to have discrepancies in the readings of the pap smears taken and the classification of cancer. What was also under question was the overall design of the study and whether any true comparisons could be drawn between women who used the diaphragm and those who took the pill. Many were similarly critical of the investigation's focus on the prevalence of the disease because it revealed little about the connection between the pill and cervical cancer.[39]

In the end editors of the *Journal of the American Medical Association* refused to publish the results of the investigation. Controversy broke out, however, when the *British Medical Journal* published the findings instead, and journalists in the lay press accused the American Medical Association of having suppressed the report because of pressure from pharmaceutical companies.[40] The FDA thought that the results of the survey did not establish a positive link between oral contraceptives and cervical cancer. Nonetheless, its officials were sufficiently worried about the findings to argue that urgent research was needed to settle the question.[41]

One of the problems that complicated the matter was the recent installation of cervical screening programmes in the United States. This made it difficult to disentangle the effects of the pill from the impact of the greater overall medical scrutiny of women. Adding to this problem was the fact that the incidence of cervical cancer differed from one social class to another and varied according to frequency of intercourse.[42] Nonetheless, the episode revealed the fact that by the late 1960s investigators were questioning Pincus's earlier assertions of the protective effect of the pill on cervical carcinoma.

By the end of the 1960s investigators had come no closer to resolving the riddle of the pill and cervical cancer, neither were they any nearer to understanding its role in other cancers.[43] To some extent research into the contraceptive and cancer had been overshadowed by the concern in the 1960s about the increasing association of the drug with cardiovascular disease. In addition, too little time had elapsed since the first marketing of the pill to make any significant long-term assessment of its carcinogenic effects. While the links between thrombotic complications and the drug were beginning to be established by the end of the first decade after the marketing of the first pill, insufficient time had passed to assess it in relation to cancer.

The 1970s and 1980s: the establishment of protective effects

During the 1960s, with anxieties focused on the pill's thrombotic complications, cancer had been far from the centre of attention. By the 1970s, however, many researchers began to focus more on the question of cancer. While a number of contraceptives were withdrawn during the early 1970s because their particular progestogen components were discovered to produce cancer in female beagles,[44] the influence of the pill on cancer remained as elusive as ever. Data collected on cervical cancer during these years, for instance, was conflicting.[45]

Despite inconclusive findings, the 1970s marked a turning point as investigators began to detect some of the positive effects of the pill and highlight it as a preventive tool in the fight against cancer. Medical experts were quick to point out the public health benefits of such findings. In many ways the news was an ideal way of deflecting previous pessimistic associations between the pill and cardiovascular problems. Now the drug could be portrayed not only as an effective contraceptive, but also as a preventive medication that was actually beneficial to women's health in general.[46]

Some of the earliest announcements about the protective effects of the oral contraceptive were made in the early 1970s in relation to breast cysts.[47] While some researchers interpreted these finding as reassuring in relation to breast cancer and the pill, few knew for certain whether the protection against breast cysts would in the long term prevent cancer.[48]

News that the pill could provide protection against ovarian and endometrial cysts reinforced the optimism sparked by the news about benign breast disease.[49] Ovarian and endometrial tumours are difficult to detect in their early stages, but are frequently fatal. The combined incidence of ovarian and endometrial cancer equals that of cervical neoplasms in many industrialized countries. For some medical experts the protection that the pill afforded against ovarian and endometrial tumours therefore counterbalanced its potential negative effects in relation to cervical cancer.[50] The finding that the pill protected against ovarian cancer was particularly welcome given the evidence that the incidence of the disease had increased in Britain and America since the 1950s. The mortality from ovarian cancer was higher in Britain than in the United States (figure 7.3). By the 1970s the condition was causing over 3,000 deaths in Britain each year, and was a more common cause of death among women over the age of 65 than cervical cancer. Ovarian cancer was the fourth most common fatal cancer among British women. In 1980 approximately 137,000 cases of ovarian cancer were diagnosed worldwide. Internationally its incidence varied from 3 to 15 per 100,000 per year. Between 1 and 2 per cent of white women were known to have a lifetime risk of developing the disease.[51] Figure 7.3 on p. 170, albeit showing scanty evidence for developing countries, illustrates the variation in

Figure 7.3 Mortality rates from ovarian cancer in selected countries, 1955–1997

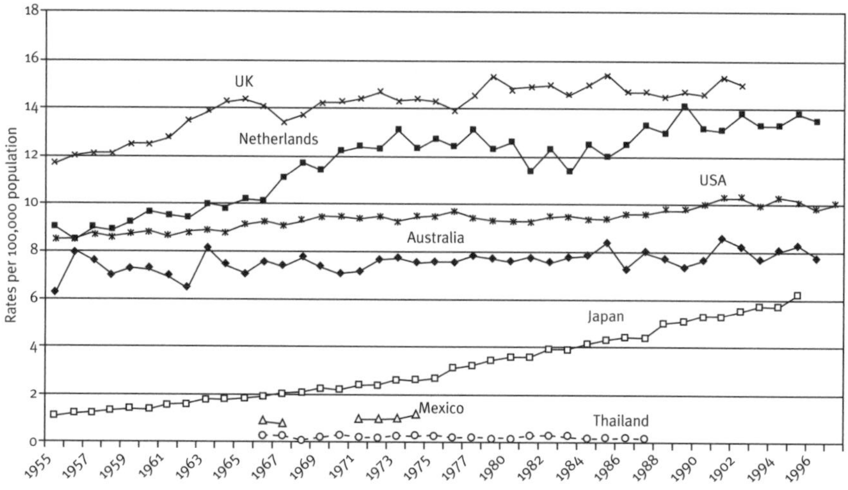

Source: WHO Mortality Database.

incidence between different countries, showing that it tended to be lower in developing countries than in more developed ones.

The first research suggesting the protective effects of the pill in relation to ovarian cancer had been carried out by the British Medical Women's Federation and 20 members of the Women's Visiting Gynaecologists Club in the 1970s. Designed as a case-control study of 300 women, the researchers reported a significant reduction in the relative risk of ovarian cancer among those who had used the contraceptive pill.[52] Following on from a theory, first proposed in 1972, that ovarian carcinogenesis could result from incessant ovulation without physiological rest among women in developed countries, the British researchers argued that the protective effect of the pill could stem from its inhibition of ovulation.[53] Some epidemiologists had also shown that pregnancy helped to protect women against ovarian cancer.[54] A further case-control study of 300 women carried out in California confirmed the British findings. The conclusions of the research were that oral contraceptives afforded the same degree of protection against ovarian cancer as pregnancy.[55]

The discovery that the pill could protect against ovarian cancer had important implications for all women's health. During the 1980s a number of studies confirmed the earlier data, showing that oral contraceptives reduced the risk of ovarian cancer by about 40 per cent and that the protection lasted for more than ten years after stopping the drug.[56] By 1989 at least 15 case-control studies had been carried out on the subject, 13 of which had shown a positive effect. The consistency of the results was particularly striking given the diversity of study designs involved and the fact that the studies had been conducted among different populations around the world.[57] One of the investigations was a multinational study conducted by the World Health Organization in five developing countries (Chile, China, Mexico, the Philippines and Thailand).[58] Moreover, the pill's substantial impact in terms of public health had been illustrated by the finding in the United States that oral contraceptives had helped prevent 1,700 cases of ovarian cancer in 1983. This, the researchers claimed, represented a 30 per cent decrease in the overall incidence of ovarian cancer amongst American women.[59]

Positive effects also began to be discovered in relation to endometrial cancer in the early 1980s. Initially this finding was surprising because during the early 1970s investigators had identified an association between oestrogens and endometrial cancer. This had been identified most clearly in the case of stilboestrol, which was shown not only to cause vaginal cancer in the daughters of women who had taken the drug but also endometrial tumours. Anxieties about the oestrogen compound in oral contraceptives were exacerbated in 1975 when a number of studies revealed that oestrogen replacement therapy, prescribed to menopausal women, appeared to increase the risk of endometrial cancer by 5 to 14 times the normal rate. The risk was higher the longer the woman was on the treatment.[60] This was announced the same year that investigations drew links between sequential oral contraceptives, which had a high content of oestrogen, and endometrial cancer. Women who took sequential pills doubled their risk of developing endometrial cancer. Introduced in the early 1960s, sequential pills involved the administration of oestrogen for the first 14 to 16 days of the menstrual cycle, followed by a combination of oestrogen and progestogen for 5 to 6 days. In 1976 a number of pharmaceutical companies, under pressure from the FDA, voluntarily withdrew sequential pills from the market because of their associations with endometrial cancer. The pills comprised 10 per cent of the American oral contraceptive market.[61]

Nonetheless, it was unclear whether other oral contraceptives had the same negative impact. Early on research into endometrial cancer in menopausal women had revealed that progestogens could reduce endometrial atrophy. On this basis some medical experts wondered whether progestogens could in fact counterbalance the problem of endometrial cancer in menopausal women who were being given oestrogen replacement therapy. Research into the combined oral contraceptives reinforced this view. Case-control studies, primarily conducted in the United States between 1979 and 1986, showed that combined oral contraceptives halved the risk of endometrial cancer. Moreover, this protective effect increased the longer a woman took the pill.[62] With this news the pill seemed to offer protection not only against ovarian cancer but also endometrial cancer.

Negative news

By the early 1980s the pessimism regarding the pill just a decade before seemed at last to belong to the past. In October 1983, however, a bombshell hit the medical profession and the rest of the world. That year, two epidemiological studies, one conducted in Los Angeles (under Dr Malcolm Pike) and the other in Oxford (under Dr Martin Vessey), indicated that the use of oral contraceptives increased the risk of cervical and breast cancer. Pike's case-control study of 314 young breast cancer patients (under the age of 32) and 314 individually matched controls was particularly worrying because it showed that women who took the pill before the age of 25 increased fourfold their risk of suffering breast cancer under the age of 37. The risk increased the longer a woman took the drug. Such news accompanied findings from a British cohort study which showed that the prolonged use of oral contraceptives could increase the risk of cervical cancer. Based on a ten-year follow-up study of just under 10,000 women (6,838 women taking oral contraceptives and 3,154 women using IUDs) who had attended family planning clinics in Britain, this research suggested that oral contraceptives might have contributed to the rise in cervical cancer in England and Wales over the previous decade.[63] Together the results of the two investigations contradicted earlier findings that failed to show a definitive risk linking the pill with cervical or breast cancer.[64]

With cervical and breast cancer causing up to 16,000 deaths in Britain a year, the news about the pill was very disturbing.[65] The new findings were particularly worrying in the case of breast cancer given the recent increase in younger women taking the drug. In Britain, for instance, among sexually active female teenagers (under the age of 20) the number taking the pill had risen from 15 per cent in 1970 to 50 per cent by 1975. By 1980 the percentage had risen even further to 80 per cent. The number of women taking the oral contraceptive under the age of 30 had also increased substantially since its first marketing. In the United States, teenage consumption of the pill, while starting later than in Britain, was also high.[66]

The most disquieting aspect of the news was that progestogens might be implicated in the cancer. This was unlike previous scares where oestrogen had been blamed for side-effects such as thrombosis. Many women who had been switched to low dose pills in the wake of the cardiovascular troubles in the late 1960s were now surprised to discover that their drug was not as safe as had previously been presumed. Pills with high doses of progestogen were now regarded as dangerous. In the light of the findings, the British Committee on Safety of Drugs (CSD) calculated that only about eight of the 45 brands of oral contraceptives were safe. Only three of the pills contained the doses of oestrogen and progestogen considered completely safe. This affected approximately 80 per cent of the 3.5 million British women then taking oral contraceptives. The committee recommended that women now be prescribed pills with the lowest suitable dose of oestrogen and progestogen, and that all long-term takers have regular cervical smears.[67]

Many were angered by the action taken by the CSD. First, many doctors were outraged that the recommendations had been made without giving them any prior warning. As had happened in the case of the thrombosis episode in 1969, local general practitioners had been forced to field a barrage of questions from concerned women without prior knowledge of the issues. Secondly, controversy soon broke out over the ways in which Pike and the committee had calculated the potency of the progestogens assumed to be carcinogenic.[68] Significantly, in February 1984 the FDA's Fertility and Maternal Health Drug Advisory Committee decided that the evidence about progestogens was still unproven. Nonetheless, the FDA decided to reaffirm the previous policy that women with a strong family history of breast cancer should be warned against the use of oral contraceptives. Where possible, the FDA recommended that patients should be prescribed pills with the lowest levels of both progestogen and oestrogen. They also advised that all pill users should receive regular breast examinations.[69]

Conflicts within the scientific community: breast cancer

While conflicts were erupting over which progestogens were con-sidered to be implicated in causing cancer, other tensions were growing within the scientific community. Just two months after the original publicity about Pike's study, another report confirmed the earlier findings. Authored by the epidemiologist Dr Klim McPherson, this report suggested that the risk of breast cancer was three times higher among women who had used oral contraceptives at least four years before their first baby. McPherson announced his results in late 1983 to a conference organized by three pharmaceutical companies with major interests in the oral contraceptive market. Attended by 800 doctors, the conference had been set up in response to Pike's publication. McPherson's news did not come as a total surprise to the audience. Nonetheless, it sparked off a fierce debate among participants. One speaker, for instance, criticized Malcolm Pike's paper in 'terms so intemperate that Pike was moved to shout, "That's libellous!" from his place in the audience ... Later, when granted the right of reply, he was emotional and close to tears.'[70]

Much of the tension of the meeting stemmed from the fact that the stakes were so high. What was on the line was not only professional reputations, but also women's lives. At least 50 million women were known to be taking the pill worldwide, with at least 20 million using it in the developing world. The new findings were particularly disturbing given the increasing incidence of breast cancer in more industrialized nations.[71] What concerned many was the thought that the putative higher risk affecting younger women taking the pill might persist into their middle age. Should this happen, medical experts feared they would witness an unprecedented rise in breast cancer in years to come. In Britain, which had one of the highest rates of breast cancer in the world, it had been estimated in 1981 that such a risk could 'eventually produce groups of women with perhaps a one-in-five chance of developing breast cancer in their lifetimes'.[72] Similar concerns surfaced among American experts.[73] The bitter personal attacks made during the 1983 conference were just a foretaste of the many conflicts that were to plague the rest of the 1980s. Indeed, fierce arguments between different camps of epidemiologists became more and more entrenched as the years wore on. Outbursts, similar to those of the meeting in 1983 were to be repeated at a conference organized in Britain in 1989. This time speakers had microphones grabbed from their hands while talking.[74]

The difficulty epidemiologists faced in understanding the data on the issue fuelled part of the battle. By the end of the 1980s dozens of epidemiological studies had looked into the question, yet their results were mystifying.[75] One of the most puzzling aspects of this research was the fact that it seemed to be younger, rather than older, women who seemed to be most at risk of breast cancer from the contraceptive pill. Early in the 1970s cohort studies had suggested a slightly increased danger of breast cancer in women under the age of 35 who took oral contraceptives over a prolonged period. Investigations during the 1980s also showed younger women to be at greater risk.[76] This did not entirely make sense in relation to the wider understanding of the relationship between hormones and the development of cancer, as the incidence of breast cancer usually increases with age. Some medical experts believed the increasing incidence of breast cancer was partly attributable to the fact that women were now living longer.

One understanding of breast cancer was that the development of breast tissue was sensitive to a woman's natural production of oestrogen during her lifetime.[77] Some experts connected the higher rate of breast cancer in older women to the decline of natural oestrogen during the menopause. Women's production of oestrogen in earlier life was also considered to be an important factor. Those who experienced early menarche, for instance, seemed to be at a slightly higher risk of getting breast cancer, as did those who became pregnant for the first time late in life. At the same time, those with mothers who had had the disease were also at a greater risk. Table 7.1 sums up the factors involved in breast cancer in a woman's reproductive cycle. The hormone progesterone was also thought to play a role in breast cancer, possibly as a protective influence. Progestogens in oral contraceptives, for instance, had been considered to be protective against benign breast disease since the early 1970s.[78]

Epidemiologists therefore began to ask how far oral contraceptives used early in a woman's life, or before her first pregnancy, might be having an

Table 7.1 Factors implicating natural hormones in the development of breast cancer

Factor	Influence on risk
Female sex	Increases risk
Age	Increases risk
Age at menarche	Inversely related to risk
Age at menopause	Directly related to risk
Surgical removal of ovary	Protection inversely related to age at surgery
Women who have never given birth	Increases risk
Age at first birth	Directly related to risk
Pregnancy	Additional children weakly protective

Source: D.B. Thomas, 'Do hormones cause breast cancer?', *Cancer,* 53 (1 Feb. 1984), supplement, 596, table 1.

effect on rates of breast cancer.[79] Much of the epidemiological data collected during the 1980s seemed to point in this direction. Research by Pike and his co-workers in Los Angeles in 1981 revealed that those most at risk of developing breast cancer at a young age were women who had taken the pill before their first full-term pregnancy. Their 1983 study showed that women taking oral contraceptives after their first pregnancy were not endangered. Nonetheless, women taking the pill before the age of 25 were found to have a high risk. This increased the longer the women took the drug. The age factor was now seen as the explanation for the earlier risk found among those taking the pill before their first pregnancy. Another study conducted by McPherson and his colleagues in Britain subsequently confirmed the Los Angeles findings in 1983 and 1987 of a strong association of breast cancer in women who had taken the pill before their first pregnancy.[80] In 1989, however, a UK national case-control study of women under the age of 36, set up by Pike, McPherson and Vessey, showed that the hazard of taking the pill appeared to be unrelated to whether women had taken it before or after their first pregnancy. The study, nonetheless, reaffirmed fears about the contraceptive in relation to breast cancer. While showing that pill use by mature women did not increase breast cancer, the investigators felt their evidence did not resolve the question about the risk to younger women.[81]

The epidemiologists had come no closer to solving the riddle by their focus on different subgroups of women. Confusing matters even further was a case-control study of breast cancer published by the Cancer and Steroid Hormone Study Group (CASH) in the United States in 1985 and 1986. This had compared 2,099 women with breast cancer and 2,065 controls of women from eight geographic regions of the United States for the period 1980 to 1982. It was one of the largest case-control investigations carried out to date, being four times the size of the studies reported by McPherson and Pike in 1983. The CASH study found no association between the use of oral contraceptives and breast cancer. This was the case even for women who had taken the pill before the age of 20 and for those who had taken the pill for a prolonged period before their first full-term pregnancy. Overall the investigators concluded that the use of the pill by young women in the United States had 'no effect on the aggregate risk of breast cancer before 45 years of age'.[82] Other investigations conducted by researchers in the United States in the 1980s had also shown no significant association between the pill and breast cancer.[83] Further research by the CASH group reconfirmed their earlier findings.[84] Nonetheless, the evidence was still inconclusive. In 1989, for instance, a reanalysis of the CASH data revealed that the oral contraceptives could be having an effect on breast cancer if taken before the first full-term pregnancy.[85]

The discrepancy in the findings among the different investigations in the 1980s provoked great discussion between epidemiologists. Geographic location and diversity of population were partly thought to explain the differing results. This was not unreasonable given that certain countries had a much lower incidence of breast cancer. Women in the United States, for instance, were four to five times more at risk of developing breast cancer than those in Japan. While diet may contribute to this difference, what is equally important is that Japanese women tend to start menstruation later, settle down to regular cycles later, and are smaller in physique.[86] Differences in childbearing patterns across the world could also not be ruled out. Others, however, argued that such factors could not be the whole explanation.[87] Some asserted that the latency effect and varying levels of pill consumption found in each country for different age groups might explain the discrepancies in the findings.[88] Yet the studies had yielded conflicting interpretations on this issue.[89] One of the problems confronting the epidemiologists throughout the 1980s was that the statistics were difficult to interpret and it was impossible to exclude problems of bias or chance.[90]

Another question in people's minds was whether the higher risk of breast cancer was linked to any particular kind of pill. McPherson and his colleagues, for instance, had found that preparations marketed before the early 1970s which contained the compound ethinyloestradiol seemed to be more hazardous. Other researchers had not found any such association. The UK National Case-Control Study also examined the effect of different pills according to their oestrogen content. Those found to be the cause of a greater risk were pills with preparations containing at least 5 mg of oestrogen. No definitive evidence, however, could be found in terms of the different progestogens contained in combined oral contraceptives.[91] By the end of the 1980s, none of the epidemiologists had uncovered any definitive evidence to prove which of the different formulations of the pill carried more risk in terms of breast cancer.[92] An additional problem was that the majority of investigations had concentrated on older higher-dose pills, and very little evidence had been collected on the newer generations of pills which now dominated the market.

The breakthrough

By 1988 over 30 epidemiological studies had been undertaken to investigate the links between oral contraceptive use and breast cancer. Yet not a single study had provided a statistically significantly answer.[93] In July 1989 a conference held at the Royal Society of Medicine in London was called to try to sort out the problem. While the conference was plagued by the conflicts between different epidemiologists which had dominated the 1980s, many of its participants realized that the only way forward was for authors of the various studies to collaborate.[94] The idea of collaboration was not new. In 1986 an editorial in the *British Medical Journal* had called for such work.[95]

Such a task was not going to be easy, however. Professional rivalry was not the only obstacle. The difficulty was bringing investigators together from a wide variety of countries and amalgamating diverse data in a uniform framework. It remained unclear how such collaboration could ever be achieved. The beginning of a breakthrough appeared with the appointment of Professor Valerie Beral to the directorship of the Imperial Cancer Research Fund Epidemiology Unit in Oxford in 1989. Replacing Malcolm Pike, who had previously held the position, Beral had extensive experience of epidemiological research into hormones and cancer, particularly in relation to pregnancy. She also had not participated in the research on breast cancer and the pill, which meant that she was more neutral than many involved in the debate over the previous decade. Moreover, Beral was in a good position to mediate between different investigators, because she had close contact with the key epidemiologists across the debate on the effect of the oral contraceptive on breast cancer.[96]

Despite her advantageous position, Beral was initially unclear about how to proceed. One of the ideas she was keen to test was whether the pill had an effect similar to hormones in pregnancy in relation to cancer. She wondered whether an extra risk of breast cancer with the pill might be strongest in young women and diminish or disappear at an older age.[97] This would be consistent with findings on the effect of pregnancy on breast cancer. The possibility nonetheless remained that prolonged use of the pill from an early age could produce a persistent and substantial increase.[98] Much of Beral's thinking was shaped by her earlier research into pregnancy and cancer in Britain, which had shown pregnancy to confer long-term protection against cancers of the breast, ovary and endometrium.[99] In one study, however, where she had compared childbearing women with those who had never been pregnant, she had discovered that those at highest risk of breast cancer were older women who had very recently had a child.[100]

Beral's original plan had been to summarize the published material. Uncertain about what methodology she should use, she spoke to the epidemiologist and statistician Professor Richard Peto, who had extensive expertise in the construction of large-scale epidemiological studies. Rather than summarizing previous studies, Peto recommended that Beral think of putting together all the original data from such research. With studies having taken place all over the world, this was not going to be easy. Her one advantage was her contact with the epidemiologists in Oxford and those who had worked on the CASH project. Once she had their collaboration, many other investigators were keen to join the research. Funded by the Imperial Cancer Research Fund, the collaboration started in 1992. By 1993 Beral and her colleagues had managed to collect epidemiological data from a wide variety of studies around the world. This was proving a major difficulty because few had attempted an analysis of data on such a large scale before. Beral and her colleagues had to analyse the data of 53,297 women and 100, 239 controls contained in 54 studies from 25 countries across the world. This represented about 90 per cent of the epidemiological information collected on breast cancer risk and the use of hormonal contraceptives over the previous two decades.[101]

When analysed, the data made apparent what no one had seen before: that the carcinogenic effect of the pill on the breast was related to its recent use. In September 1993, Beral and her colleagues announced the results to a gathering of epidemiologists. Their results were greeted with a stunned silence. After years of debate it seemed that the answer was finally to hand. It was clear that the results of all the previous studies, rather than contradicting each other, showed a uniform pattern: that the raised mortality from breast cancer occurred among those who were using or had recently used the pill and for ten years thereafter, but that users who had stopped the pill more than ten years before showed no excess of mortality. In the case of women taking the pill, the risk was only slight. Tumours that were diagnosed in women taking oral contraceptives tended to be localized to the breast and were less clinically advanced. This contrasted with women who had never used oral contraceptives, where the cancer was more likely to spread to other parts of the body. The tumours diagnosed in women taking the pill were therefore potentially easier to treat. A woman's family history of breast cancer made no impact on the results. The data also indicated that risk was unrelated to any particular oestrogen or progesto-gen. Interestingly the higher doses of hormones were seen to be associated with less risk.[102]

Resolving a problem that had intrigued epidemiologists for decades, Beral and her colleagues set about refining their results. In 1996 the study was officially published in the British medical journal the *Lancet*.[103] Publi-cation, however, was greeted with uproar by the media. One headline in the British *Sunday Times* read 'Pill users face 10-year tumour risk'. Others talked of a 'new scare over breast cancer'. Such negative publicity had occurred despite the precautions taken by the medical community to release the full data early to the press and the fact that the risk was very small in absolute terms. Measures had also been taken to warn doctors of the results so that they could reassure their patients.[104]

Despite the media hype over breast cancer and the pill in 1996, many medical practitioners took the results of the study to be positive. While women on the pill faced a slightly increased risk, any tumour that developed was likely to be clinically less advanced than in women not taking the pill. More importantly, the carcinogenic effect of the pill on the breast diminished after ten years of stopping the drug. It was therefore unlikely that the medical profession would witness an epidemic of breast cancer in future years among older women who had taken the contracep-tive. Physicians were once again reassured in January 1999 when a 25-year follow-up of its cohort of 46,000 women by the British Royal College of General Practitioners confirmed the earlier findings of the collaborative study.[105]

Conclusion

The results of the studies on breast cancer and the pill in the 1990s put to rest for the moment concerns that had weighed on people's minds for years. Breast cancer was the one factor that many had feared might tip the odds against the safety of the pill overall. The extent to which it was of major public concern was highlighted by data from France and the United States in the 1990s, which showed that breast cancer reduced women's life expectancy by ten years. As one epidemiologist pointed out in 1991, shortly before the collaborative study was launched, breast cancer was so common that 'any increase in risk associated with a widely used method of contraception would be a serious concern'. He went on to point out that

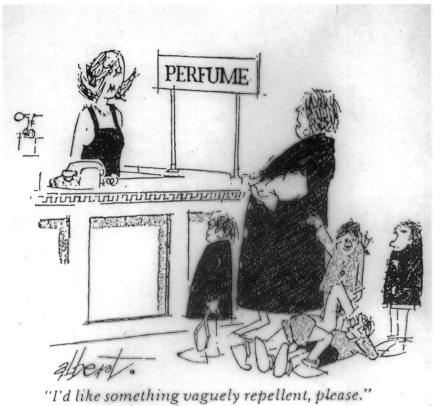

"I'd like something vaguely repellent, please."

1. Cartoon from the 1950s. How women coped before the pill.

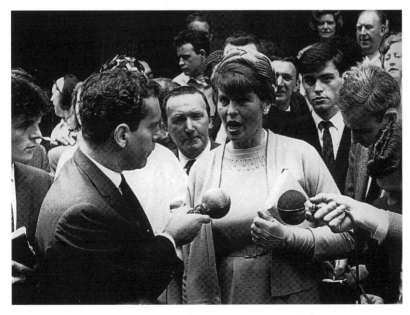

2. Dr Anne Biezanek, greeted by reporters after successfully challenging her bishop to give her communion even though she was taking the pill, May 1964.

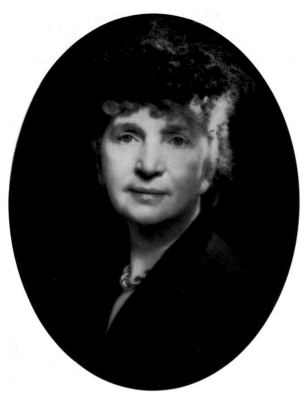

3. Margaret Sanger, 1945.

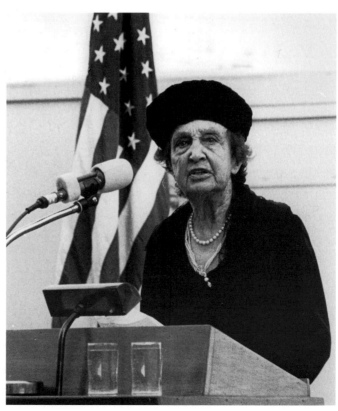

4. Katherine McCormick, at the dedication of Stanley McCormick Hall, MIT Women's Housing, October 1963.

5. Gregory Pincus, *c.* 1930s.

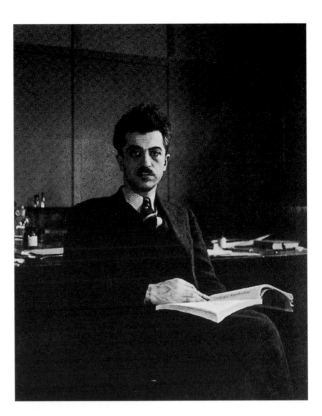

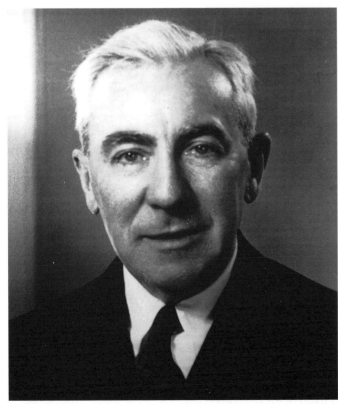

6. John Rock.

7. Farmer extracting Mexican yam from the earth, near the city of Orizaba, 1977–8.

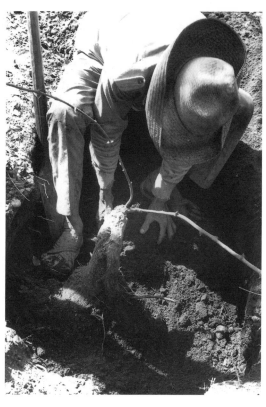

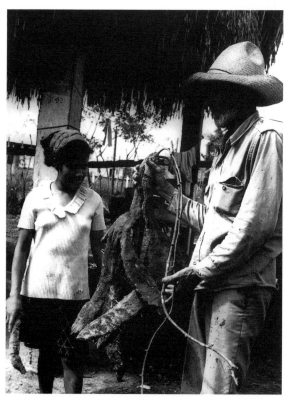

8. Farmer with Mexican yam, near the city of Orizaba, 1977–8.

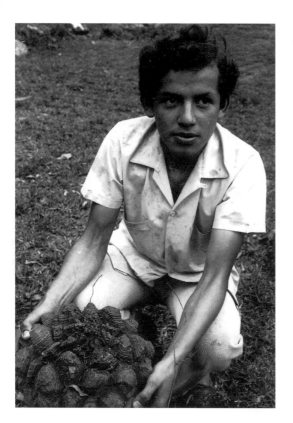

9. Boy with Mexican yam, near the city of Orizaba, 1977–8.

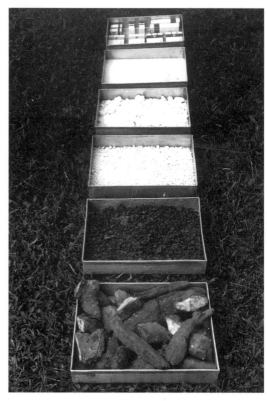

10. From the Mexican yam to the pill: different stages of production, near the city of Orizaba, 1977–8.

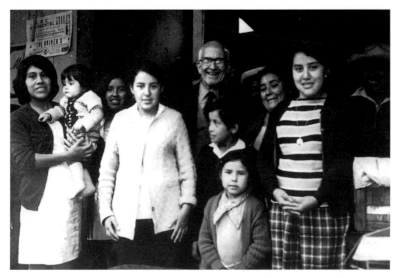

11. Russell Marker with the storekeeper and family who helped him whilst he produced the first progesterone.

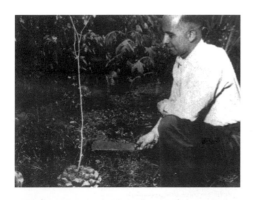

12. Russell Marker was the first to identify the Mexican yam as a source of diosgenin, the substance needed to produce steroid hormones.

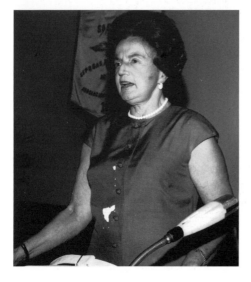

13. Edris Rice-Wray, speaking at a Medical Association of Puerto Rico meeting on the problem of population growth, 1974.

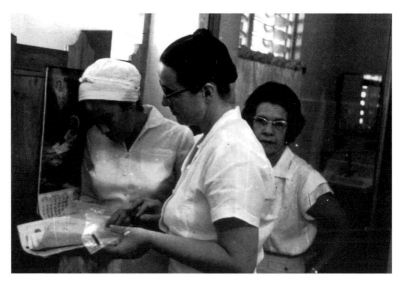

14. Adaline Satterthwaite checking details for the clinical trials of the pill, Humacao, Puerto Rico, late 1950s. Note the Catholic image on the calendar on the wall. Puerto Rico was a strongly Catholic country.

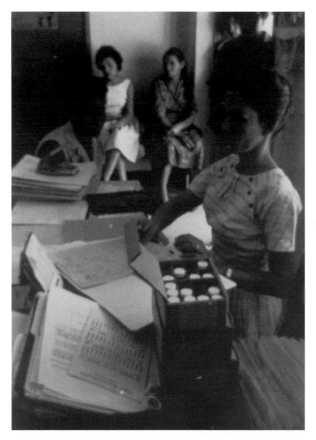

15. A health worker organizing pills for distribution for the clinical trials of the pill, Humacao, Puerto Rico, late 1950s.

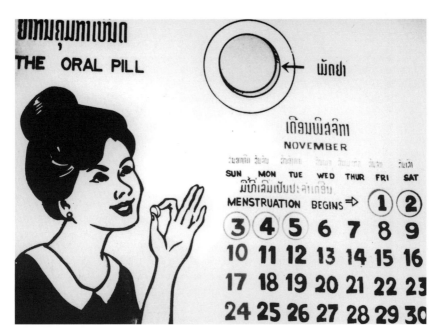

16. Malaysian poster explaining pill use.

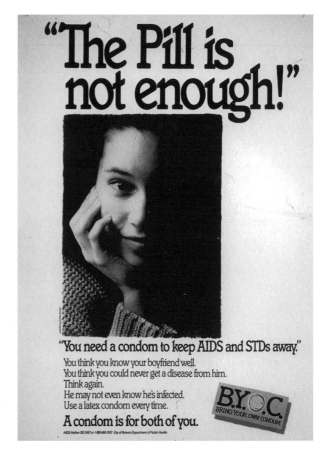

17. City of Toronto Department of
Public Health advertising
campaign.

'Breast cancer also happens to be a disease that women and their families particularly fear, so any increase in risk might carry a disproportionate weight when choices of contraception are being made.'[106] For women living in the more developed world where breast cancer has recently been increasing, the findings of the collaborative studies done in the 1990s have come as a tremendous relief. In addition to breast cancer, recent research has also shown that the overall excess of mortality from the pill (apart from breast cancer) is also restricted to its current and recent users and that this disappears ten years after ceasing to take the drug.[107]

Yet certain riddles about the pill and cancer remain. The Royal College of General Practitioners' study of 1999 suggests that the patterns observed for breast cancer and other forms of mortality might be similar in the case of cancers of other female reproductive organs. They suggest that cancer of these organs 'may also be affected by current and recent use of oral contraceptives but may wear off after use stops'.[108] Nonetheless, evidence is still to be collected to prove this assertion.

In the case of cervical cancer, this is a particularly important question. While this is a cancer which affects only a small proportion of women in the developed world, in more deprived socioeconomic parts of the world it is a major public health concern. The main problem in examining this issue is the difficulty of disentangling the effects of the pill from socioeconomic factors, as well as sexual behaviour, such as age at first intercourse and the number of sexual partners the male partner has previously had. Equally important is the effect of screening programmes.

No conclusive evidence has been collected anywhere to date on the connections between the pill and cervical cancer.[109] At present Beral and her colleagues are investigating the effect of oral contraceptives on cancer of the cervix, endometrium and ovaries using the same meta-analysis techniques they used for exploring the issue of breast cancer. This research, which reanalyses old studies, is funded by World Health Organization.[110] Whatever the outcome of this study and future research, it will have a major impact in assessing whether the risks of the pill outweigh its benefits for women living in the less developed world.

While the puzzle of cancer continues, epidemiologists and medical practitioners have nonetheless come a long way in terms of understanding some of the relationships between oral contraceptives and the pill. The debate has gone through many twists and turns. At the time of its first marketing many medical experts feared the worst in terms of cancer; others were more optimistic, arguing that it might have protective effects.

During the initial years many of the anxieties about the carcinogenic effects of the drug were overshadowed by reports of its cardiovascular complications. By the late 1970s many medical practitioners began to change their tune about the dangers of the pill as increasing numbers of investigations revealed that it protected against ovarian and endometrial cancer.

In the light of this evidence many medical practitioners began to see the pill as more than just a contraceptive and to embrace it as a weapon to fight cancer. One medical expert has pointed out that oral contraceptives might be the 'only prescription drug that increases life expectancy'.[111] Dr Joseph Goldzieher went even further in the 1990s to argue that all women of reproductive age and even older should be using oral contraceptives for at least two years of their lives because of their 'anticancer effect'.[112]

Such views stem from the discovery that the pill can protect against ovarian cancer, one of the leading causes of gynaecological malignancy among women in many developed countries. Studies estimate that use of the pill may have reduced the risk of ovarian cancer by about 40 per cent. The reduction in the incidence of cancer increases the longer a woman takes oral contraceptives. Women taking the pill for at least 12 years can reduce their risk of ovarian cancer by 80 per cent. In the case of endometrial cancer the pill is thought to reduce the incidence of the disease by about 50 per cent. Moreover, the protective effects against endometrial and ovarian cancer continue long after women discontinue taking the drug.[113]

It is unlikely, however, that the arguments are over. To date most of the research has been conducted on the effects of the old formulations of oral contraceptives, but little has been done on the constituents of newer pills. One of the questions currently being asked is whether the older and higher doses of oral contraceptives gave better protection against cancer than the newer low dose pills. Given the need for a long period to elapse before carcinogenic effects can be fully assessed, the effect of the pill on cancer will continue to be debated for many years to come. One advantage scientists will have is the novel approaches opened up for conducting epidemiological research in the wake of the 1993 study into oral contraceptives and breast cancer. New methodological and statistical techniques as well as the computer have been invaluable in this process. Much of the research on the pill has taken place against an increasing emphasis in medicine on the need for evidence-based studies and meta-analysis.[114] What will remain controversial, however, is how the evidence collected by these methods should be interpreted.

8

'A Dream Come True': The Reception of the Pill

In 1922 Margaret Sanger wrote, 'No woman can call herself free who does not own and control her own body ... It is for women the key to liberty.'[1] This belief had been the driving force in Sanger's search for a contraceptive pill. From her perspective the contraceptive pill represented the means for women to free themselves from the continual burden of reproduction. She was not alone: in 1928, the British birth control campaigner Marie Stopes commented that 'the demand for a simple pill or drug' for contraception was 'astonishingly widespread'.[2] A woman who joined one of the first clinical trials for the pill in Britain summed up the feeling of many when she said that for her the appearance of the pill had been 'a dream come true'.[3] In 1969 an American female journalist on the *Los Angeles Times* also captured the feeling of the time when she said, 'Modern woman is at last free, as a man is free, to dispose of her own body, to earn her living, to pursue the improvement of her mind, to try a successful career.'[4]

The rapid take-up of the pill when it was first launched on the market in the early 1960s highlights the strong desire for such a contraceptive. Within five years of its launch in the United States, nearly 11 million women across the world were taking the pill every year, over 5 million of them American (see table 8.1).[5] The swift popularity of the drug was most prominent in developed countries such as Australia, New Zealand, the United States and Britain. By 1968 at least 34 per cent of married women of childbearing age in Australia and New Zealand were currently taking the pill. By 1969 the percentage of married women aged 15 to 44 years

Table 8.1 Estimated number of oral contraceptives produced and sold around the world, 1965–1967

Region	January 1965	July 1966	July 1967
Developed countries	5,205,600	7,235,000	9,960,000
USA	4,000,000	5,000,000	6,500,000
Canada	260,000	450,000	750,000
United Kingdom	275,000	415,000	700,000
Australia, New Zealand	380,000	590,000	670,000
Europe, including USSR			
(excluding SIDA purchases)[1]	250,000	690,000	1,200,000
Japan	50,000	90,000	140,000
Developing Countries	795,000	2,330,000	2,883,000
Latin America	500,000	1,600,000	1,934,999
Mexico	55,000	170,000	270,000
Brazil	–	646,000	750,000
Argentina	–	260,000	340,000
Colombia	37,000	64,000	75,000
Other Latin America	–	460,000	499,000
Far East	100,000	367,000	587,000
Singapore	25,000	60,000	73,000
Malaysia	15,000	37,000	46,000
Hong Kong[2]	20,000	30,000	53,000
South Korea	6,000	32,000	58,000
Thailand	–	19,000	97,000
India	–	35,000	70,000
Other, Far East	34,000	94,000	110,000
Near East and UAR	145,0000	273,000	320,000
United Arab Republic	–	200,000	220,000
Turkey	–	45,000	60,000
Iran	–	15,000	18,000
Iraq	–	13,000	22,000
Africa	50,000	100,000	122,000
World	6,000,000	9,515,000	12,843,000

Figures consolidated from reports of actual sales and production by the individual manufacturers of oral tablets throughout the world, cross-checked against regular marketing research surveys and government import records. The number of users was calculated by dividing the number of pills used in an area over a 12-month period by 13. These figures, however, do not represent the actual numbers of women taking the pill.

1 SIDA is the Swedish International Development Authority which gives substantial numbers of oral tablets to developing countries.

2 Some of the pills were apparently destined for export.

Source: Population Council, *Studies in Family Planning*, Dec. 1967, cited in US Congress, Senate *World Population and Food Crisis: Hearings before the Consultative Subcommittee on Economic and Social Affairs of the Committee on Foreign Relations*, 90th Congress, Feb. 1968, 523.

currently taking the pill was just under 25 per cent in the United States (9 million) and over 15 per cent in Britain (1.5 million). Worldwide the figure was 18 to 19 million (excluding China and Eastern Europe), representing about 2 per cent of the world's female population.[6]

Such unexpected and unprecedented usage not only surprised the pharmaceutical industry, but also amazed physicians, family planners, social reformers and politicians. The overwhelming popularity of the pill could be attributed to the clever marketing strategy of its manufacturers, who, in order to overcome the social and political taboos surrounding contraception, deftly linked the drug to the fight against population growth and poverty.[7] Such an explanation, however, ignores the fact that by 1968 it was largely middle-class women in the developed countries who took the pill rather than impoverished women in Latin America, Africa and Asia for whom the drug was originally intended (figure 8.1).

From the perspective of a middle-class woman living in a country like the United States or Britain, the pill was not so much an instrument for curbing population growth as the long sought tool for family planning. A letter written to Gregory Pincus in 1958 by a British woman sums up the delight with which many women greeted the coming of the pill.

> Having just read the most heartening news I have ever seen in a newspaper ever – that is an article in the Daily Mail on your research into [the] anti-pregnancy pill. May I offer heartfelt and grateful thanks – I'm sure on behalf of millions of women in this country too, for your work.

Figure 8.1 Pill users as a percentage of married women aged 15–44, worldwide, 1968

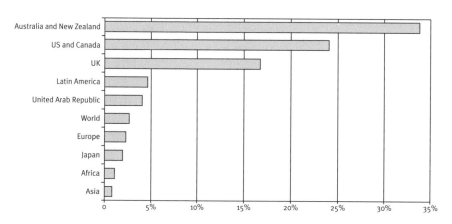

Source: J. Peel and J. Potts, *Textbook of Contraceptive Practice* (Cambridge, 1969), 127.

> To one who has suffered unbelievable mental and physical agony on account of unwanted pregnancy, I speak with deep personal gratitude on your work. I'm sure it will add immeasurably to the happiness of women on earth. May God bless your efforts.[8]

Yet the benefits the pill brought were double-edged. From the beginning women began to experience nausea, weight gain, headaches and other reactions on taking the drug. While oral contraceptives were gradually reformulated to minimize such side-effects, many problems persisted. For some women the reactions were enough to discourage them from continuing the medication. Others, however, were willing to put up with any side-effects because of the ability to enjoy sex without worrying about the consequences.

Enthusiasm for the pill plummeted dramatically in the late 1960s, however, when the medical profession began to link the pill with more serious health problems, such as cardiovascular complications like blood clots. By the early 1970s, within a decade of its availability, the contraceptive had fallen from its pedestal as a wonder drug. Now women had to balance the freedom from pregnancy offered by the pill against the risks it posed to their health. In this context many women, particularly those in the United States, began to question the control the contraceptive gave them over their reproductive cycle and to challenge the ideas put forward by those such as Margaret Sanger. For these women the swallowing of a pill represented not so much a liberty as the imposition of a control over their bodies by the medical profession and the pharmaceutical industry.

The decision to take the oral contraceptive was as much bound by the wider social and political attitudes towards sexual relationships, motherhood and female employment as by an individual woman's expectations and physiological reactions to the drug. As this chapter shows, women's responses to the pill were complex and changed over time. Much depended on a woman's age, class and marital status, as it did on where she lived, the types of contraceptive she had used before the appearance of the pill and the kind of relationship she had with her male partner. Added to these factors were changing medical opinions regarding the safety of the drug and the degree to which she understood and paid attention to such issues. Moreover, a woman's decision to take the pill was not only subject to influences, but it had important consequences: for her own health and her expectations about sex and contraception, and for men as well.

Contraception before the arrival of the pill

When examining the initial response to the oral contraceptive it is important to understand the types of contraceptive techniques available before its release. Ranging from rudimentary methods such as abstinence, withdrawal and abortion, to appliances such as the condom, diaphragm, sponges and syringes that had become increasingly popular since the 1920s, these straightforward contraceptive devices were important in shaping the initial response to the pill. While it is difficult to find accurate statistics on the choice of contraceptive techniques and individual preferences before the emergence of the oral contraceptive, some trends were discernible. These had important repercussions not only for the reception of the pill, but also on the degree to which it challenged prevailing norms about who was to take responsibility for contraception.[9]

One of the most important determinants of contraceptive choice was geographic location. In 1959, on the eve of the release of the pill, for instance, couples in Britain and the United States showed a distinctive preference for certain kinds of contraceptives. Table 8.2 provides an estimate of the types of contraceptives used by British and American couples who married in the years between 1930 and 1960. In both countries the condom was overwhelmingly the most popular method. This was in part a consequence of the development of latex and the emergence

Table 8.2 Comparative popularity of specific contraceptive methods among married women in the UK and the USA, 1959 (percentages)

Contraceptive methods (all users)	UK wives married in 1930–60	US wives married in 1935–55
Condom	49	43
Withdrawal	44	15
Safe period	16	34
Chemicals	16	10
Pessaries	10	4
Diaphragm	11	36
Douche	3	28
Other methods	6	4

Percentages add up to more than 100 per cent, possibly because couples combined several methods.
Sources: E. Draper, *Birth Control in the Modern World* (London, 1972), p.308; J. Peel and M. Potts, *Textbook of Contraceptive Practice* (Cambridge, 1969), 26, table 2.

of thinner, disposable condoms in the 1930s. No longer made from thick rubber, these new condoms not only allowed greater sensitivity during intercourse, but were also considerably cheaper than their predecessors. The provision of free condoms to troops during the Second World War to prevent the spread of venereal disease had similarly encouraged their use, and their popularity had grown rapidly in Britain and the United States after the war. One British survey suggested that as many as 51 per cent of couples who had married between 1950 and 1960 had used the condom, while another indicated that at least 61 per cent of those married between 1941 and 1967 had used it.[10]

One of the striking features of table 8.2 is the fact that the Americans had a greater preference than the British for female-oriented contraceptives, such as the diaphragm and the douche.[11] This can be explained in part by the fact that female devices had been developed and marketed much earlier in the United States. Despite stringent legal restrictions, female contraceptive appliances had become big business since the years of the Great Depression: by the late 1930s their sales outnumbered those of condoms by five to one. While the diaphragm and jelly remained too expensive for many women, contraceptives such as douches and suppositories were less costly. Manufacturers had created a large trade in bargain-priced female contraceptives, marketing them along the lines that they gave women freedom from fear of pregnancy. Many of these contraceptives were of doubtful efficacy and could be dangerous to women's health, but they rapidly became equated in the consumer mind with the ideal of the 'modern woman'.[12]

The growth of the female contraceptive industry in the United States helped promote a culture in which female contraception became the norm rather than the exception. This continued after the Second World War; by the 1950s it was estimated that one in three American wives were using diaphragms and contraceptive cream. Obtained from family planning clinics or private medical practitioners, the diaphragm was more commonly used by middle-class women. The growing popularity of the diaphragm not only showed the increasing preference for female contraception, but also the ever greater reliance of many women on medical experts to supply their contraceptive needs.[13]

In Britain, by contrast, the mass marketing of female contraceptives took longer to develop. Those using female contraceptives tended to be the better off. Evidence collected by birth control clinics in Britain indicates that the percentage of middle-class couples using female contraceptive appliances grew from 9 to 40 per cent, while among working class couples it rose from only 1 per cent to 28 per cent between 1910 and 1930.[14] More-over, traditional methods of contraception, particularly those involving male responsibility, remained the norm in Britain much longer than in the United States, even as late as 1959. One of the most popular male forms of contraception in Britain up to the 1950s was the withdrawal method, coitus interruptus, which required the man to withdraw his penis before ejacula-tion.[15] The prevalence of the withdrawal method can be deduced from a British marriage survey conducted in 1959–60, which indicated that about 43 per cent of the informants had used coitus interruptus at some point in their marriage and between 21 and 32 per cent had relied on nothing else.[16] The high incidence of the withdrawal method can partly be explained by the very long-standing tradition of its use, especially in British working-class communities.[17]

Oral interviews with British working-class couples who were sexually active between 1925 and 1950 indicate that overall contraception was perceived to be a male rather than a female affair. Men were thought to know more about sex and had better links with networks where they could pick up information on sex and contraception. Male responsibility for contraception was also connected to particular notions of masculinity in which men were perceived to be the active partners pursuing sex. Just as importantly, men tended to associate contraception with certain roles and obligations within the family. Many men, for example, saw withdrawal as a mark of their strength and manhood.[18]

Reception of the pill and its impact on contraceptive and sexual behaviour

The distinctive contraceptive patterns in Britain and the United States had important consequences for the ways in which the pill was received in each country.[19] As table 8.1 and figure 8.1 indicate, by the mid-1960s a third of all American wives had used an oral contraceptive, and at least a quarter of them preferred it above other methods. This figure was to climb even further in the following years. By the late 1960s the majority of American women had taken the pill. In 1970 the US National Fertility Survey indi-cated that at least 36 per cent of all married couples using contraception were using the pill.[20] Similarly by 1973 at least a quarter of American married women were using oral contraceptives, and two-thirds of them had tried them at some point in their lives.[21]

By contrast in Britain only 16 per cent of British married women were prescribed the oral contraceptive by 1968. To some extent the swifter and higher uptake of the pill in the United States reflected the earlier marketing of the drug, as well as the long-established disposition towards female methods and medically prescribed techniques in the country.[22] In this context the pill was seen as merely another option for women. Interestingly, however, the pill seemed to become the contraceptive of choice in the United States between 1950 and 1970, overtaking the diaphragm and the condom as the most popular method (table 8.3).[23]

Table 8.3 Most recent method of contraception at time of survey among married women in the USA (percentages)

Contraceptive	1950	1960	1970
Condom	27	18	14
Diaphragm	25	10	6
Pill	–	27	34
Surgical sterilization	–	–	16
IUD	–	–	7

Source: United States National Fertility survey 1955, 1960, 1970, cited in E. Watkins, *On the Pill* (Baltimore, 1998), 61–2.

While the pill may have found an earlier and more receptive audience in America because of the earlier preference for female contraception, it nonetheless rapidly grew in popularity in Britain. Table 8.4 indicates the change in preferences of couples married before 1945 and after 1964. Based on a survey of 6,306 once-married women, one of the noticeable features of this table is the decline in the use of withdrawal and the rise in the use of the pill among couples married after 1964 compared with the choices made by couples married before 1945.

Those who were first to try the oral contraceptive in Britain tended to be women from the higher social classes.[24] Nonetheless, it was not long before the pill became universally accepted among all social groups. A survey of 2,300 British couples in the late 1960s, for instance, showed that 25 per cent of working-class couples married between 1961 and 1965 were using oral contraceptives. This was slightly more than the percentage for couples not in the working class, which was 22 per cent. The same survey showed a decline in withdrawal, which had been the original method of preference

Table 8.4 Patterns of contraceptive methods used by couples married before 1945 and after 1964 in England and Wales

	Percentages married	
Last method used	*Before 1945*	*After 1964*
Condom	40	41
Withdrawal	45	29
Pill	2	24
Safe period	4	10
Diaphragm and Jelly	6	10
Suppositories	4	2
Abstinence	6	3
IUD	–	2

Source: General Register Office survey of 6,306 once-married women, 1967, cited in E. Draper, *Birth Control in the Modern World*, (Harmondsworth, 1972) Appendix 2.

among working-class couples.[25] Table 8.5 indicates that the trend towards the pill and away from coitus interruptus continued through into the 1980s.[26] Other male methods, such as the condom, also began to decline in these years, in the same way as they had done a decade earlier in the United States.[27] By 1975 the pill had overtaken the condom as the most

Table 8.5 Trends in the use of contraception: current method used by ever-married British women aged 16–40, 1967–1983 (percentages)

	1967	*1970*	*1976*	*1983*
Pill	13	19	32	29
IUD	2	4	8	9
Sterilization (female and male)	–	4	15	24
Condom	28	28	16	15
Withdrawal	17	14	5	4
Total	69	75	77	81
Sample size	4,211	2,520	3,378	2,850
Average use ineffectiveness[1]	7.5%	6.2%	3.2%	2.8%

1 This is the measure of the effectiveness of each method of contraception in preventing pregnancy. Of the methods used the pill is regarded as the most effective and withdrawal as the least effective. Thus the substantial decrease in average use ineffectiveness from 6.2 to 3.2 per cent between 1970 and 1976 is partly reflected by the fact that more women were choosing the pill. This is discussed in detail in Murphy.
Sources: M. Murphy, 'The contraceptive pill and women's employment as factors in fertility change in Britain, 1963–80: a challenge to the conventional view', *Population Studies*, 47 (1992), 223, table 2; *General Household Survey* (London, 1983), table 8.5.

popular form of contraception among married British women.[28] The appearance of the oral contraceptive in Britain, therefore, marked a radical turning point in working-class contraceptive culture, whereby women, rather than men, now took responsibility for contraception, a phenomenon that had occurred much earlier in the United States.[29]

The question of who should take responsibility for birth control is only one feature among many in understanding contraceptive behaviour and how this affected the reception of the pill. Before the pill most contraceptive techniques were only moderately effective unless used with great care. This level of risk would have been important in shaping people's attitudes towards contraception generally and their expectations about fertility control. Prior to oral contraceptives, few couples believed they could effectively control fertility and thus did not expect to exercise any firm planning of their family size. Most couples accepted that there was an element of risk in all of the contraceptive techniques they used.[30] The introduction of the pill dramatically altered this view.

From the beginning the pharmaceutical companies and birth control campaigners promoted the pill as at least 99 per cent effective. Such a promise was fundamental to people's attitudes towards oral contraception, for family planning no longer seemed to be a question of Russian roulette. Indeed, the efficacy of the pill raised people's expectations of the efficacy of contraceptive techniques in general. From that point on people began to measure the efficacy of other contraceptives against the standard set by the pill.[31] Within this context the level of risk of pregnancy became a much more important question in contraceptive choice. The ability to plan the size of families enabled couples to devote themselves to other priorities such as education, the pursuit of a woman's career, and material acquisition, without foregoing sexual intercourse.[32] In reshaping people's attitudes as to what was now possible the pill not only altered contraceptive conduct but also influenced reproductive behaviour. Now women, particularly those from the middle-class, could delay having children until it was convenient, and more successfully combine a family with a career. They could also plan with greater confidence when and how to have children, deciding, for instance, to have longer spaces between births, or confining their childbearing years to a restricted set period to limit the expense of childcare and time spent away from work.[33]

In reality the effectiveness of the pill was dependent on a woman's ability to adhere to instructions on taking it. Nonetheless, the allure of its reliability was a powerful attraction for women wanting to have both a family life and a career. One survey of 1,484 women from 12 areas in England and Wales in the late 1960s indicated that 63 per cent believed the pill to be the most reliable form of contraception. This was way ahead of any other form of contraception; only 14 per cent of women, for example, believed the sheath to be trustworthy (the contraceptive technique perceived to be the most reliable after the pill). The dependability of other methods was regarded with even more suspicion. One woman's comment about the pill summed up the thinking of many when she said, 'It's 100 per cent. You simply can't get caught.'[34]

The pill not only changed people's attitudes about the effectiveness of contraception, it also affected the extent to which they were willing to allow contraception to intrude on their sexual life. Taken by mouth at a time independent of intercourse, the innovative feature of the pill was that it was sexually unobtrusive. This was unlike most other current forms of contraception, which coincided with, and indeed often interrupted, sexual intercourse. The novelty of separating contraception from intercourse in fact confused a number of women who first took the pill. A British family planning doctor recalled the bewilderment of some of her patients over its use. One woman, for instance, put the drug in her vagina, and another confused the term 'oral' with 'aural' and placed the pill in her ear. Others assumed they only had to take the drug at the moment of intercourse. [35] This was not surprising given that previous forms of contraception had often necessitated use at the very moment of intercourse and usually involved the genital area. The idea of a contraceptive 'pill' was itself unfamiliar; as one British pill-taker commented, 'people weren't as sophisticated then about taking drugs ... things like penicillin ... weren't available until after the War, so, therefore [taking the pill] was a fairly unknown thing to be doing, a bit Space Agey.'[36]

Many women chose the pill precisely because it involved no fiddling around and they could feel more 'natural' during the sexual act. As one woman commented to the British survey of 1967–8, the use of the pill during sex was 'just like not using anything', which made her more relaxed and able to enjoy the sexual experience.[37] Another woman, who had married in 1955 and started taking the pill as part of a clinical trial after conceiving two children, highlighted the ease of using the contraceptive by comparison with the Dutch cap (the diaphragm). She recalled that using the cap was a 'terrible affair, you used to have to coat it with cream, and squeeze it to get it in, and often it used to just fly out of your hand, so after a few moments of chasing round the bedroom all sexual desire had gone'.[38] One woman similarly called the cap 'a passion-killer'.[39] The pill allowed for greater spontaneity between couples in terms of when and where they had sex.[40] The cap was not only messy, it could also be awkward. In the case of one couple, who preferred to have sex in the morning, the woman had to wear the cap for at least eight hours. This often caused great discomfort, and meant she would try to put off having sex till a more convenient moment.[41] Comparing the pill with other forms of contraception, one woman reflected the feelings of many when she noted that the pill felt a 'much cleaner' and much more 'efficient' form of contraception.[42]

Not all women felt the same, however. Dr Jean Infield, a British family planning expert, remembered that a number of her patients in the early 1960s lost their libido after replacing the condom with the pill because they did not like the fact that they now had semen in their vagina. In these cases the women felt the pill had made the sexual act much messier and less attractive.[43] Some women paradoxically found that the effectiveness of the pill diminished the pleasure of the sexual act. Two, for instance, who began to take the pill during a clinical trial in Slough in the early 1960s, discontinued its use because they felt it was too safe and missed the gamble of not knowing whether or not they would have their period each month. For some women this element of surprise had spiced up their sexual enjoyment.[44] Women who were unsure about whether to have any future children might also have been put off by the very safety of the pill. By taking the pill, women were denied the element of risk and the natural process.[45]

The contraceptive pill thus had important consequences for sex as a whole. For a number of women, it provided the opportunity to enjoy intercourse for the first time.[46] The recollections of one woman highlight the freedom it gave many. Having suffered the discomfort and inconvenience of the cap, she felt the pill gave her a sense of 'marvellous freedom', because it allowed her to enjoy sex for the first time. As she said, 'I can still remember that feeling of elation, you know, it was marvellous! It was like winning the pools!' Now she could have sexual intercourse without any premeditation.[47] Her reaction was not uncommon. Many women felt that in reducing the fear of pregnancy, the pill allowed them to feel more comfortable about sex and to achieve their full sexual potential for the first time.[48]

The torment that many went through before the arrival of the pill is illustrated by the story of Mrs A.C. who had borne three sons by the age of 25. None of her pregnancies had been planned. Part of the reason for the pregnancies was because neither she nor her husband had enjoyed using condoms, the Dutch cap or the rhythm method and had resorted to the withdrawal technique. After her third child, Mrs A.C. became 'a nervous wreck' whenever her 'husband wanted to make love'. As she recalled 'it got to the stage where if ever my husband came near me, I just froze ... in fact it was threatening our marriage'. Keen to find a remedy, she sought help from a doctor. Unfortunately, the doctor turned out to be a Catholic who did not approve of family planning. The only advice Mrs A.C. received was that she 'indulge in a glass of sherry before going to bed to relax'. While the sherry certainly relaxed Mrs A.C., it also resulted in a fourth pregnancy. Nonetheless, the pregnancy allowed Mrs A.C. to enjoy sex again for a while precisely because she was no longer afraid of falling pregnant. From her perspective the pill provided the sexual freedom she had only experienced when actually pregnant.[49]

The risk of pregnancy not only inhibited women psychologically, it could also affect men. Dr Denise Pullen, a family planning doctor working in the 1950s who helped conduct some of the first British clinical trials for the pill, recollected the case of one British man 'who was so frightened of his wife conceiving again that he had become totally impotent'. His potency only returned once his wife started taking the oral contraceptive.[50] The pill therefore not only freed women sexually, it also helped some men.[51]

Unlike male methods of contraception, most female forms necessitated women making an active decision immediately prior to sexual intercourse. This was not easy given the social and cultural inhibitions about women initiating sexual activity. Indeed, many British working-class women had previously preferred the male methods of contraception, such as the condom and coitus interruptus, precisely because they could escape responsibility for contraception and maintain the aura of passivity.[52] A survey conducted in Britain in 1967–8 suggests that many working-class women continued to prefer contraceptive methods controlled by men well into the 1960s, after the advent of pill.[53]

Taken at a time separate from that of sexual intercourse, the pill was revolutionary in that it allowed women to preserve the appearance of passivity while taking some precaution. The case of a British woman, married to a policeman, who joined a pill trial in Birmingham in 1962 illustrates the passive attitude some women adopted when thinking about contraception and the convenience of the oral contraceptive. Commenting on the pill she recalled:

Oh it was very good because – for him ... being in the police force his hours were very erratic, and it was difficult for us because he used to sort of sometimes go on nights and come in at four o'clock, two o'clock in the morning, and you know I mean my last was a total surprise to me because I think I conceived him while I was asleep. I don't think I feel like I had anything to do with that at all, and so it was a relief to both of us to feel that you know should accidents happen, I wasn't going to get pregnant ...[54]

A further advantage was the fact that the oral contraceptive could be swallowed. This was particularly appealing for women who disliked touching their vagina, which other forms of female contraception required. Such inhibitions were not uncommon, particularly among British working-class women. As the British family planning doctor Denise Pullen recalled about women involved in the pill trials of the early 1960s, they 'were delighted to have a method of contraception which was dissociated from sex. They could pop their pill in their mouth, and forget they had anything below their waist.' Many of these women had previously been reluctant to visit the family planning clinic precisely because they did not want to have their 'private parts' touched even by their doctors.[55]

The pill was also unique, and significant, in that unlike any other form of contraception women could use it without the knowledge of their partners. Women no longer had to depend on the cooperation of men in order to control their fertility. This had particular advantages for women whose husbands refused to have anything to do with family planning. The psychological relief that the pill provided is shown by the case of Mrs M.D., whose husband, even after three children, 'absolutely refused to have anything to do with planning a family at all'. She considered the pill 'marvellous' because it allowed her total control over her fertility without having to negotiate with her husband, which had previously proved fruitless. Indeed, she started taking the pill after performing an illegal abortion on herself, which had resulted in her being rushed to hospital for a 'massive transfusion of blood'.[56]

Such an experience was far from unique and highlights the attraction of the pill at a time when abortions were often difficult to procure and dangerous to women's health.[57] Similarly, the reaction of Mrs M.D.'s husband was not unusual. Many women recalled the difficulty of getting their husbands to take contraception seriously. The comments of one American woman, married to a lawyer, reveals the difficulty some women experienced with their husbands:

I certainly can't count on Evan to use precautions. I can't even count on him to give me enough time to use a diaphragm. The IUD? Well, I don't know whether they have proven them reliable enough yet. Besides, Evan is just the type who might pull it out for a joke. Some men do that you know. As a voluntary social worker, I've seen it.[58]

The suffering women experienced on account of the lack of cooperation of their husbands is summed up by the case of Mrs C.H., a British woman, who took the pill in the 1960s. Years later, she remembered:

I tried to make him use condoms as we call them now, and he would sometimes and not others which was totally unsatisfactory, and I felt as if he'd only got to sort of look at me and I'd become pregnant. Of course I got caught and soon after I had my daughter I became pregnant again, so I just didn't want the hass[le] – I mean ... it was a worry, it was a nightmare really ... waiting every month to make sure you came on, I mean now, it seems such a long time ago, but even now I can conjure up how I felt.[59]

She was so enthusiastic about the pill that she endured the difficulty of travelling with two small toddlers all the way to Birmingham, a long and difficult journey from where she lived at the time, in order to obtain it as a volunteer in a clinical trial. In later years she continued to travel to Birmingham to get the contraceptive when her doctor refused to prescribe it for her on account of his concerns about thrombosis and other side-effects.[60]

The control that the oral contraceptive offered over fertility provided many women with a new sense of independence in other parts of their lives. Mrs M.D., for example, stressed that the freedom the pill gave her to control her fertility freed her psychologically from being so reliant on her husband. This gave her a new sense of autonomy in all aspects of her life. She saw the pill as 'an opening up, a beautiful breath of fresh air that fell into your life or swept through it'.[61] Similarly Mrs C.H. felt that the pill not only helped the sexual side of her relationship with her husband, making her a lot less tense, it also enabled her to return to work and to become financially independent. Her conclusion about the pill was that it had definitely 'liberated' her. The confidence it had given her had stemmed from the release she felt from the constant anxiety of becoming pregnant.[62] Such feelings were not uncommon. Mrs R.T., for instance, commented that before taking the pill all she could 'see in the future was one baby after another'. This had been particularly troubling to her given that her previous three births had been difficult and she was tormented by the financial restraints already imposed by her existing children.[63]

While many women welcomed the new freedoms, this was not always the case with men. In some instances men felt that the pill undermined their responsibility for contraception and challenged their masculine identity, particularly as the initiators of sexual activity. One of their deepest anxieties was that the pill would allow women to be unfaithful more easily. Such fears were not new and had been evident in response to earlier female contraceptives. Denise Pullen, for instance, recalled sailors taking their wives' diaphragms to sea or deliberately puncturing them, in order to keep their wives on 'the straight and narrow'. Such behaviour survived the pill. As Pullen recollected, it was not uncommon in the early 1960s for men to flush their wives' oral contraceptives down the toilet. The difference between the pill and other female contraceptives, however, was that it could be more easily reissued. It took only a matter of seconds to prescribe an oral contraceptive again; the replacement of a cap would have involved not only a physical examination, but a number of follow-up visits to ensure it was the right fit and being inserted properly. It was also easier for women to hide the pill than other contraceptives, since it was dissociated from intercourse.[64]

The hidden nature of the oral contraceptive also gave women a greater ability to control when and with whom they had sex. As Pullen points out, because men were unable to check whether or not a woman had taken a pill, they were more reliant on the cooperation of women in pursuing sex without the risk of pregnancy.[65] Yet, for the women taking the pill, the freedom it gave them over the control of fertility could be double-edged. By diminishing the risk of pregnancy, the oral contraceptive undermined the powerful psychological weapon women had previously possessed to deny sexual intercourse. After all, men could now argue that as there was no risk in having intercourse why should they not do so. Within this context the pill changed expectations about sexual behaviour. Now sexual intercourse was much higher on the agenda for some couples than other forms of sexual activity, such as heavy petting, which had been one way of avoiding pregnancy. This is particularly ironic given that the pill was the first contraceptive deployed at a time separate from intercourse. For some women the enhanced status of sexual intercourse may have increased their sexual pleasure, but this was not necessarily the case.

Nonetheless, the fact that the contraceptive enabled women to have a greater ability to accept or deny sexual relations challenged the traditional passive role assumed of women within the sexual relationship.[66] At the same time, it allowed women greater control over fertility than ever before. Some men disliked the pill precisely because it allowed women to control their fertility without any discussion. For example, a woman could now trick a man into making her pregnant by pretending to be on the pill. One man interviewed in the 1960s confirmed he preferred male methods precisely because 'then I would know exactly what was happening'. This was clearly important because, as he said, his wife could unilaterally decide to have another child merely by stopping the pill without informing him.[67]

The arrival of the pill also transformed perceptions about who should take responsibility for contraception. Interestingly, some men who initially objected to women taking the pill were quick to change their minds once they realized it released them from the responsibility for contraception and the ease it gave them during the sexual act. To some extent it could be argued that the growing use of the pill led to complacency among men that contraception should be the responsibility of women.[68] This attitude is summed up by the comments of a young American man in the late 1960s, who stated: 'Once a guy has had a taste of sex on the pill, he just won't settle for anything else.'[69]

Many women increasingly assumed responsibility for contraception. A study conducted in 1965 in England and Wales of 6,300 married women indicated that an increasing proportion was taking the lead in contraception. This was particularly noticeable among the younger women and those married after 1964.[70] By the early 1970s, however, with the growing publicity about the contraceptive's side-effects, many women were increasingly unhappy about the responsibility the pill placed on them. They began to question the fact that they should be the ones to take responsibility for contraception when the sexual act itself was of obvious benefit not just to themselves but also to men. Moreover, some began to feel that this responsibility had enabled men to become more detached and non-committed in a vital part of the sexual relationship. In this context some women began to feel not so much that they had control over their own bodies, but rather that they were being used. This is summed up by the experience of one California woman who, in the mid-1970s, fell pregnant when she deliberately decided against using any precautions because of the alienation she had felt when using the pill. As she admitted, when she had used the pill she felt it had allowed her boyfriend to have sexual intercourse without any explicit thought of her welfare. This had left her with the sense that it had been 'a one-way street for his benefit' and not for her. Where women did fall pregnant, they were also often left with the feeling that they were socially to blame.[71]

The changing user of the pill

Just as there were shifts in attitudes relating to the purpose of contraception and where the responsibility for it should rest, so too were there changes in the types of women who took the pill. Originally aimed at older women with children, the oral contraceptive was rapidly to become the contraceptive of choice among young women with no children. Indeed, one of the features of the pill was the youthfulness of its early takers. As one American study pointed out, the popularity of the pill among younger women partly reflected the fact that young people were more attracted to innovation than their elders, who often kept to familiar methods with which they were already satisfied.[72] In 1965, two-fifths of American women under the age of 30 were using the pill, yet only one-tenth of those aged over 40 had ever used it. Similarly 'among couples where the wife was under 25 and had used some method of contraception, almost half were on the Pill'. The same study declared that couples seemed to have adopted the pill 'as a way of life'.[73] Figures from Britain showed a similar preference for the pill among younger married women. Many of these women had in fact known no other form of contraception.[74]

What is interesting about the pill is the fact that it seemed to coincide with a more general rise in the use of contraception among the younger generation. In 1955, for instance, only 68 per cent of American women aged 18–24 used contraception; by 1965 the proportion had risen to 84 per cent. It is difficult to assess the influence of the pill on the greater adoption of contraception among the young. Nonetheless, it is clear that most of the younger women who were using contraception in the 1960s were opting for the pill as their method of first choice.[75]

Age was not the only determinant of who was likely to take the pill. Education was also vital. In 1965 better educated American women were more likely to take the pill than those less educated, perhaps reflecting the fact that the more educated people were, the more likely they were to hear of new ideas and to adopt them. Early enthusiasm for the pill was also related to where a woman was living and her ethnicity. Interestingly, in the United States, the earliest adopters of the oral contraceptive were based in the west. Part of this may have reflected a less traditional and more open Californian lifestyle. The early popularity of the pill in the west contrasted with its reception among blacks in the southern United States, a substantial proportion of whom (14 per cent) had not even heard of the pill by 1965. African-American women, regardless of their educational background, adopted the pill less readily than white women.[76] In later years, however, this pattern was to change. One survey in the 1970s indicated that the number of African-American wives between the ages of 15 and 29 using the pill increased substantially between 1965 and 1973, jumping from 31 to 65 per cent. The increase was in part attributable to the growth of subsidized family planning programmes which made access to the pill easier.[77]

Educational and social background also played a part in who took the pill in Britain. University-educated women, for example, were much more likely to be aware of the pill and to use it in the mid-1960s than those with an unskilled background. Similarly those living in more middle-class and urban areas tended to have a greater knowledge of and access to the pill.[78] From the early 1970s, however, the socioeconomic profile of British women taking the pill changed dramatically. A number of studies carried out between 1967 and 1985 showed that by the latter date the greatest proportion of women taking the pill tended to come from lower down the socioeconomic scale. This shift in the profile of the British pill-taker occurred most conspicuously between 1967–8 and 1973, the years when the cardiovascular problems associated with the pill were making most public impact. It would therefore appear that the more educated and skilled women were faster to react to these anxieties. Thus, while women in the higher socioeconomic and educated category had adopted the pill earlier, they were also the least likely to use it once health hazards were announced. By contrast the less educated and least skilled were slower to be prescribed the pill and also slower to react to new information on its side-effects. Similar patterns were observed in Finland. In Britain the decline in usage by women from higher socioeconomic groups in later years might also have reflected the fact that they tended to be demographically older than those from lower classes. One survey carried out in 1975 indicated that women over the age of 30 accounted for at least 30 per cent of women from the two higher social groups and only 16 per cent of those from the three lower social groups. This was particularly important given that the thrombotic hazards were more commonly associated with women over the age of 35.[79]

One of the marked features of the earliest users of the pill in both Britain and the United States was that they were married. In part this reflected the social expectations surrounding sex and marriage. At the time of the pill's introduction, premarital sex was widely frowned on. Reflecting this attitude, clinical trials of the pill in Britain, for instance, specified that it should only be given to married women with at least one living child.[80] One reason for insisting that the women should already have had children was the need to ensure that those who took it had proven fertility. This was important not only for verifying the drug's efficacy, but also because of the fear that it could cause long-term infertility.[81]

Proof of marriage continued to be important when the oral contraceptive was publicly introduced in both Britain and the United States.[82] All patients who were seen at a British family planning clinic in the early 1960s were questioned about their marital status before they were given the pill.[83] Husbands were also expected to sign a consent form when a woman took the contraceptive on a trial basis. This was stipulated so as to ensure that the decision was a dual one and that husbands had understood the potential side-effects. Women were denied the drug where husbands had not given their consent or where they could not prove marriage.[84]

Nonetheless, attitudes were changing. As early as 1963 a number of American birth control clinics were giving the pill to unmarried mothers receiving welfare relief because of its potential to reduce public expenditure on social welfare.[85] Unwed mothers with children, however, were not the only ones obtaining the pill in these years. By the mid-1960s increasing numbers of single women, without children, in both the United States and Britain were finding ways to get hold of the pill. An intrepid single woman, for instance, could obtain the drug from a family planning clinic by pre-tending to be married. One British doctor remembered seeing the same cheap wedding ring being produced by a number of women, it having passed it around the waiting room of the family planning clinic.[86] After 1964, however, single British women began to have access to family planning services through the establishment of special clinics serving their needs.[87]

A large proportion of educated single women also came into contact with the pill for the first time through college and university health centres. The importance of the university for the provision of the pill should not be underestimated, as the 1960s was a period when an unprecedented number of women were admitted to university in Britain, the United States and elsewhere. In university life the pill was often part of a wider flouting of traditional conventions. Magazines and books captured the prevalent mood, with frequent articles about the new modern single woman who, unlike her predecessors, was free to experiment sexually without condemnation or the fear of pregnancy. Now single women could play the field just as freely as single men. The pill was to play a major part in shaping this new image of the single woman.[88]

Yet it would be a mistake to associate the oral contraceptive with a revolution in sexual behaviour among single women. Indeed there is plenty of evidence to suggest that single women were engaging in premarital sex well before the introduction of the pill. This can be seen, for instance, in the rise in extramarital births before the 1960s. In Britain the extramarital birth-rate had risen dramatically during the Second World War and continued to do so throughout the 1950s and into the 1960s. Many of these births were occurring among increasingly younger women, reflecting the fact that more women were engaging in sex earlier.[89] Evidence from one British national survey indicates that about 46 per cent of women who were born in the early 1930s and who married in the 1950s were single when they first experienced sexual intercourse.[90] Similar patterns were observed in the United States. Approximately 36 per cent of American women who became sexually mature during the years 1920 to 1950 had sexual intercourse before marriage.[91] The increase in sex outside marriage after the Second World War was not unique to either Britain or the United States, but could be observed in many other countries.[92]

While the pill may not necessarily have triggered more sexual activity among the unmarried, it is important not to under-rate the psychological impact it had on single women. Just as with her married sister, the oral contraceptive provided a vital release from the age-old torment of possible pregnancy. Given the social and financial difficulties many single women experienced on having a baby, the possibility of pregnancy provoked substantial fear. Money worries and the question of reputation were not the only considerations. Well into the 1950s it was not unusual for a British unwed mother to be regarded as sexually deviant and to be sent to a psychiatric institution.[93] Helen Gurley Brown, an American journalist who wrote *Sex and the Single Girl*, a book that caused a sensation in 1962 for its promotion of sex among single women, and who became editor of the British edition of *Cosmopolitan* magazine in 1965, highlighted the fact that prior to the pill single motherhood was not even an option for most women because of what it could do to their standing in the community. According to her, the revolution the pill brought was not so much about allowing single women to have sex for the first time, as enabling them to *enjoy* sex for the first time.[94]

With the introduction of the pill women could now indulge in sex not only without the anxiety of pregnancy, but without the prospect of what conventionally came with it, such as marriage and the loss of a career. One single British woman, who started taking the pill when she went to university in 1969, recalled that the pill 'freed sex from being a commitment to settling down and having babies', which she had never wanted to do. From her perspective the pill enabled her 'to be outrageous and to be accepted as a person' in her 'own right'. Indeed, she argued, the contraceptive gave her the freedom 'to behave just like men'. As she saw it, 'men could have sex without worrying about the consequences and I didn't see why I should not be the same'.[95] This was a freedom she felt men had always taken for granted. As she put it, 'Men do what they want, they are not always counting the price and computing what they would have to cope with, with children.'[96] Summing up what the pill had done for her and other single women, she commented, 'It made us more equal. We were able to choose what we did or did not do with our own bodies. It was no longer the case that we were forced automatically into marriage and childbearing. It became a fairly respectable thing to be a single woman and to have your own life. ... You were not a man's appendage.'[97]

Such attitudes were becoming increasingly common among the younger generation. G. M. Carstairs, a professor of psychological medicine, summed up the view of many when he spoke in his Reith Lectures in 1962, broadcast on the radio, of the rise of a new concept of sexual relations. According to him sexual relations had now become not only 'a source of pleasure but also a mutual encountering of personalities in which each explores the other and at the same time discovers new depths in himself or herself'. In his view premarital sex and the use of contraception was a judicious way for couples to discover if they were suitable for marriage without the burden of a potential unwanted pregnancy.[98] His views were not isolated. Many psychologists and social reformers in the United States were also promoting sexual relations as a means of self-growth and exploration.[99] Such ideas were not new to the 1960s, but access to reliable contraception gave single people greater freedom to have such sexual relations.

One of the interesting aspects of the single pill-taker was that she was becoming increasingly younger by the decade. By the mid-1970s the young teenage girl had joined her older sisters in taking the pill on a regular basis.

In part this reflected changes in the age at which women were first having sex, which had been decreasing steadily since the Second World War.[100] By 1962 more than 1,000 girls under 16 were giving birth to illegitimate children each year in Britain. Indeed, the illegitimacy rate among girls under 16 had risen rapidly since 1954.[101] Such figures fuelled a moral panic in the early 1960s about a rise in teenage sex.[102]

What was novel about the new young woman was that she could now discuss sex more frankly and had a greater awareness of contraception. Part of this was related to the more open public discussion of sex and contraception that had accompanied the introduction of the pill. Indeed it was difficult for schoolchildren to avoid media debates about the pill. One British family planning expert, Dr Aviva Wiseman, was surprised to find herself, in 1966, being questioned by pupils at a high school in North London about the validity of the oral contraceptive only being given to married women. Many of these girls linked the use of the pill to the planning of families and their ability to have careers.[103] Such awareness was not unique to Britain. One American family planning doctor, Dr Mary Calderone, remembered being astonished in 1966 to see a packet of birth control pills fall from the handbag of a schoolgirl in a crowded corridor of a New York City junior high school. The girl had managed to obtain the pills from her married sister.[104]

Younger women were not only gaining a greater awareness of the pill, they were also gaining more access to it. By the mid-1960s, for instance, some American birth control clinics were issuing contraceptive pills to young girls who were thought to be in trouble and whose sexual impulses were thought to be uncontrollable. By 1966 Dr Edward Tyler, who ran some of the earliest clinical trials of the pill in Los Angeles, was providing the contraceptive to girls who had either had a baby or to those whose mothers feared they would soon become pregnant. Planned Parenthood clinics in New York followed a similar rule. Girls given the pill either had to be accompanied by a parent or guardian or be referred to the clinic by a social worker, a health agency, a clergyman or a physician. Some young women were also able to gain oral contraceptives through their family doctors at home, or through a prescription for their married sisters or friends. Others would wear an engagement ring in order to persuade doctors to give them the drug in preparation for marriage.[105]

Yet, while some were able to get hold of the pill, the vast majority found it difficult. It required a great deal of nerve on the part of a teenage girl to come forward to get the contraceptive from a family planning clinic catering primarily for married women. Reflecting this difficulty, many teenage girls in the United States continued to rely on their male partner to take responsibility for contraception.[106] This was to change dramatically as a result of the increasing public provision of the pill from the late 1960s to the mid-1970s. Between 1971 and 1976 the proportion of unmarried American women aged between 15 and 19 years taking the oral contraceptive increased from 15 to 31 per cent. Part of this growth in pill use stemmed from the greater utilization of family planning clinics by teenagers. The number of adolescents using such clinics rose from 453,000 in 1971 to 1.1 million in 1975. The importance of these clinics in determining the use of the pill among young women can be seen from the fact that only 32 per cent of the women coming to them for the first time were taking the drug, but 80 per cent started taking it once counselled at the clinic.[107] Oral contraceptives were also on the rise among young women in Britain. Between 1970 and 1975 the number of sexually active female British teenagers (under the age of 20) taking the pill rose from 15 to 50 per cent. By 1980 the percentage had risen even further to 80 per cent.[108]

Within 15 years of the pill's appearance, the profile of its average user had changed dramatically. A British survey of 7,792 women in 1976 indicated that the overwhelming majority of married women taking the pill were under the age of 30. Indeed the proportion of women taking the pill increased the younger they were. At least 61 per cent of women between the ages of 16 and 19 were choosing the pill over other forms of contraception. This compared with 66 per cent for the age group 20 to 24, 46 per cent for those aged 25 to 29 and 30 per cent for those aged 30 to 34. The youthfulness of the pill taker was not confined to married women. The same survey showed single women to have a greater preference for the pill over other forms of contraception. Indeed, the pill had become the contraceptive of choice for single young women.[109] This was not a phenomenon confined to Britain but could be found in many other developed countries across the world.[110]

The user of the oral contraceptive in the late 1970s was therefore very different from those of the very early 1960s, when a married woman with at least one child was the targeted recipient. By the 1980s, for instance, the predominant consumers of the pill in the United States were unmarried women. A survey conducted in 1987, for instance, indicated that 48 per cent of unmarried sexually active American women aged 18–44 used oral contraceptives. This was much higher than the national average for all women of this age, which was 24 per cent.[111] Such a shift towards the unmarried woman had been accompanied by a change in the use to which the pill was being put. By the 1980s oral contraceptives were being used primarily to avoid premarital pregnancies or to delay first pregnancies in marriage rather than as a means of timing subsequent births and ending childbearing.[112]

Attitudes about the side-effects and safety of the pill

One of the reasons for the increasing youthfulness of the pill-taker was the growing concern from the late 1960s over the higher risk of cardiovascular complications resulting from oral contraception for those over the age of 35.[113] The fear of health hazards, however, was not confined to those aged over 35, or restricted to concerns about thrombosis. How a woman viewed the safety of the drug was partly dependent on the historical moment at which she was taking the pill and what role it was to play in her sexual life and relationships.

Many of the women who took the drug in its earliest days were very aware of the potential risks they were taking, but thought nothing of it. Some women dismissed such dangers by weighing them against other factors. The reasoning of such women is exemplified by the case of Mrs J.A. who took the pill as part of a British trial in the early 1960s. She dismissed people who saw the pill as something unnatural and dangerous. As she commented:

> perhaps I was naive but I don't think I was, I thought well people – my mother-in-law had eleven pregnancies, and nine children came out of that, and if you were sort of artificially pregnant it's only what you would have been if you hadn't been on the pill, wasn't it? And that's the way I looked at [it and] people said to me, 'it isn't natural', but what is natural? To have a baby every year, isn't [is] it? [114]

Another British woman, Mrs M.F., a midwife and health visitor who took the pill on a trial basis after falling pregnant three times while using a diaphragm, remembered weighing up the risks of the oral contraceptive against the fact that at least 800 Puerto Rican women had taken it before her. This did not necessarily reassure her, because, as she admitted, Puerto Rico was a long way from England, which made her question the validity of the studies for her own safety. Despite these qualms she remembered that she never felt nervous about taking the pill even though she did experience some minor side effects such as spotting. All she remembered was that she did not think about the consequences very much and had only occasional 'vague feelings' of concern. From her perspective she was helped by the fact that there was little literature in the early days that would have prompted fears.[115]

Such reactions were not uncommon. Indeed many women were prepared to put up with very debilitating side-effects because of the benefits that the pill promised. This is captured by the attitude of one British woman, Betty Vincent, who started taking the pill on a trial basis after having conceived four children in quick succession and been forced to abandon nurse training. After the trial she had continued to take one of the earliest and strongest oral contraceptives for 17 years with no ill-effects. From her perspective she would have continued to take the drug whatever the costs to her health. As she put it, 'I wouldn't have cared if I had [had problems]. I would have put up with headaches and things like that because the alternative was to keep getting pregnant every year.'[116] Such a response was not unique. One American woman, when asked by a doctor in the late 1960s to stop using the pill because of the risk of cancer, retorted:

> Look, I don't care if you *promise* me cancer in five years, I'm staying on the pill. At least I'll enjoy five years I have left. For the first time in eighteen years of married life I can put my feet up for an hour and read a magazine. I can watch my favorite TV program without having to catch up on my ironing at the same time. I can usually get a full night's sleep because there is no baby to feed or toddler to take to the toilet. If you refuse to give me the pill, I'll go get it from someone else.[117]

Even where women suffered side-effects they were willing to take the risk of continuing the medication. Some American women interviewed in the late 1960s, for instance, who had experienced side-effects such as bloated breasts, were reluctant to give up the pill because they felt their increased breast size had increased their feminine attractiveness. Others were also keen on the pill because it had improved their complexion. One medical librarian who had tried six different oral contraceptives during a three-year period in the 1960s refused to give up the pill despite suffering constant headaches, nausea and leg cramps that would wake her sometimes five times a night, indicating that she was willing to put up with such effects because, as she put it, 'my complexion had never looked so beautiful. All the little pores disappeared. I hardly needed make-up.'[118]

Mrs R.T., who had previously had three children went on the pill as part of a clinical trial in Birmingham, UK in 1962. She experienced terrible migraines, but bore the pain because she believed that having volunteered to take the pill she should put up with the bad as well as the good. Part of the way she coped with the drawbacks of the pill was by reminding herself that after a month she could swap the one she had for another with potentially fewer side-effects. She also overcame her misgivings because the doctors seemed to brush her symptoms aside. At that time it also seemed to her that the benefits of the pill 'far outweighed the thoughts of any ill-effects, or side-effects, or long-term effects that the pill may well have had'.[119]

Not all women, however, accepted the reactions they experienced on taking the pill. From the beginning of the clinical trials women had been coming off the pill following nausea, weight gain, break-through bleeding and headaches.[120] The discomfort experienced by some women is illustrated by the following experience of a British woman:

> The pill made me extremely lethargic, especially in the evening. Along with the tiredness, there was a bloated sensation, which was very unpleasant, as I felt as though I was bursting out of my clothes. I began to get very severe headaches which interfered with my life. I then moved house, and a different pill was recommended by the new doctor. This one was dreadful. I experienced severe breast tenderness, and recurrent thrush – which was death to my sex life.[121]

One of the side-effects women complained of in the early years of the pill was the loss of their sexual drive. This was a particularly disturbing phenomenon for those who had looked to the drug as a means of enhancing their sex lives. In some cases women on the contraceptive were unable to achieve orgasm. Others merely became bored with sex. As a fashion coordinator for a Los Angeles department store put it in the 1960s, 'It was getting so that I was sure that even an orgy wouldn't turn me on.'[122] Some women by contrast found that the drug made them more desirous of sex. This was not always pleasant as it could leave them with 'a driving hunger that leaves them no peace'.[123] Others found that the pill dried up their natural vaginal secretions and made sex painful.[124]

What is revealing is the way in which some sections of the medical profession tended to dismiss such experiences writing them off as psychosomatic. The distress this caused women should not be underestimated, as can be seen by the following testimony of a single British woman writing about her experiences with the pill during the 1970s and 1980s:

> I hated the pill, I felt nauseous each morning and irritable, dopey, depressed and nagging (quite unusual for me). Remembering my bad experience with the last GP, I went to a different one, a woman. I'd been on the pill for two months, and I was hoping that this GP would agree with me not to wait out the three-month trial period, and to stop taking it immediately, as my symptoms were annoying and persistent. However, she was completely convinced before I opened my mouth that the pill had few, if any, side effects. My complaints were 'psychological' according to her. She then attempted to penetrate to the depths of my psyche to discover the mental problems I was having ... depression.[125]

Yet she had always been happy prior to taking the pill.[126] Such an experience was not that uncommon. Another British woman recalled:

> The pill left me towards the end of each cycle feeling half way through a pregnancy – bloated, heavy, weary, with splitting headaches I never normally suffer. No doctor expressed the faintest interest but murmured something about having to take minor inconveniences in place of a major one – i.e. an actual pregnancy.[127]

Many women found their encounters with the doctor left them dissatisfied and questioning the authority the medical profession as a whole.[128] Such dissatisfaction was not confined to Britain. The American journalist Barbara Seaman, whose book, *The Doctor's Case against the Pill*, inspired public protest about the health hazards of the pill and the Gaylord Nelson hearings in 1970 (which resulted in the inclusion of warnings of the side-effects of the pill on the label) had been galvanized to write her book partly because of the number of letters she had received from women who felt that doctors had ignored their complaints about the oral contraceptive.[129]

In a number of cases women's encounters with the medical profession made them feel guilty about complaining. This is illustrated by the recollections of another British woman:

> The pill gave me feelings of depression. Very slowly, I began to put on weight. I felt like a balloon full of water. I got depressed for no apparent

reason. This was unlike me – I'm a cheerful person. [At the FPA] they had occasionally mentioned that I seemed to have put on weight – but that was my fault for eating too much – I should go on a diet. When they asked me if I had any problems I felt that being depressed and liquid retention would sound stupid and I didn't think they were caused by the pill. I thought it was my fault.[130]

Even where doctors did make an attempt to ask whether women had complaints about the pill, many women refused to talk about them. One British woman, for instance, remembered lying to the doctor about the reactions she experienced on taking the pill. As she said:

At every visit, the doctor asked if I had any problems. I lied. I said no. I hadn't any way of explaining and I wanted to be a sensible woman, not a 'neurotic' who blamed the pill for emotional difficulties. For the next two years I got steadily worse – depressed, irritable, jumpy, subject to violent and unpredictable mood swings, and in the end, thought a lot about suicide, and concluded that I just had a morbid personality. Then I lost my pills, and found myself suddenly cheerful.[131]

For some women these adverse reactions were to have a dramatic effect on the rest of their lives. This was particularly the case for those who suffered cardiovascular complications from taking the high oestrogen pills in the early 1960s. In some cases the pill resulted in death. Others were left maimed and incapacitated, the most unfortunate having to have limbs amputated. In many cases these effects led not only to poor health but social isolation and difficulties with carrying on a normal life. The case of Betty H., an American woman who suffered painful blood clots in both her legs and her left arm after having taken the pill in the early 1960s, illustrates the difficulties. After her initial treatment Betty was to spend the next few years in and out of hospital. Her therapy consisted of anti-coagulants, surgery and a waist-high elastic stocking which not only made her hot and sweaty, but required an hour to put on in the morning and the same amount of time to take off at night. To add to her suffering her partner left her because he could not take the strain of her illness. While Betty was to become resigned to her situation, not everyone was as amenable. Anita, an American woman who had also suffered blood clots after taking the pill in her early twenties, was much more resentful: 'Even when I feel okay, I never know when I'll have a flareup. I have to think about it all the time. I can't sit in one position too long. I can't exercise or risk getting too tired. When the clots are bad, I'm not allowed to drive. Even when they don't bother me, I can't drive for more than an hour.' She concluded, 'I don't think my life has ever really been in danger, but it's been one big mess.'[132]

Such cases not only contrast strikingly with the dry statistics with which the scientists were wrestling in connection with the adverse reactions of the pill, as revealed in previous chapters; they also did little to alleviate the fears of other women. Neither did the increasingly negative publicity emerging about the contraceptive from the late 1960s. Mrs R.T., for instance, who had initially continued to take the pill despite experiencing side-effects such as headaches, eventually gave up the contraceptive because of the growing publicity about adverse reactions to the drug and the fears she began to have about what it could do to her health in the long term.[133] Fears about the dangers of the drug increased over the years as the media increasingly drew attention to the hazards. A survey undertaken in Britain between 1967 and 1970 indicates how married mothers were becoming increasingly aware of the health hazards associated with the contraceptive. This survey is particularly interesting because it was begun at the very moment when the issue of thrombosis was beginning to surface in the media and ended when the British government warned doctors to cease prescribing high oestrogen pills associated with the problem. In 1967, 37 per cent of the women interviewed spontaneously mentioned the possibility that the pill might cause heart disease, thrombosis or even death. By 1970 the proportion had gone up to 58 per cent. Similarly the numbers of mothers who thought there was a definite risk of thrombosis or heart attack also increased from 25 to 58 per cent in these years.[134]

What effect the increasing awareness of the risks of the pill had on women's decision to take it is hard to measure. Much depended on how they were alerted to its risks and how these were balanced against other factors in their lives. Clearly a woman's choice to take the pill was a very individual decision, based on the type of relationship she had, her family circumstances, her medical history and the alternative contraceptives available to her. The society in which she lived was also an important factor. This can be seen, for instance, in the cases of Britain and the United States shown in figure 8.2, which indicates that, from the early 1970s, American women dropped the contraceptive much more rapidly and consistently than in Britain.

While demographic trends might account for this difference, the dramatic fall in the percentages for certain years indicates that this was not the main reason. From figure 8.2 we can see that the percentage of American women taking the pill first dropped in the light of the news about thrombosis and the pill in the late 1960s, and was to decline even more in the light of possible carcinogenic effects. A survey conducted in the United States in 1985 indicated that at least 76 per cent of American women believed there were substantial risks associated with the pill.[135] While some British women exhibited similar patterns, the decline was less dramatic, and in fact the percentage taking the pill continued to rise overall despite publicized risks.

What is particularly interesting is how slow British women were to discontinue the contraceptive, given the prominence of British medical scientists in reporting the risks of both thrombosis and cancer. This contrasted with the Netherlands, Australia and the United States, where scientists were slower to connect adverse reactions with the pill. Yet US women tended to be more vocal and protested much more publicly about the side effects of the pill. In the 1970s some led an effective campaign to have such contra-indications marked on pill labels. Their actions may therefore have been instrumental in swaying public opinion. In Britain protests

Figure 8.2 Minimum percentage of women aged 15–44 supplied with oral contraceptives through commercial channels in four countries, 1964–1981

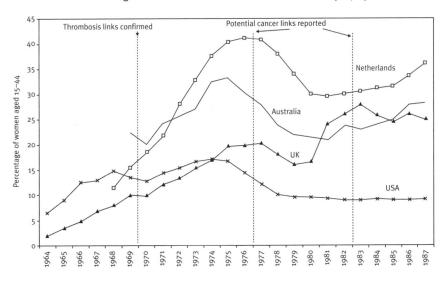

Source: E. Ketting and A. P. Visser, 'Contraception in the Netherlands: low abortion explained', *Patient Education and Counseling*, 23 (1994), 165–6, figs 1 and 2.

by women were virtually non-existent, partly reflecting their deferential attitudes towards the medical profession as a whole, as well as the absence of a strong consumer lobby within the National Health Service.[136] Another explanation for the different response in the United States was that the American public tend to be both faster overall than the British in adopting technological innovation as well as slightly quicker in absorbing scientific information about its risks. This might also have been true for Australia and the Netherlands. Studies in the United States during the 1970s and 1980s indicated that much of the discontinuation of the pill in these years was correlated with the media reports of the drug's adverse effects.[137]

Conclusion

While the pill had clearly fallen from its pedestal by the 1970s, its remarkable feature was its continued widespread diffusion in many parts of the world up to the end of the twentieth century.[138] In the United States, for example, despite the fact that the number of current users had sharply declined by 1982, at least 80 per cent of married women had used the pill at some point in their lives.[139] Elsewhere the exposure to the pill was similar, if not higher, with at least 90% of married women using it at some time.[140]

Even where the pill was taken for only a short time, its widespread use had set a standard by which all other forms of contraception were to be judged. One of the key questions it had raised was the efficacy of contraception in general. Prior to the emergence of the pill many couples as well as family planners and governments had accepted the fact that all contraceptives carried a risk of pregnancy. The introduction of the pill, however, had radically shaken this belief and raised the standard for the acceptability of other contraceptives. Swallowed by mouth and taken at a time other than during intercourse, the pill had also challenged people's acceptance of the need for contraceptives to interfere with sexual intercourse and spontaneity. The hidden nature of the pill also gave women the possibility of maintaining an aura of passivity while protecting themselves from the risk of pregnancy.

Yet the pill had brought about a double-edged liberation. What was seen at first as a miraculous and convenient method of contraception that would bring happiness to women was, by the late 1960s, no longer held in the same esteem. An American woman who gave up the pill in the late 1960s sums up the dilemma women began to face on taking the pill:

We're all doing so many terrible things to our bodies. Up to a point, medicine and science made great advances. But now things are getting all mixed up. What can you do when you're caught up in this swirl of convenience-and-pollution? Air pollution. Water pollution. Body pollution. Additives to foods that may be poisonous. What do you do? Move to Tahiti? Grow your own vegetables in the backyard or on the roof? The pill is part of the whole picture. Once you agree to live in a civilized, 'convenient' life, where do you draw the line?[141]

Such a vision of the pill was a very long way from the ideas put forward by Margaret Sanger in the early twentieth century.

While oral contraceptives had fallen out of favour by the 1970s, they were to have a lasting influence on the kinds of contraceptive choices people were to make in the following years. This can be seen most clearly from the rapid adoption of voluntary sterilization in the wake of the pill's decline. Between 1970 and 1980 there was a fivefold increase in reliance on female sterilization worldwide. In some countries, such as the United States, Canada and New Zealand, sterilization had become the most widespread contraceptive method. One of the factors contributing to this increase was the introduction of a simpler surgical procedure, which reduced not only the cost but also the discomfort of the operation for women. [142]

Worldwide, by the 1980s sterilization had become more common than the pill and the IUD put together. Many scholars attribute this dramatic increase in the use of voluntary sterilization during the last quarter of the twentieth century to the widespread availability and adoption of oral contraceptives in former years. An American woman's comment in the 1960s summarizes an attitude inspired by the pill that was to become dominant for many decades to follow: 'as far as sex goes, well we want to be able to do it in unexpected times and places. That's half the fun. We're finished with that greasy kid stuff forever. If my doctor forced me to give up the pill ... I'd just go ahead and get my tubes tied. Or Jim would have a vasectomy.'[143] In the light of the health scares, people also became increasingly selective about the risks they were willing to accept as well as the side-effects they would be prepared to suffer from a contraceptive.[144] On this basis voluntary sterilization was the most obvious alternative for those who had previously used oral contraceptives, especially for those no longer planning to have children. The pill therefore had a lasting impact on people's contraceptive choices even where it was no longer used.

9
Divisive Device: The Pill and the Catholic Church

In 1968 Pope Paul VI astonished the world when he reaffirmed in his encyclical *Humanae Vitae* (Of Human Life) the old Catholic doctrine that the use of artificial contraception was forbidden. He made it clear that any use of the pill for contraception would be regarded as immoral and against the will of God. As he stated it, 'The moment has not come for man to entrust to his reason and his will, rather than to the biological rhythms of his organism, the task of regulating birth.'[1] The encyclical came after years of earnest debate about marriage and contraception within the Catholic community. It also occurred at a time when the church was beginning to reach out to its lay members and begin a process of reform embodied by the establishment of the Vatican Council (1962–5). Aimed at modernizing the church, the Council changed many of the age-old characteristics and practices that had come to be accepted as the norm within the church. Indeed it changed the very way in which the Catholic church was run, allowing lay people more of a voice alongside bishops and priests. Among the changes the Council had instituted was saying mass in the vernacular as opposed to Latin, and removing the obligation to abstain from meat on Fridays. In taking such steps the church showed not only that it was willing to listen to its lay members, but that it wanted to engage with the wider world.[2]

Within this context, the pill exemplified the path towards modernization. While, however, many welcomed the pill as the symbol of change, others saw it as a threat to the status quo. Any debate about the pill could not escape the wider tensions then occurring within the church leadership between the more orthodox members who sought a continuation of tradition and the liberals who were eager to embrace a policy of reform. What was at stake was not only an acceptance of the contraceptive pill, but the basis on which the church should maintain its authority in the world. For many Catholics the pill proved one of the most divisive issues the church had had to confront since Galileo was tried for heresy in 1633 for publishing a book which argued that the earth revolved round the sun. Just as Galileo had challenged the foundations of people's ideas about the world, so the pill threatened fundamental ideas about reproduction and its control. As the Chicago-based priest and sociologist Father Andrew Greeley commented, the pill controversy in many ways exceeded that of Galileo: 'The Galileo controversy, as important as it was to intellectuals, had nothing to do with what goes on in the beds of married people two or three nights a week, every week of the year.'3

The pill and the church's stand on contraception

The pill was unlike any other form of artificial contraception that the Catholic church had encountered before. Much of the church's stance on artificial contraception had been established in the first centuries after the death of Jesus in response to the growth of anti-marriage and anti-procreation movements, which had emerged out of a belief that the second coming of Christ was imminent and that the world would soon come to an end. Once people realized that the end of the world was not so near, attitudes began to change. Clement of Alexandria, in the second century, was the first Christian theologian to argue officially that the purpose of marriage was procreation. From his perspective the Christian law was for 'husbands to use their wives moderately and only for the raising up of children'. He went on to state: 'To have coition other than to procreate children is to do injury to nature.'4 This was to be the foundation on which the Catholic church established its policy for contraception. Echoing these beliefs, in 1930 Pope Pius XI in his encyclical *Casti Connubii* made it clear that artificial contraception should be regarded as 'base', 'indecent', a 'sin against nature' and 'intrinsically vicious'.5 In accordance with this, all artificial contraception was believed to be the taking of an intended life. Any use of the diaphragm, douche, spermicidal jelly or condom was seen as tantamount to frustrating God's will and ultimately to murder. The church, however, always made a distinction between contraception and abortion. The only method couples could use if there was a serious problem was periodic abstinence.[6]

Remaining strong within the church establishment up to the 1950s, such beliefs were to meet an unprecedented challenge with the development of the pill. First, unlike earlier forms of contraception the church had opposed, the oral contraceptive was not mechanical, neither did it kill or hinder the passage of sperm. Secondly, it seemed to mimic the natural functions of the female human body. Indeed, the pill appeared to accord with the Catholic faith's approval of 'natural' contraceptive techniques such as the rhythm method, authorized by Pope Pius XII in 1951.[7] Moreover, when approving this method, the pope had made it clear that the church would welcome any scientific improvement in the technique.[8] This endorsement of the rhythm method resulted in part from new scientific means devised during the 1930s to calculate the incidence and length of a woman's sterile period. For many Catholics the pill represented no more than a further manifestation of such advances in science. From their perspective the use of hormones to control a woman's cycle was no different from the use of mucous tests in determining her sterile period for the rhythm method.[9]

Nonetheless, by contrast with the 20 years of peaceful theological debate that had preceded the acceptance of the rhythm method, the oral contraceptive provoked a much more public response from the church. Indeed the chemical action of the pill meant that it could not be regarded as merely a theological matter. Any debate on the issue within the church could not avoid engaging directly with questions about reproductive biology and endocrinology. In this context contraception could no longer be seen as just an issue of morality.[10] Never before had the elite of the church discussed sex and female physiology in so detailed and frank a manner. This was witnessed not only during the debates within the Vatican Council, but also in the public discussions among lay Catholics and in the burgeoning literature on the issue.[11] Responding to this heated argument, in the early 1960s 182 Catholic scholars from the European and American continents petitioned the Pope and the Vatican Council for a 'far-reaching reappraisal' of the contraception issue.[12]

The issue of the contraceptive pill was not confined merely to questions of science and morality. It had major repercussions for the future membership of the church. As many bishops and priests pointed out, the church was losing many of its married worshippers over the matter. Forced to choose between obeying the commands of the church and satisfying the needs of conjugal and parental love, many people were choosing the pill over the church. The question at the heart of the debate was whether Catholics could continue to attend communion if they used a contraceptive technique other than the rhythm method.[13]

The very fact that the pill needed to be taken every day and worked in the body physiologically made it a particularly fraught issue for some observant Catholic women. As Dr Anne Biezanek, an English Catholic convert with seven children, pointed out, 'If you're using a condom or something like that, you hold your breath, dash off to church, confess, and get communion, and then sigh and fall back again into your sinful way of living.' This was the way she felt most Catholics had managed with the church's teaching on contraception up to the 1950s.[14] However, the fact that the pill had to be taken on a regular basis meant that women were being reminded that they were continuously preventing pregnancy and therefore, in the church's eyes, living in a 'chronic state of sinfulness'.[15]

In March 1963 Willem Bekkers, Bishop of S-Hertogen-Bosch, publicly aired his misgivings about the choice people were being forced to make. Moreover, in his broadcast on a Catholic station in the Netherlands, he pointed out that while the church's teaching might be set, 'the context of a dogma' could 'change'. As he explained, 'The people have troubles. They are inquiring. And so I argue this way. If I see people in the church not going to communion because they feel guilty in violating the ban on contraception, and I know they are the kind of people who would otherwise go to communion, then I say this is a reason for reconsidering the entire question.' His broadcast brought the matter of the pill and what it was doing to people's consciences to the forefront of the Vatican Council.[16]

An article in *Newsweek* captured the mood of the time: 'Not since the Copernicans suggested in the sixteenth century that the sun was the center of the planetary system has the Roman Catholic Church found itself on such a perilous collision course with a new body of knowledge while all about swirl dangerous currents.'[17] Similar remarks were made by the primate of Belgium, Cardinal Leo Josephs Suenens, a liberal Catholic, when he entreated the Vatican Council not to be afraid of re-examining the traditional position on contraception when considering the issue of marriage. He concluded that they did not 'want another Galileo case' on their hands. As he exclaimed, one was certainly enough in the history of the church.[18] Suenens was backed in his plea by the 87-year old Greek patriarch Maximos, who stressed birth control to be 'an urgent problem because it lies at the root of a great crisis in Catholic conscience'. He went on to argue: 'There is a question here of a break between the official doctrine of the Church and the contrary practices of the immense majority of Christian couples. Are we not entitled to ask if certain positions [of the church] are not the outcome of outmoded ideas, and, perhaps, a bachelor psychosis on the part of those unacquainted with this sector of life!'[19]

The church had already proved it was not totally resistant to change on contraception. As early as 1958, two years prior to the official marketing of the pill as a contraceptive, Pope Pius XII, addressing the Seventh International Congress of Hematology, formally recognized the pill's use for therapeutic purposes.[20] By agreeing to its use for the treatment of conditions such as endometriosis and excessive and painful menstrual bleeding, Pius XII, while not agreeing to its utilization as a contraceptive, had effectively implied that it could be used to regulate irregular menstrual cycles. Many within the church took this as a sign that it could be taken to strengthen the reliability of the rhythm method.[21] Reflecting this sentiment, a Catholic priest in the Chancery office of New York Archdiocese indicated that the 'church would not consider it a sin if a Catholic woman regulated her menstrual period with such pills and thereby increased the rhythm method's effectiveness'.[22] Nonetheless, it was clear that the pill was considered immoral if used openly for fertility control. One of the reasons the Pope had condemned its use for this purpose was that the effects of the contraceptive were regarded as tantamount to sterilization, a practice strictly forbidden by the church.[23]

Debating the merits of the pill

Pius XII died barely a month after making his 1958 statement on the pill, and left behind him a debate that was to continue with ever increasing intensity. The issue at the heart of the discussion was whether the pill could indeed cause permanent sterility. One of the most prominent individuals to challenge this idea was Dr John Rock, the obstetrician who had played a key role in the first clinical trials of the pill. Rock was a devout Catholic who not only had a crucifix hanging above his desk but also attended Mass every day. His interest in the pill was more than merely medical. Wrestling for years about how to preserve the strength and stability of the family, Rock had initially been conservative about birth control, seeing it as something only to be prescribed where a woman's health was at stake. Co-authoring a handbook in the 1930s entitled *Voluntary Parenthood*, Rock cautioned against postponing pregnancy in early marriage because of the possibilities of infertility in later life. During these years he was a firm supporter of the Catholic teaching that the purpose of sex was procreation. Moreover, as he argued to the Committee on Maternal Health, 'Nature intended motherhood to be woman's career, and her proper career, she should start right away ... Anything which diverts her from her prime purpose is socially wrong.' He ended his speech by declaring that sex could not 'be made an end in itself without dire consequences'.[24] Similarly in 1943 he had challenged the idea that legal restrictions on medically prescribed contraception should be lifted, noting:

> I hold no brief for those young or even older husbands and wives who for no good reason refuse to bear as many children as they can properly rear and as society can properly engross. Ignorant of the fact that sustained happiness comes only from dutiful sacrifice, such deluded mates are perhaps doing society a backhanded favor. Whatever genetic trait may contribute to the intellectual deficiency which permits them selfishly to seek more immediate comfort, is at least kept from the inheritable common pool, and in time their kind is thus bred out.[25]

In 1954 when Margaret Sanger, a lapsed Catholic herself, first heard Rock was to be involved with the development of the pill she not surprisingly opposed his involvement on the grounds that 'he would not dare advance the cause of contraceptive research and remain a Catholic'.[26] Rock, however, had changed his views towards contraception by the early 1950s as a result of growing anxieties about overpopulation and its potential for economic and social upheaval.[27] Moreover, Rock had admitted to McCormick that he 'was a "reformed Catholic" whose position is that religion has nothing to do with medicine or the practice of it and that if the Church does not interfere with him he will not interfere with it – whatever that might mean'.[28] Sanger herself soon realized that, as a Catholic, Rock would be a useful ally in gaining acceptance for the pill. As she later remarked in 1960, 'Being a good R.C. and as handsome as a god, he can just get away with anything.'[29]

Despite his original declaration to McCormick, Rock soon changed his position towards the church. As he later confided to a supporter, he was convinced that the official church attitude towards contraception was 'bunk'.[30] An expert on the oral contraceptive as well as on infertility, Rock was in a strong position to dispute the church's belief that the pill caused sterility. He countered this idea by pointing out that the drug merely mimicked a woman's own physiology, imitating her natural endocrine chemistry to prevent her egg from maturing. Moreover, he stressed that the oral contraceptive had a rebound effect and that, by giving the ovary a temporary rest, it could actually enhance a woman's fertility. Rock also highlighted the fact that because the pill was taken at a time divorced from intercourse, it actually preserved the integrity of the sexual act, criteria established by the church for the acceptance of contraception.[31]

Measured by these various yardsticks, Rock felt that the church should not equate the pill with earlier contraceptive methods that it had condemned, such as the condom and diaphragm.[32] The following sums up his position:

It is my confident hope that the medication will prove acceptable to my church, since it merely gives to the human intellect the means to suppress ovulation; these means have heretofore come only from the ovary and, during pregnancy, from the placenta. These unthinking organs supply their hormone, progesterone, at those times when nature seeks to protect a fertilized ovum or growing foetus from competition for the woman's resources. The oral contraceptive simply duplicates the action of this natural hormone, when the woman herself feels the necessity for protection of her young – present or prospective.[33]

From Rock's perspective the pill was merely putting the rhythm method on to the scientific basis endorsed by Pope Pius XII in 1951.[34] As he later reiterated,

The rhythm method, which is sanctioned by the Church, depends precisely on the secretion of progesterones from the ovaries, which action these compounds merely duplicate. It is progesterone, in the healthy woman, that prevents ovulation and establishes the pre- and post-menstrual 'safe period'. The physiology underlying the spontaneous 'safe period' is identical to that initiated by the steroid compounds and is equally harmless to the individual. Indeed, the use of the compounds for fertility control may be characterized as a 'pill-established safe period' and would seem to carry the same implications.[35]

Rock first openly articulated his beliefs at a meeting of the American Society for the Study of Sterility in April 1960, a month before the Food

and Drug Administration officially approved Enovid as the first oral contraceptive. During this meeting he made it clear that he viewed the pill as a
'morally permissible variant of the rhythm method'.[36] This marked the
beginning of a long campaign. Aged 70, and in good health, Rock was
particularly well suited for his battle against the church. Not only had he
helped to develop the first pill, but he was also confident and candid about
speaking his mind. Appearing several times on television and writing
countless articles for leading journals and newspapers, Rock soon attracted
widespread attention.[37] As he wrote to Katherine McCormick in 1961, 'I
find myself more than ever in the forefront of the gradually increasing
efforts of many to weaken the traditional opposition of my Church's
officials to rational methods of birth control.' Such a position was, he
admitted, 'bound to advance' him 'to the firing line, if not to the wall'.[38] In
the spring of 1963, after having nursed his wife who was dying of cancer,
Rock became even more prominent with the publication of his book, *The
Time Has Come: A Catholic Doctor's Proposals to End the Battle over Birth
Control*. Swiftly translated into French, German and Dutch, the book sold
widely around the world and was taken as a straightforward challenge to
the Catholic church.[39] In fact the precise wording and arguments made in
the *Humanae Vitae* encyclical of 1968 can be read as a direct answer to
many of the issues raised by Rock in his book.

Rock's book was greeted with immediate hostility by Catholics in the
United States. One such was the Reverend Monsignor Francis W. Carney,
director of the Family Life Bureau of Cleveland Catholic diocese, who went
so far as to refer to Rock as a 'moral rapist, using his strength as a man of
science to assault the faith of his fellow Catholics'.[40] In Europe Rock
encountered more sympathy. In August 1963, five months after the publication of his book, seven Dutch bishops issued an official statement calling
on the Vatican to reconsider its stand on contraception, given the advent of
the pill and new views on marriage and sexual matters. Indeed they felt that
the pill should be approved for use in special circumstances, such as to
provide protection to those who were in danger of rape. Many theologians
around Europe supported these sentiments.[41]

Among those who backed John Rock was Pope Paul VI's own private
theologian, Father Benard Häring. As Häring put it in 1964, the pill 'unlike
[other] contraceptives, does not interfere with the act of conjugal intercourse. They affect the functions of nature, an altogether different thing.'
He went on to comment, 'We have a right to help nature.' On this basis,
therefore, he saw no reason for women not to take the pill to 'obtain a

normal cycle'. While there was still some uncertainty as to whether the current pill would adequately satisfy the church's requirements, he and many others were sure that science would soon perfect a 'Catholic pill'. For these reasons he was sure that the church should treat the pill differently from other contraceptives.[42]

The Vatican examines the merits of the pill

The Vatican's initial detailed investigation of the pill was confined to a small commission composed of six members, two demographers, two economists and two physicians. One of the physicians was the British doctor John Marshall who had pioneered the rhythm method using body temperatures.[43] Meeting secretly in 1963 the members of this commission were handicapped by their inadequate scientific expertise. This made it difficult for them to assess not only how the pill worked and whether it could be considered as natural as the rhythm method, but also whether it caused sterility. In the wake of the thalidomide disaster, members of the commission were also concerned about approving a method of contraception that might prove to be yet another medical catastrophe. Their anxieties had some foundation, given that this was the time when the pill was beginning to be suspected of causing thrombotic reactions, and its long-term consequences were still far from certain. In addition to these problems, the scientists on the commission quickly recognized that there was another dimension to the issue. As John Marshall remembered, there came a critical moment when 'those of us who were scientists approaching it from a scientific point of view ... realized that the man and woman in the street – or the man and woman in bed – ought also to have a say in the matter. It wasn't just high theology or science, it was human involvement and feelings and experience as well.'[44] On this basis the small commission was cautious in its final recommendation to the Pope, indicating that he should not make any definitive statement about the pill at that particular time.[45]

In 1965 Pope Paul VI extended the small commission in an attempt to gain greater clarity. Known as the Pontifical Commission on Population, Family and Birth, it was highly unusual in the history of the church in that it included lay men and women. Never before in the history of the Catholic church had the laity been given such a prominent role in advising on Catholic doctrine.[46] Among the lay advisers were three married couples. Included in order to represent the views of those with personal experience of the church's teachings on marriage and contraception, these couples were probably picked because they were considered to be safe by the establishment.[47] However, they were to prove vital in providing the celibate clerics on the commission with an understanding of the very personal and real dilemmas ordinary Catholics faced as a result of the church's rulings.

Two people who had a leading influence on the commission were Pat and Patty Crowley, a middle-aged, middle-class couple from Chicago. They had played a pioneering role in an international organization called the Christian Family Movement that organized groups to study ways of making the Christian message relevant to modern marriage.[48] Using the network of the Christian Family Movement, the Crowleys were instrumental in setting up a survey for the commission to gather testimonies from couples about the daily experience of the church's teachings on contraception. Most of the couples interviewed had at least six children and some had as many as 13. This was the first time that the church had ever attempted to hear what ordinary Catholics had to say about the rhythm method. Moreover it was the widest investigation ever made of lay Catholic beliefs on such a sensitive matter.[49] Evidence collected for the survey indicated that many couples saw the rhythm method as not only distasteful but also very difficult to practise. They felt that the method often endangered the harmony of married life. Some of the painful problems these couples faced can be gauged from the following excerpts taken from the letters to the Crowleys:

I bend over backwards to avoid raising false hopes on my husband's part. This sounds ridiculous, but I stiffen at a kiss on the cheek, instantly reminded that I must be discreet. I withdraw in other ways too, afraid to be an interesting companion, gay or witty or charming, hesitant about being sympathetic.

The slightest upset, mental or physical, appears to change the cycle and thereby renders this method of family planning useless. ... My husband has a terrible weakness when it comes to self-control in sex and unless his demands are met in every way when he feels this way, he is a very dangerous man to me and my daughters.

We have three sick kids at home, another kicking in my stomach, and a husband full of booze. I have lived on hope, hope in God, hope in taking a long time for the next pregnancy, hope that someone understands my problem.[50]

Summing up the evidence, Patty Crowley stressed that:

> No amount of theory by men will convince women that periodic continence is natural. We have heard some men, both married and celibate, argue that rhythm is a way to develop love. But we have heard few women who agree. Over and over, we hear women say that the physical and psychological implications of rhythm are not adequately understood by the male church. ... The wife who is unsure, who is afraid of another pregnancy, is not a true love-mate and can come to resent her husband, intercourse, in fact, her whole life ... Couples want children and will have them generously and love them. They do not need the impetus of legislation to procreate. It is the very instinct of life, love and sexuality.[51]

The experiences highlighted by the survey, and by the couples who sat on the commission, not only emphasized the pain and sacrifice many were being forced to suffer in order to obey their church's teaching, but made it clear to the majority of the members of the commission that a new approach on marriage and contraception was needed.[52] For many of the celibate academics sitting on the commission the survey came as a revelation of the distress experienced by ordinary Catholics. As John Marshall recalled, 'Those who had come to [the question of contraception and marriage] from a purely academic point of view, either in terms of population statistics or theology in the abstract, were increasingly astonished at the openness of these people who were willing to share their experiences.'[53] The power of the evidence also lay in the fact that it had been collected not from dissidents but from those most loyal to the teachings of the church.[54] A leak to an American Catholic paper indicated that 60 of the 64 theological experts and 9 of the 15 cardinals sitting on the commission favoured a change, and that some were willing to approve not only the pill but also the recently developed intrauterine device for contraception.[55] Moreover, the commission made it clear that the majority did not see contraception as intrinsically evil, or consider that the church's acceptance of contraception would go against its teachings and tradition. Similarly members made it clear that the issue needed to be resolved as soon as possible.[56]

While not resulting in a revolution in Catholic doctrine, the commission took a major step in acknowledging that sex was as important as an expression of love between spouses as it was in furthering procreation.[57] At the same time it made it clear that while couples should not resort to sterilization, they had a right to limit the size of their families and to select the contraceptive method most suited to their needs. The commission recommended that contraception should be effective and that it should take into account 'the biological, hygienic and psychological aspects, and personal dignity of the spouses, and the possibility of expressing sufficiently and aptly the interpersonal relation of conjugal love'. The ultimate decision, however, should be left up to individual couples.[58] There was much in the commission's statement that was surprisingly close to the wording and arguments first articulated by John Rock in his book.[59]

Humanae Vitae and its aftermath

In weighing up the findings of the commission, Paul VI felt that he faced an impossible task. For him the decision rested not only on questions about Catholic teachings on marriage and contraception, but also on whether he believed that he really had the power to change a doctrine that had been maintained for so long. Within this context he felt that his views were valueless when weighed against the history of the institution. His final choice, some have argued, was therefore made not on the basis of arrogance and authoritarianism, but more as a result of an excess of modesty about his own powers.[60]

After considering the question for over two years, Paul VI finally decided to ignore the Papal Commission's findings and recommendations. Publishing his encyclical, the *Humanae Vitae*, the Pope made it clear that the church would maintain its prohibition on all mechanical and chemical means of contraception. The only approved form of contraception remained the rhythm method, and this was restricted to couples who had 'well-grounded reasons for spacing births, arising from the physical or psychological condition of husband or wife, or from external circumstances'.[61] Overall the encyclical revealed a deeply conservative approach to artificial contraception. It disputed many of the points made by Rock and indicated that approval of contraception 'could open wide the way for marital infidelity and a general lowering of moral standards'. Moreover the Pope's statement reasoned, 'Not much experience is needed to be fully aware of human weakness and to understand that human beings – and especially the young, who are so exposed to temptation – need incentives to keep the moral law, and it is an evil thing to make it easy for them to break that law.' The Pope also made it clear that he feared that the proliferation of contraceptives might lead to abuse. As he put it, 'a man who grows accustomed to the use of contraceptive methods may forget the reverence due to a woman, and, disregarding her physical and emotional equilibrium, reduce her to being a mere instrument for the satisfaction of his own desires, no longer considering her as his partner whom he should surround with care and affection'.[62]

Much of the conservative attitudes expressed in the encyclical reflected the strong role played in its final preparation by Cardinal Alfredo Ottaviani. Through his position as the Secretary of the Holy Office, Cardinal Ottaviani had a powerful voice within the Vatican. He had not only chaired the Papal Commission on Population, Family and Birth in 1965, he was also put in charge of the secret commission set up by the Pope to draw up the final encyclical. Early in the 1960s Ottaviani had indicated that he regarded the contraceptive pill as different from the rhythm method, not only because he saw it as directly impeding 'the course of the conjugal act' and disrupting the 'biological integrity of the act of intercourse', but also because it might 'favour hedonism'.[63] The eleventh of 12 children, and the son of a poor baker, Ottaviani made it clear that 'the freedom granted couples by the [Vatican Council] to determine for themselves the number of their children cannot possibly be approved'.[64] Moreover, Ottaviani had made it obvious that he did not agree with the findings of the Papal Commission. John Marshall went so far as to suggest that Ottaviani regarded the commission 'as a kind of aberration in the life of the Church'. During much of the proceedings Ottaviani had in fact spent the time snoozing. As Patty Crowley recalled of Ottiavani's part in the commission, 'He really just sat there, I don't think he participated very much. ... They'd have to end meetings because he was asleep.'[65]

Ottaviani was not alone in his reservations about the pill and was backed by many orthodox members of the church. Their argument was not based on any real consideration about birth control; rather it was based on the fact that any change in the traditional teaching of the church on contraception would be severely embarrassing politically because it would rescind a position defended by the Catholic church in the outside world for so long. From their perspective, it was a question of the church's authority. Such reasoning was crucial in getting the Pope to agree that such a reform would effectively repudiate centuries of policy which had condemned contraception as a mortal sin worthy of excommunication.[66]

Ottaviani's obdurate stance must be seen in the context of his overall opposition to the reforms instigated by the Vatican Council. In his role as the guardian of the faith within the church, the motto on his coat of arms, *Semper idem* (always the same), summed up his overall position. From its inception Ottaviani had been a severe critic of the Vatican Council, using his position within the Holy See to prevent any moves for reform. During the debate on the abandonment of the Latin Mass, for instance, he had stormed out of the session. Angered that anyone could even think of changing a teaching that had not been altered since the seventh century, Ottaviani did not return to the council's deliberations for a fortnight. In some ways the *Humanae Vitae* could be seen as the compensation offered to Ottaviani and his conservative allies for the more liberal acts that had been passed in other areas during the Vatican Council. As Peter Hebblethwaite, biographer of Pope Paul VI, put it, the *Humanae Vitae* might be seen as 'Ottaviani's I-told-you-so revenge' for the Vatican Council.[67]

Nonetheless, while conservative forces may have gained a victory in the wording of the final encyclical, the issue of contraception and the Catholic church was far from resolved. Quite against its intention to bring the community together, the encyclical effectively split the church in two. For many it came as a total shock. John Rock, not surprisingly, greeted the Pope's encyclical with horror, arguing that the position of the encyclical was 'no longer valid' and that it was far from 'purely traditional' in its attitude. Such a stance, he pointed out, was particularly disappointing 'at a time when the Church has publicly absolved Galileo of his misjudged so-called error in declaring that the earth revolves round the sun'. Furthermore, he stressed, 'We can't wait another 300 years for the Church to admit it's made another mistake when we're been dealing with something like population.'[68]

Rock was not alone in such views. Around the world the Pope's message was greeted with dismay. One liberal Catholic newspaper in the United States summed up the popular mood when it commented that 'to say that this is a bitter disappointment is an understatement. It will plunge whole sections of the Church into gloom.'[69] Within a day of the encyclical's publication, huge numbers of Catholic priests and members of their congregations started to protest by walking out publicly from Mass. For many this protest did not come without pain. A letter from Denis Hurley, Archbishop of Durban, South Africa, illustrates the tension that many felt at the time. Interviewed by a Catholic weekly in Cape Town, Hurley admitted that while the Pope 'had a right to make the decision', he had 'never felt so torn in half'. Indeed, he felt the episode was one of most painful experiences in his life as a bishop.[70] Similarly, a petition mounted by over 600 American Catholic theology teachers declared the encyclical to be invalid and 'incompatible with the Church's authentic self-awareness as expressed at Vatican II'. Moreover, they claimed, it showed 'an almost total disregard for the dignity of millions of human beings brought into the world without the slightest possibility of being fed and educated decently'. It went on to state that the encyclical had paid 'insufficient attention to the ethical import of science'.[71]

For many Catholics the encyclical was the turning point in their faith, with some deciding to leave the church altogether. Indeed the pronouncement on contraception was a defining moment for the Catholic church and membership plummeted drastically.[72] Remarkably, however, John Rock, when commenting on the encyclical, indicated that he was prepared to stand by the church, stating, 'I have utter and complete confidence in the Catholic Church, I believe it could be about as dependable a transmitter of the mind of God as man can evolve. And until I see better, I stand by this one.'[73] Even those who decided to remain within the church crossed a threshold in their perception of the Pope's authority. Concluding that neither the Pope nor celibate clergymen had any clear idea about sex and marital life, Catholics for the first time began to disobey the traditional restrictions on contraception. Prior to the Pope's pronouncement many observant Catholics had been reluctant to use the pill and other forms of contraception apart from the rhythm method. After 1968 many otherwise devout Catholics began to adopt the pill and practise contraception in large numbers.[74]

By the late 1970s Catholics were using contraceptives with almost the same frequency as other religious groups.[75] Figures from a sample of seven non-Catholic countries and 12 Catholic countries suggest that while the overall uptake of the pill tended on average to be lower in Catholic countries, it did not seem to be directly affected by the publication of *Humanae Vitae*. As figure 9.1 indicates, the average percentage of women taking the pill in fact increased steadily after the encyclical. Women in European Catholic countries, however, seem to have been much more in favour of using the pill than those in Latin America (figure 9.2). Part of this difference may be accounted for by the very different ways in which Catholicism was understood and practised in each area. However, the lower uptake of the pill in the Latin American nations may also have reflected the lower consumption of the pill found more generally in developing regions.[76]

By the late 1970s the pill had become one of the most popular methods of contraception among many Catholic women all over the world, and far

Figure 9.1 Average percentage of women aged 15–44 buying oral contraceptives from pharmacies in selected Catholic and non-Catholic countries around the world, 1964–1987

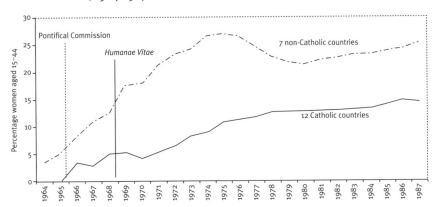

Catholic countries: Austria, Belgium, Brazil, Colombia, France, Ireland, Italy, Mexico, Peru, Portugal, Puerto Rico, Spain.
Non-Catholic countries: Australia, Canada, West Germany, Netherlands, New Zealand, UK, USA

The percentages in the graph are calculated as follows: (1) Pharmacy sales of oral contraceptives were divided by 13 to give the maximum number of women taking them for one full year – or woman years of use; (2) Woman years were divided by the female population aged 15–44 x 100 to give the minimum % of women aged 15–44 buying them in sufficient quantity for one year of use. No attempt is made in these data to account for non-fertile women or women not married, not at risk of pregnancy or already pregnant. These figures represent the minimum number of users because the woman-year concept counts, for example, two women using oral contraceptives for six months apiece as one woman year. On the other hand, pharmacy purchases from wholesalers include supplies in inventory and thus may overcount actual users during a period of inventory build-up.

Source: Population Reports, Series A, no. 5 (Jan. 1979) and no. 7 (Nov. 1988).

Figure 9.2 Average percentage of women aged 15–44 buying oral contraceptives from pharmacies in selected Catholic countries in Europe, and Latin America, 1966–1987

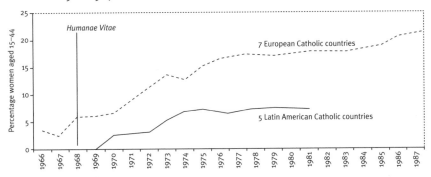

European Catholic countries: Austria, Belgium, France, Ireland, Italy, Portugal, Spain.
Latin American Catholic countries: Brazil, Colmbia, Mexico, Peru, Puerto Rico.

Data calculated as in figure 9.1

Source: Population Reports, Series A, no. 5 (Jan. 1979) and no. 7 (Nov. 1988).

exceeded the rhythm method. Table 9.1 suggests that during the 1970s and 1980s the pill was much more favoured than the rhythm method in many European countries, including Austria, Belgium, France, Italy, Portugal and Spain. The one exception was Poland, where the rhythm method continued to be highly popular into the 1980s. This may, in part, have reflected the particular Catholic culture of the country, which was very traditional, as well as the lack of availability of the pill in Poland overall.[77] During the same period, the rhythm method also fell in popularity in Latin America. Even in Peru, where the rhythm method was more popular than the pill during the 1970s and 1980s, the pill had become one of the most favoured methods by the 1990s. In practice, therefore, the encyclical had little overall impact on the contraceptive decisions of most Catholics around the world. As one Catholic woman in the United States commented, 'If all the women who take the pill stopped going to church, there would hardly be any women there, only men and children.'[78]

The widespread expectation of imminent change during the early 1960s had in itself led many Catholics to decide to use the pill before the encyclical was published. One survey by the American magazine *Newsweek* in 1965 indicated that 38 per cent of American Catholics were currently using the pill or another artificial contraceptive method. Of those under the age of 35, at least 60 per cent were using such contraception, and at least eight out of ten of them were eager to see the church approve the pill. Similarly, in the largely Catholic country of Italy at least 7 million packets of oral contraceptives were sold in 1965. The pill was also one of most widely marketed pharmaceutical products in the overwhelmingly Catholic region of Latin America, where at least 1.5 million women, mostly from the upper- and middle-classes, were taking it by 1965.[79]

As Father Andrew Greeley pointed out, the encyclical had in fact come too late: the people had 'already made their decision'. From his perspective the episode had been a fiasco for the church. 'It was a peculiar thing. The pill came along and the Church hesitated and vacillated, while people were making up their own minds. Had the Church acted more quickly, perhaps the outcome would have been different. But as it was, the people reacted by saying, you're wrong on the pill, maybe you're wrong on a lot of things.'[80] In this respect the Pope had fallen in Catholic estimations and no longer seemed infallible. Exemplifying this, two surveys undertaken by Greeley and his co-workers indicated that the number of Catholics who believed that the Pope derived his authority directly from Jesus declined between 1963 and 1974 from 70 to 42 per cent.[81]

Table 9.1 Average percentage of women of reproductive age using the pill or the rhythm method in selected Catholic and non-Catholic countries, 1966–1991

	Year	Rhythm method	Pill
Catholic countries: European			
Austria	1981	8.7	40
Belgium	1966	16	5
	1975	7	30
	1991	2.1	46.4
France	1972	9	11
	1978	6.4	26.6
	1988	6.4	29.7
Italy	1979	9	14
Poland	1972	20	2
	1977	30	7
Portugal	1979	4	19.1
Spain	1977	6	13
	1985	3.6	15.5
Catholic countries: Latin America			
Colombia	1969	–	4.8
	1976	5.1	13.3
	1980	4.9	17.4
Mexico	1976	3.1	10.8
	1982	3.8	14.2
	1987	4.4	9.8
Peru	1969	7	3
	1977	10.9	4.1
	1981	17	5
	1986	17.7	6.5
	1991	5.7	20.7
Puerto Rico	1968	1.7	11.3
Non-Catholic countries			
Australia	1986	2	24
Canada	1984	2.2	11
Netherlands	1969	11	27
	1975	3	50
New Zealand	1976	1.5	28.6
UK	1970	5	19
	1975	1	30
	1986	2	19
USA	1965	6.8	15.1
	1973	2.8	25.1
	1976	3.4	22.5
	1982	3.2	13.4
	1988	2.1	15.1

Figures pertain to current contraceptive use as reported in interviews with women married or in consensual sexual relationships.

Source: UN, Levels and Trends of Contraceptive Users Assessed in 1994 (New York, 1996), table A6.

What changed in 1968 was that people no longer worried about abstaining from communion when using contraception. The shift in attitude is captured by the comments of a Mexican Catholic woman who, within weeks of the encyclical, remarked, 'Well, like my husband says, "Pray to God and go to Mass, but keep taking the pills because if we have any more children the Pope isn't going to give us a hand to educate them.'[82] Her response was not unusual. Indeed many liberal priests and bishops themselves decided to turn a blind eye to the practice and began to give communion even to those openly taking the pill.[83]

Conclusion

The Pope's encyclical of 1968 not only disappointed Catholics around the world but also disheartened many within the wider community. Nowhere was this more apparent than among those who looked to the pill as the weapon against population growth. It would be wrong, however, to view the Vatican's encyclical as a decision not to get involved with the population question. As early as 1954, Pope Pius XII had indicated that the church should be considering population issues, pointing to the rhythm method as one solution. His successor, John XXIII, also engaged with the issue of population growth in two of his major encyclicals, *Mater et Magistra* and *Pacem in Terris*.[84] There was much concern within the Catholic church about the anti-clerical sentiments and hostility to the church then being manifested in places such as Latin America.[85] Many associated such tensions with social upheaval and pressures on resources caused by population growth. Pope Paul VI summed up the potential in his Christmas message of 1963 which ended: 'Hunger can become a subversive force with incalculable results.'[86] Significantly the Pontifical Commission on Population, Family and Birth had included 11 delegates from developing countries in its proceedings. These representatives had also represented the church at a population conference in Delhi in 1963.[87]

Despite its concern over population growth, the church was uncertain as to the policy line it should take.[88] Some within the Catholic community, such as John Rock, believed that population growth could be tackled only through the church's acceptance of contraception, pointing out that large family size led directly to poverty. But not everyone agreed.[89] One Jesuit demographer, Father Clement Mertens, pointed out to an American journalist covering Vatican II, Robert Kaiser, in 1963 that 'the pill is not the solution to the problems in the Third World countries'.[90] *Humanae Vitae* took a similar line. Repeating the words of John XXIII, the encyclical stated:

> No statement of the problem and no solution to it is acceptable which does violence to man's essential dignity; those who propose such solutions base them on an utterly materialistic conception of man himself and his life. The only possible solution to this question is one which envisages the social and economic progress both of individuals and of the whole of human society, and which respects and promotes true human values.

Within this context, contraception, rather than being seen as an answer, was viewed as providing the potential power to public authorities to 'impose their use on everyone' and 'to intervene in the most personal and intimate responsibility of husband and wife'.[91]

Whatever the merits of the argument, the Pope's decision to reject the findings of the Pontifical Commission on Population, Family and Birth and ban the contraceptive pill fragmented the church. While many opted to continue to attend services despite deviating from the church's teachings, others simply left altogether. In the longer term however, the church itself turned a blind eye. The pill, more than any other focus of debate during the Second Vatican Council, had shown that the church was no longer the all-powerful organization of past centuries. The issuing of edicts, moreover, no longer seemed a viable way of enforcing control over the church's lay community. Interestingly, Paul VI himself was so traumatized by the aftermath of *Humanae Vitae* that he never wrote another encyclical. As the author and journalist Edward Stourton, points out, 'it was as if his capacity to offer moral guidance had been exhausted'.[92]

In 1997, 30 years after the encyclical, Pope John Paul II finally issued a document which, although continuing to reaffirm the church's opposition to artificial contraception, advised priests to be compassionate in the confessional box when dealing with couples who practised contraception.[93] In a real sense this signalled a quiet conclusion to a revolution that had begun in the 1960s.

The Catholic church's decision not to approve the pill illustrates the fact that the uptake of the contraceptive was largely determined by wide cultural and religious factors. Its resistance to the pill was not unique. The next chapter shows how governments and couples in developing countries also chose not to adopt the oral contraceptive as a solution to the perceived population explosion. The Catholic church's response to the pill shows that rather than bringing the world together as the developers of the oral contraceptive first envisioned, it in fact opened new wounds and reinforced old divisions.

10
Panacea or Poisoned Chalice?

'Not since the sulfa tablets emerged in the 1930's to conquer pneumonia and a host of other infections, has a little tablet exerted such far-reaching influence upon the world's people. It may, in fact be the most popular pill since aspirin. It is certainly relieving bigger headaches – both family and global.'[1] These words, written by an American journalist just six years after the pill had been released in the United States, underline the revolutionary qualities contemporaries attributed to the pill within a short time of its appearance. Not everyone, however, viewed the pill in such a positive light. Indeed, some went so far as to suggest that its effects were more 'devastating than the nuclear bomb', attributing to it the sexual revolution and a wave of promiscuity.[2]

Whatever the conclusions to this debate, it is clear that the acceptance of the pill was not uniform across the world and was closely intertwined with the social, political and economic issues of the day. As this chapter shows, the slow adoption of the pill in many developing countries by comparison with those considered more developed highlights the fact that the contraceptive was far from the neutral product that would be accepted in every culture as had been hoped for by its original makers.

Pill consumption around the world

One of the noticeable features of the pill today is that its highest consumption is in the developed world. By 1979 commercial sales of oral contraceptives in developing regions accounted for about 56 million monthly cycles, which was less than one-fifth of the figure in the more developed world.[3] This contrast continues: table 10.1 and figures 10.1 and 10.2 indicate that, while the actual numbers of women taking the pill were almost identical in the developing and developed world, by the late 1980s and 1990s the overall percentage of people using the pill was greater in more developed parts of the world, where it was one of the most commonly used methods. The percentage of the population using oral contraceptives was most marked in northern and western Europe and least on the Indian subcontinent, in China and within Africa. Significantly today the pill is one of the least popular contraceptive methods in China and India, the world's two most populated countries where governments have promoted some of the most active family planning programmes. Here sterilization and the IUD had become the dominant forms of contraception by the 1990s.[4]

Table 10.1 Oral contraceptive use among married women of reproductive age, worldwide, 1988

	Estimated percentage of women	Estimated number (millions)
Developed Areas		
Australia and New Zealand	30	0.9
Europe and USSR		
East (includes USSR)	6	3.5
North (Scandinavia)	21	0.6
South	14	2.8
West	29	8.8
Japan	1	0.2
North America	18	7.0
South Africa	15	0.6
Total	14	24.4
Developing areas		
Asia		
China	5	10.1
Indian subcontinent	2	3.2
Other Asian	13	9.2
Latin America and Caribbean	16	8.3
Near East and North Africa	12	4.4
Tropical Africa	5	3.3
Total	6	38.5
Grand total	8	62.9

Source: 'Lower-dose pills', *Population Reports*, Series A, no. 7 (Nov. 1988), 6, table 1.

Figure 10.1 Percentage of population using different contraceptive methods in developing and developed countries, 1990–1991

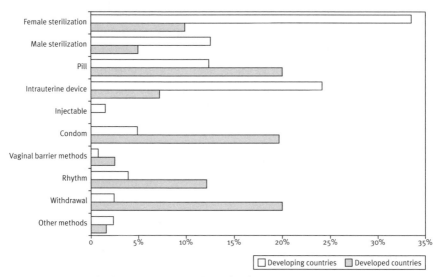

Source: IPPF, *Meeting the Challenges: Promoting Choices* (1992), 9.

Figure 10.2 Estimated number of users of specific contraceptive methods in developed and developing countries, 1990 (millions)

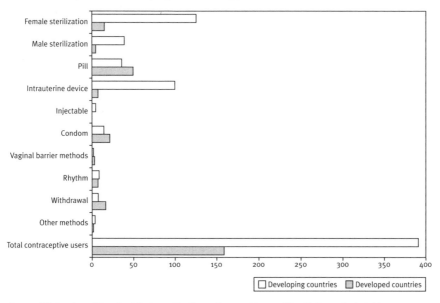

Source: UN, *Levels and Trends of Contraceptive Use as Assessed in 1994* (New York, 1996), 61, table 17.

Female sterilization has in fact increased worldwide, accounting for 15 per cent of all contraception in 1983 and 20 per cent in 1994. Indeed, no other form of contraception showed so significant an increase in the period.[5]

The disparity in the uptake of the contraceptive pill in differently developed regions is particularly striking when we consider the early emphasis its developers placed on its usefulness in curbing world population growth and their specific marketing efforts in the developing world. Gregory Pincus was especially active in promoting the oral contraceptive in developing countries. His efforts in this field were funded by Katherine McCormick and achieved in collaboration with G. D. Searle and the Population Council. Much of his initiative involved urging non-Western governments to adopt the oral contraceptive as part of their social policies. He and G. D. Searle also lobbied international organizations such as the United Nations Population Agency and the World Health Organization to promote the pill.[6]

Links with international agencies were considered important in view of the need to subsidize the cost of contraceptive provision in poorer nations. This was seen to be vital because in the early 1960s the cost of the pill was regarded as a major obstacle to its use in those countries.[7] The infrastructure of the international bodies also made distribution of the drug easier, because their involvement lent it a 'global seal of approval' and diminished the negative connotations of an American export.[8] From the perspective of the pharmaceutical companies, alliances with international organizations were also attractive from a commercial point of view, not only providing important business opportunities but also enhancing their corporate image.[9]

From 1968 onwards international aid organizations, such as the United States Agency for International Development (USAID), the Swedish International Development Authority (SIDA) and the United Nations Children's Education Fund (UNICEF), began to supply oral contraceptives free of charge to family planning programmes in developing countries. Between 1968 and 1974 these agencies shipped nearly 150 million cycles of oral contraceptives to both government and privately sponsored family-planning programmes. SIDA itself donated the drug to 13 countries and acted as a purchasing agent for another 24, negotiating the buying of the contraceptive at low bulk prices. Similarly UNICEF contributed either pills or raw materials to at least six countries. By far the greatest provider was USAID, which supplied at least 65 nations.[10] Together the shipments by USAID, SIDA and UNICEF represented about 10 per cent of the total of oral contraceptive sales in the major world markets during 1972. Moreover, donations to Asia, Africa and Latin America almost equalled the sale of the contraceptive through other commercial channels in these places.[11]

This huge charitable effort had some effect on the overall uptake of the pill in developing regions: from 1970 sales of the pill increased greatly in developing countries. While hard statistics are difficult to gather on this issue, sales of the oral contraceptive tripled in Asia and doubled in Latin America between 1972 and 1979. Family planning programmes assisted by international organizations supplied a substantial number of these pills. By 1979 such provision accounted for more than double the amount sold through commercial channels in developing countries.[12]

Overall, however, pill consumption remained low in developing regions. In 1977 only about 10 per cent of women of reproductive age, for instance, were purchasing oral contraceptives on a regular basis in Brazil and Puerto Rico, countries with some of the highest rates of pill use in the developing world. This contrasts with figures from more developed countries, where in the same year the rates ranged from 20 per cent in Britain to 30 per cent in Australia and above 40 per cent in the Netherlands. The distribution of oral contraceptives in developing countries continued to be firmly in the hands of international organizations.[13] Table 10.2 indicates the disparate ways in which the oral contraceptive was distributed around the world in 1977. Donor agencies continued to be important in the distribution of the pill into the following decade. Between 1985 and 1988 donor agencies were shipping an average of 74.3 million cycles a year to developing countries, enough to provide for 5.7 million women of reproductive age. This accounted for approximately one-sixth of all oral contraceptives consumed in developing countries.[14]

Table 10.2 Estimated numbers of women using oral contraceptives in developed and developing countries according to commercial or governmental source, worldwide, 1977 (millions)

	Developed countries	Developing countries
Commercial sales (IMS Health Inc)	21	4
Other commercial sales*	3	1
Government programmes	4	9

* Calculated by Population Council and US Agency for International Development, 1977.

Source: 'OCs – Update on usage, safety, and side effects', Population Reports, Series A, no. 5 (Jan. 1979), A-144, table 9.

Obstacles to the uptake of the pill

Obstacles that prevented the early uptake of the pill in developing countries are best illustrated by the difficulties that Pincus and his collaborators encountered in India. Here, despite accepting the necessity of a policy on population, the government strongly opposed the pill. Part of this stemmed from a belief that the pill represented yet another form of Western oppression.[15] Questions of safety, however, also played a significant role in the decision. Like many within the Catholic church, Indian regulators feared that the pill might disrupt nature. In addition they were hesitant about accepting the American scientific data on the drug without first testing it according to their own criteria. This astounded Pincus and his colleagues, who initially assumed it would be simple to persuade India to test the pill on a clinical basis. India was to go to far greater lengths than almost any other country to place obstacles in the way of the pill, opting instead for contraceptive methods such as the IUD and sterilization.[16]

The reaction of the Indian government was not unique. Indeed hostility to the pill could be found closer to home. During the late 1960s major tensions over the pill surfaced within the African-American community in the United States. Against the background of the black civil rights movement, much of the domestic debate over the contraceptive was concerned with whether it was a tool of genocide designed by the white man to eliminate the African American race in America, or really a route to liberation. Their reaction was shaped in part by the increasing scepticism of the scientific community as a whole, a group with a reputation already tarnished by its promotion of genetic explanations for racial differences in the context of intelligence testing. Moreover, during the 1960s and 1970s, thousands of poor African-American women were coercively sterilized through federally funded family programmes across America. Unease over the pill was not diminished by the fact that state legislators had considered a number of sterilization bills primarily targeted at black women on public assistance.[17] Some of the most violent reactions to the pill came from militant black men who castigated black women at political meetings for using the pill and called on them to throw it away in order to 'breed revolutionaries'. Some went so far as to threaten to firebomb a Planned Parenthood clinic in Pittsburgh. But the hostility was not universal. Many black women embraced the pill, seeing it as an effective means of controlling their fertility and escaping the trap of poverty.[18]

The contraceptive pill was therefore far from a neutral product. Significantly the Soviet Union also reacted against its use at first, probably as a result of its associations with the United States and Cold War tensions. Ideology, however, was not the only critical factor against the adoption of the pill. A number of European nations, for instance, whose researchers had little experience of the pill, initially hesitated to approve it. Questions of safety were an overriding consideration. The pill was, for example, withdrawn in Norway in 1962 when its thrombotic complications were first reported, and only remarketed in 1964.[19] Japan, a highly industrialized country, also proved very resistant and continued to reject the use of the pill as a contraceptive until 1999. Up to that time only the high dose pill was available to Japanese women, and this was restricted to medical cases. A similar story prevailed in North Korea.

Acceptance of the pill was clearly dependent not only on considerations of safety, but on a range of other social, political, cultural and economic factors. Japan illustrates the complex dynamics involved in the adoption of the pill particularly well. As early as 1953 Japanese scientists had begun to collaborate with Pincus in human trials of some of the experimental compounds used for contraceptive purposes, and by the mid 1950s the Japanese Ministry of Welfare was providing funds for the testing of progesterone as part of the pill's development. As it happened, Pincus made his first public announcement of the possibility of creating an oral contraceptive at the Fifth International Conference on Planned Parenthood in Tokyo in 1955. A number of Japanese gynaecologists also conducted trials from the late 1950s in a number of different Japanese hospitals. Despite this, however, the Japanese government blocked the eventual sale of the pill.[20] As with India, the government did not trust the scientific criteria presented by the American scientists. More importantly they were hesitant about the introduction of the contraceptive because they had no way of enforcing a restriction on its sale to prescription channels alone. What worried them most was that the pill might fall into the hands of young unmarried women.[21]

The Japanese government's refusal to approve the sale of oral contraceptives hardened over the years. Part of the hostility was influenced by the long-standing opposition from doctors and the rubber industry, who feared that any acceptance of the drug would result in the loss of billions of yen in revenues, on the one hand from performing legal abortions, and on the other from the sale of condoms. The sum collected from such services was substantial. The condom industry, which commanded 86 per cent of the contraceptive market, produced $573 million in sales revenue in 1997. At the same time, Japan had one of the highest rates of abortion in the world, with 343,000 cases reported in 1995. Legalized during the 1950s, abortion was until very recently one of the main forms of (female) fertility control in Japan. The ban on oral contraceptives was, of course, a contributory factor to the high use of condoms and the need for abortion.[22]

In addition to the opposition of the medical profession and the rubber industry, the Japanese government was loath to approve the pill. During the 1960s this reluctance stemmed from caution over the product's safety, but in later years the government's concern centred more on the pill's potential to escalate sexual promiscuity and from the 1980s its inability to protect against diseases such as AIDS. It was also feared that the pill might exacerbate the decline in the country's birth-rate, already below replacement level, with consequent implications for the nation's manpower and economy.[23]

During the thirty years of the Japanese government's vacillation, feminist groups in the country also grew increasingly opposed to the drug, seeing it as invasive, destroying the natural rhythm of the female body and depriving it of the power to control and heal itself. The rejection of the contraceptive also stemmed from a fear that it might repress a woman's sexuality because of its daily regimen. Moreover Japanese feminists disliked the fact that it placed full responsibility for contraception on women. While very few in number, the feminist protestors, together with continuing publicity over the negative side-effects of the pill in the West, clearly adversely affected the attitude of Japanese women in general. The pill was finally approved in Japan only in the wake of criticism of the obvious double standard when Viagra gained official sanction there in the 1990s, only six months after it had appeared on the American market.[24]

Japan's response to the pill and the varying levels of its uptake in the rest of the world once again illustrates the fact that, as had been the case with the Catholic church, acceptance of the pill can not be separated from wider social and political concerns. Moreover, like many other technologies, the pill was loaded with notions of gender and other cultural values. Formulated on the basis of the hormones that all women were thought to possess, it was regarded by many of its original developers as a drug suitable for women across the globe, and a weapon to combat the world population explosion in every country. The reality however was very different. One of the reasons the Indian government had decided against the pill was because it was regarded as ill-suited to its female population. Many sociologists, demographers and activists in the Indian family planning movement believed the contraceptive required too much medical surveillance and intelligent cooperation from the patient to be attractive to Indian women.[25]

They were not the only ones to draw this conclusion. In 1973 the central medical committee of the International Planned Parenthood Federation pointed out that a major obstacle to the uptake of the pill in less developed countries was the fact that it necessitated medical guidance and a prescription. On this basis they felt that the oral contraceptive was not only 'geographically, economically, and sometimes culturally inaccessible to many women', but that such a requirement amounted to 'discrimination against the many [who were] urgently in need of protection against unplanned pregnancy'.[26] The fact that family planning organizations insisted on medical supervision and prescription was seen as particularly questionable in countries where women who could afford to get the pill privately could do so over the counter without seeing either a doctor or obtaining a prescription.[27]

By the middle of the 1970s some countries had tried to tackle these problems through schemes to distribute the pill through community-based health-care schemes whereby women could gain supplies without the presence of a doctor or the necessity of a prescription. This step significantly boosted its uptake. By 1979 the pill had increasingly been accepted in places where community-based programmes were in place. This included Thailand and Malaysia, where it was now being distributed through paramedical personnel such as midwives, and Colombia and Indonesia, where it was given out by community workers and village leaders. Distribution of the contraceptive also rose in countries such as Tunisia and Sri Lanka, in which it was being sold at subsidized rates without medical supervision in pharmacies or local shops and bazaars.[28]

Packaging the pill

In addition to experimenting with new ways to distribute the pill, manufacturers also developed new regimes for actually taking it. As the early trials in Puerto Rico and Haiti had shown, women found it difficult to remember when to take the pill. What was particularly confusing was the fact that they had to start the medication, stop it and resume it at certain points in their cycle. This was especially difficult to remember for women who could not read or count. In Puerto Rico investigators had tried to get round this problem by supplying the women with rosary beads to aid their memories. Elsewhere other methods were also explored. In Pakistan, for instance, investigators tried to get women to coordinate the taking and stopping of the pill in accordance with the cycles of the moon. But these techniques were far from successful.[29]

Even when women were able to read, the pill was not easy to use. American and British women, who were often more literate than those in the developing world, also battled with confusion about when to start and stop the drug. Part of this stemmed from its packaging. Initially the pill was dispensed in bottles together with written instructions. It was therefore very difficult for women to remember whether they had taken the pill each day, how many they had taken since the start of their menstrual cycle and how many remained. Neither did this always make for harmonious marital relations. David Wagner, an American who later designed special packaging for the pill, commented: 'There was a lot of room for error in whether "the Pill" was actually taken on a given day. I found I was just as concerned as [my wife] was in whether she had taken her pill or not. I was constantly asking her whether she had taken "the pill" and this led to some irritation and a marital row or two.'[30]

In fact the distinctive packaging that exists for the pill today is a by-product of these rows between Wagner and his wife. One of the ways he tried to resolve the argument was to put on the dresser a piece of paper listing the days of the week with a pill on each day. This was designed so they could see at a glance whether a pill had been taken each day. While the scheme did wonders for their relationship for a time, two to three weeks later it was totally ruined when something fell on to the dresser and scattered the paper and the pills all over the floor.[31] The system and the experience inspired Wagner to invent a container that could keep the pills according to days of the week without spilling, and that could be easily carried around in a woman's handbag. In designing this he had the advantage that he had worked as a product engineer.[32]

In July 1962 Wagner applied for a patent for the box he had devised for packaging the pill. Known as Dialpak, it was circular in shape and could be moved around to show which day of the week it was and when the last pill had been taken. Shortly after patenting his invention he sent Dialpak to G. D. Searle and Ortho Pharmaceutical for their consideration. While neither of these companies responded to Wagner, within a short time they were selling their pills in replica dispensers designed to aid patient memory. Later awarded compensation for this pirating, Wagner had designed a box that was to become an important marketing device for the pill in years to come, and a fashionable feminine accessory.[33]

What is interesting about Dialpak is that it was invented by the spouse of a patient who had struggled to remember to take the pill and had not orig- inated from the pharmaceutical companies themselves. Moreover it marked the first time a prescriptive medication was specifically packaged to aid patient memory. Prior to its appearance patients were expected to rely on their own memory or to buy special separate boxes as a way of remembering. The incorporation of a reminder with the packaging of the oral contraceptive was therefore a novelty in the history of drugs.[34]

In later years, pharmaceutical companies began to devise new methods of packaging. In part this stemmed from a desire to find a way round Wagner's patent, but it also became an important means of distinguishing themselves from their competitors. Neither were the changes confined to the packaging; they also involved reforms to the regimen of taking the pill. Originally women were expected to take the first pill on the fifth day, and to continue until the twenty-first day, of their cycle. This involved swallow- ing 20 tablets and meant that a woman stopped and started her medication at different times of the week. In the mid-1960s, Searle revolutionized this regimen when it brought out Ovulen-21 which added an extra pill to the cycle. The product was marketed along the lines that it allowed women to stop and start the pill more easily. The advertisement of Ovulen-21 to doctors highlights the novelty of this regimen, 'Ovulen-21 works the way a woman thinks by weekdays ... not "cycle days". Ovulen-21 lets her remem- ber the natural way. Once established, her starting day is always the same day of the week ... because it is fixed at three weeks on–one week off.'[35]

Other pharmaceutical companies followed suit, adding yet more pills to the regimen. In 1968 Organon Laboratories of England devised a 22-day regimen for their oral contraceptive called Lyndiol. This regimen, they argued, allowed for 'maximum patient reliability' because 'each course of tablets always begins and ends on the same fixed day of the week. ... Thus, if the "last" tablet is taken on a Friday evening, then the first tablet from the next pack is taken on the next Friday evening.'[36] In 1965 Mead Johnson issued a 28-day regimen with its sequential oral contraceptive called Oracon. Because of its ease of instruction, medical personnel quickly favoured this 28-day regimen. Now women did not have to be told to remember when to start and stop the pill, but could continue to take it throughout the month without any breaks. Moreover, they could choose on which day of the week to start the contraceptive. Sunday proved particularly popular because it replicated the weekly calendar and allowed for 'period-free weekends'.[37]

The 28-day regimen proved popular not only among medical practitioners and their patients, but also among pharmaceutical companies, who soon began to copy Oracon's formula. One of the advantages of the regimen was that companies could move away from the calendar format instituted by the Dialpak dispenser. Now pills could be placed in a rectangular arrangement within a blister pack, and women were guided to the correct order of taking the pills by the use of graphic arrows marked on the packaging.

Yet such packaging was not foolproof. Some women, for instance, have been found to ignore the arrows on the packets, removing pills from the pack at random, or vertically instead of horizontally. This is particularly problematic where the pack contains placebos and the pills need to be taken in a certain order to prevent pregnancy.[38] These difficulties have not been made any easier by the appearance of new generation lower dose pills, which need to be taken not only daily but at an exact time every day. Moreover the potential for falling pregnant when forgetting to take just one of the new generation pills is much greater than with the pills of the past.[39]

Initially much of the change to the packaging and the regimen had been motivated by a desire to circumvent Wagner's original patent. It soon became apparent, however, that alterations might be made to make the product more attractive to users in other ways, such as introducing iron supplements in the package. Using iron as placebos within the 28-day regimen was seen as particularly useful for replacing the mineral loss many women experience during menstrual bleeding. And there were other additions. In 1991, for instance, one oral contraceptive package also included a mechanism for reminding women to self-examine their breasts at the appropriate time of their cycle.[40] The inclusion of iron supplements and patient reminders show how the packaging of the pill helped to turn the contraceptive into more than a device aimed at preventing pregnancy. Now it could be used as a vehicle for improving women's health overall. Significantly these measures were undertaken in the wake of alerts about the safety of the pill and growing concerns over issues such as breast cancer in the developed world from the 1980s.

Changes to packaging were also made with the aim of enticing more users in the developing world. During the late 1960s, for instance,

G. D. Searle, through the sponsorship of USAID, began to offer a 28-day package explicitly to attract women in developing countries. The introduction of iron supplements in the package was also regarded as a particularly useful aid for marketing in less developed regions where nutritional deficiencies were seen more frequently and anaemia was a common problem.[41] At the same time the packaging was further improved by a foil-lining that was heat and moisture proof, an important protection against the climate of many developing countries. In addition the packaging included a symbol designed to strengthen consumer recognition among the illiterate, and graphic illustrations were also often included. Illustration 16 shows one of the pictorial ways Malaysian women were taught to use the pill. At the same time, three-month supplies began to be distributed in one packet in order to save women having to return to the clinic every month. This change was particularly important given that regular visits to a doctor in developing countries were expensive, very infrequent and often not part of the culture.[42] In China, other innovations were introduced in the 1970s, such as paper pills, in which the steroid hormones were impregnated into sheets of rice paper. Such paper pills were considered more suitable for transportation and for women to carry around.[43]

Informing women about the use and hazards of the pill across the world

By the 1970s oral contraceptive packaging incorporated standard warnings about the potential risks of the medication. Known as the patient package insert, this had been inspired partly by the protests of American women during the Nelson hearings regarding the issue of thrombosis and the pill in 1970.[44] Such a warning was unusual in the history of prescribed medications. Before the pill the only other drug application for which the FDA required a patient package insert was isoproterenol inhalators. Isoproterenol is a bronchodilator which works by relaxing muscles in the airways to improve breathing. It is used to treat conditions such as asthma, bronchitis and emphysema. Among its most serious side-effects are an allergic reaction (difficulty in breathing; tightening of the throat; swelling of lips, tongue or face; or hives), chest pains or an irregular heartbeat.[45] Unlike today when inserts have become standard practice for many prescribed drugs, until the 1970s most patients received warnings about their drugs from their doctor. The addition of such inserts to the packaging of the oral contraceptive pill can be partly attributed to its ubiquitous use, and the expectations it raised among American consumers about pharmaceutical products overall.

While the patient package insert has become an established feature of the pill, the wording used in such inserts has been the subject of much controversy. In the United States, for instance, the insert is regarded today by many consumers and medical practitioners as a legal document designed to protect manufacturers rather than to provide information for users. This is very different from the original intention of those who campaigned for such an insert in the 1970s. Initially the main aim was to supply instructions on use and basic warnings about risks such as thrombosis so that the patient could decide whether or not to take the medication on an informed basis. Until the early 1990s, however, the insert was far too long and too linguistically complex for most women to understand. Indeed, the format of the document was pitched at a much higher educational level than was considered appropriate for most health education materials in the United States.[46]

One survey of American patient package inserts demonstrated serious difficulties with the instructions before 1992, when the FDA attempted to standardize and simplify the content. Most of the inserts were unreadable because they had been printed in extremely small type on pastel-coloured paper. Instructions were also difficult to find because there were virtually no headings within the text. In addition to these problems, information for physicians was printed before instructions to patients.[47] The latter were in themselves very difficult to follow. Most manufacturers also gave instructions for all their oral contraceptive brands on one insert. This could include information on up to 13 different brands. As each pill has a different formulation and regimen, it was difficult for the user to ascertain which instructions were appropriate for the brand they were taking. One of the problems, for instance, was working out when to start a particular brand, whether to stop it at certain times or to continue to take it continuously throughout the month. This was not particularly helpful for those women choosing to switch between different formulations or brands of the pill. The directions were particularly baffling when explaining to women what to do if they missed taking three or more pills (see table 10.3 below). Most important of all, the recommendations for back-up contraception when a pill had been forgotten, and instructions as to how long it should be used, were very confusing. In some cases it seemed that the instructions actually increased the woman's risk of an accidental pregnancy.[48]

If the fairly well educated American woman was battling to make sense of the instructions, this was equally the case for women in less developed countries. An added difficulty for women in developing regions was that the instructions were not always translated into the local language. Moreover donors and manufacturers did not always supply instructions with the pill packs.[49] In addition, warnings attached to oral contraceptives varied greatly according to where the product was distributed. As is the case for other medications, the warning attached to the oral contraceptive was dependent on the standards set by each country. Inevitably the standards were applied with varying degrees of strictness so package inserts were not uniform across the world.[50]

Table 10.3   Number of pill brands in the USA giving various instructions in the patient package inserts on what to do after three missed pills

Instructions	No. brands
Begin taking pills again as soon as you remember	15
Wait until you have a period or until doctor determines not pregnant[1]	8
Begin a new pack on first day of bleeding	4
Wait until first Sunday after the last pill taken, then begin a new pack	12
Wait 4 more days, then begin a new pack (on 8th day after last pill was taken)[2]	5
No information for 3 or more missed pills	12

1 It is unclear in these instructions whether the user should resume using the current pack or begin a new one.
2 For no more than three missed pills.

Source: M. Williams-Deane and L. S. Potter, 'Current oral contraceptive use instructions', *Family Planning Perspectives*, 24/3 (May/June 1992), 113, table 4.

Not only did the standards expected of such warnings vary, but much of the advice given on serious reactions to the pill was also based on information collected from studies of women in more developed regions of the world.[51] This is particularly questionable if applied to women in less developed countries who do not share the same 'diet, lifestyle, genetic heritage, exposure to disease vectors and environmental contaminants, [or] smoking habits ...'[52] The relevance of the data collected in the developed world for women in less developed regions is illustrated best in the case of cardiovascular disease. First, the overall incidence of circulatory problems, with the exception of hypertension, is much lower in developing nations than in the developed world, where as much as a third of the female population of reproductive age is predisposed to circulatory disease. Secondly, many of the associated risk factors, such as high cholesterol and smoking, are markedly less prevalent in the developing world. Women in the developing world, however, may face other risks that are currently unrecognized and that may be an important consideration when taking the pill. Given this situation and the paucity of studies on the effects of the oral contraceptive on women in developing regions, it is quite possible that risk factors that have been isolated for cardiovascular disease in more westernized societies are not universal.[53]

It is difficult to know what implications such differences have for the safe distribution of the pill worldwide. A report by the Population Information Program in the United States in 1979 argued that oral contraceptives might pose no serious threat in the long run to most women in developing areas and that the risk of pregnancy and childbirth far outweighed any of the hazards identified for women in developed countries. In making this claim the authors highlighted the case of Bangladesh, where, of 100,000 women under the age of 40, almost 200 were expected to die in childbirth, compared with about 10 to 20 deaths among those taking oral contraceptives. They went on to argue: 'Even in developing countries where maternal mortality is lower than in Bangladesh, [oral contraceptives] are much safer than childbirth at all ages below 40.' On this basis they concluded that 'the continued increase in [oral contraceptive] use in the developing world and the spread of community-based distribution systems are well justified from a public health point of view, contributing as they do not only to lower birth rates but also to improved maternal health and survival.'[54]

Clearly the differing risk of maternal mortality between the developed and developing world makes a great difference to the decision as to whether to take the pill and whether it necessitates strict medical supervision. The number of women dying in childbirth in less developed countries in the 1990s was in excess of 500 per 100,000 live births compared with an average of 25 deaths in more industrialized countries. Indeed, in some parts of the world complications from childbirth account for a major proportion of overall deaths among women of reproductive age. In parts of Asia, Africa and Latin America, for instance, between 10 and 30 per cent of deaths among these women result from problems during pregnancy or childbirth. By contrast such deaths account for less than 2 per cent of all mortality among women of reproductive age in the United States and

Europe. While much of this difference is attributable to differing standards of maternity care, access to contraception and safe abortion and varying levels of income, such statistics highlight the very different risks women have to assess when considering whether or not to take the pill. Table 10.4 indicates some of the different risks faced by women in developing and developed countries calculated in 1975. No leaflet designed to warn about the pill's side-effects could hope to capture these variations in mortality and their implications for understanding the risks in relation to the pill. Moreover, as chapters 6 and 7 illustrated, the medical profession itself is constantly having difficulties in evaluating the safety of the pill.

One of the major problems in discussing the hazards of the pill is the fact that these risks are often shaped by more general cultural frameworks. The importance of cultural perceptions about health and the body are highlighted by the evidence collected by medical anthropologists in Sri Lanka, which revealed that people explain the effects and risks of the pill within the context of their own beliefs and ideas about reproductive physiology. As the anthropologists commented, 'A pervasive notion among informants was that the pill worked because of its heating effects in the body.' Indeed, this was how the problems caused by the pill were understood. Some informants, for instance, 'noted that taking these pills every day raised the heat level of the body to such an extent that male and female *dhatu*, a substance associated with vitality and strength, was burned up'. This was seen as having potentially harmful effects. Some claimed that 'the excess heat in a woman's body caused by taking a pill rendered the womb dry [and that] over time a dry womb becomes incapable of accepting a male seed'.[55] One of the challenges, therefore, is to find a means of explaining the action and side-effects of the pill in cultural terms that can be understood by local populations.

In addition to their difficulties in understanding the kinds of risks they face, women have access to very different versions of the pill across the world. This results not only from the marketing strategies of different pharmaceutical companies in each country, but also from the policies pursued by individual governments. This is most clearly demonstrated in the context of the high oestrogen pill in Britain and the United States. As we have seen in chapter 6, high oestrogen pills were phased out after 1970 in Britain on account of their cardiovascular complications, but remained in circulation in the United States until 1988. Elsewhere there were similar variations. During the 1980s, there was a dramatic shift towards lower

Table 10.4 Mortality associated with pregnancy and contraception in developed and developing countries, 1975

Method of fertility control	Estimated method failures per 100 woman-years (developed + developing)	No. pregnancies from method failure (developed + developing)	Estimated no. of deaths from method (developed + developing)	No. deaths from pregnancy Developed (25 per 100,000 births)	Developing (500 per 100,000 births)	Total deaths from pregnancy and method Developed	Developing
No contraception	0	60,000	0	15	300	15	300
Oral contraception	1	1,000	3	<1	10	<4	13
IUDs	3	3,000	1	<1	15	2	16
Condom and diaphragm	2	15,000	0	4	75	4	75

This table represents a model of mortality based on the estimates of method failures in column 1 and estimates of mortality from specific methods in column 3. Column 1 is adapted from US Food and Drug Administration estimates and a similar but not identical Population Council analysis. Column 3 is based on estimated mortality in the USA, primarily from thromboembolism. In developing countries where thromboembolic disorders are rare, mortality associated with use of oral contraceptives may be lower than in the USA. Also mortality may be lower with lower dosage pills. The differences between oral contraception and IUDs in the last two columns are not statistically significant.

Source: 'Advantages and disadvantages of orals outweigh disadvantages', *Population Reports*, Series A, no. 2 (Mar. 1975), A-35, table 1.

oestrogen pills worldwide, but some countries were quicker to adopt them than others. One survey of 37 countries in 1987 showed that while low oestrogen pills accounted for up to 85 per cent of all pharmacy purchases of combined oral contraceptives in 18 developed countries, it constituted only 60 per cent in 19 developing areas. Moreover sales of oral contraceptives with over 5 mg of oestrogen retained a large proportion of the market in certain places. These included Brazil, Central America, Colombia, Franco-phone Africa, Morocco, Pakistan, the Philippines, Taiwan and Turkey.[56] Given the side-effects associated with different pills, such variations have important consequences for women and the risks they face.

Government policies and cost in the distribution of the pill

One of the overriding determinants of the pill's availability is the type of family planning service that exists in each country. In the developed world, for instance, with the exception of the Republic of Ireland, pill use is greatest in places where women are more likely to seek their family planning provision from general practitioners, such as Britain. Family doctors are more likely to offer the pill because of the ease with which they can prescribe it compared with the IUD, diaphragm or sterilization, all of which necessitate greater training and skill on the part of the medical practitioner.[57] This contrasts with countries such as Finland, Norway and Sweden, where IUD use is greater because of the dominance of family planning clinics in the provision of contraception. Uptake of the pill is lowest in areas where family planning is generally set apart from the main health-care structure, and chiefly provided through specialists such as obstetricians and gynaecologists, as in the United States. The considerable sums these specialists charge for their services partly explains the lower uptake of the pill in these countries.

The key to pill use is determined not only by who provides the contraception, but also how much women are charged for it. From early on, the pill's developers were concerned that the high costs involved in its production would make it prohibitively expensive for women in less developed areas. This gave them an impetus to reduce the content of the hormones in each pill.[58] While in later years manufacturers found a cheaper way of producing oral contraceptives, this did not necessarily make them any more affordable. By 1974 the retail price of the drug varied across the world, from as high as $2.50 per cycle in the United States to between $0.50 and $1 elsewhere. Even at its lower price the oral contraceptive frequently remained way beyond the budget of many women in developing countries.[59] The fact that it had to be constantly purchased on a regular basis also rendered it economically problematic. This made it much less attractive than sterilization or the IUD, which only necessitated a single payment. It is therefore not surprising that in later years sterilization and the IUD became more popular than the pill in less developed regions. Even in the United States the price of oral contraceptives was a disincentive. Here the price in fact began to rise during the 1970s in the wake of increasing liability claims against pharmaceutical companies supplying contraceptives and the increased expenses that manufacturers had to face in terms of insurance and legal defence. Many of these costs were recouped by raising the price of the drug.[60]

Couples did not always have to shoulder the costs of the pill, however. The contraceptive was not only heavily subsidized in many developing nations through the donations of international organizations and government family planning programmes, it was also subsidized in many developed countries, where access was via family planning programmes under the umbrella of national health schemes. By the late 1980s, for instance, women in Britain, Italy, the Netherlands, Portugal and Sweden could obtain both the prescription and their supplies free of charge, regardless of income. In other countries, while no charge is made for the prescription, pill supplies have to be bought (Canada, Switzerland, Australia, Belgium, Denmark, France, Germany, New Zealand, Finland and Norway). By contrast, most women in the United States, Austria, Greece, Ireland and Spain, even those on low incomes, are expected to pay for both the prescription and the supplies of the pill. Only those who have no money at all may expect some help in bearing the economic costs of contraception in these five countries.[61]

Such differences in the costs women are expected to bear in relation to the pill have an important bearing on its uptake. A survey in 1988 of 20 different developed countries not surprisingly indicated that women were less likely to use the oral contraceptive in places where they were expected to pay for the prescription, such as in Greece and Spain, and more likely to use it in places where they were not, as in Italy and Portugal. Similarly women's use of the contraceptive tended to be lower in places where they were also expected to pay for the drug itself, as in the United States, where up to 1998 they could not even recoup such costs from health insurance.[62] The negative effect of charges for prescriptions and supplies is particularly strong among older women, perhaps in part because older women have already had their children and have a greater range of possibilities available to them, including sterilization, which is less expensive.[63]

Much of the cost women have to bear in relation to the pill is determined by the priority governments have given to family planning and the way they have balanced this against other questions of social policy.[64] Britain is particularly interesting in this context. Today the pill is one of the few prescription drugs in Britain provided free of charge. Indeed, it is one of the few medications to have escaped the raising of charges in recent years. In 1998 the British government faced uproar from backbenchers and opposition parties in the House of Commons when it was rumoured that charges would be made for the pill.[65] Yet in the early 1960s oral contraceptives were among the few drugs for which patients had to pay. Such a change in policy illuminates not only the increasing acceptance of contraception in the past three decades, but also growing anxiety over the issue of population and changing priorities within the context of social policy.

In Britain during the 1960s women could only obtain free prescriptions and supplies of the pill from family planning clinics which had funding for this purpose from their local authority. Where women went to general practitioners or hospital consultants for their pill, the free provision of such a contraceptive was dependent on the discretion of an individual doctor. Even patients at family planning clinics faced possible charges if they were considered to be able to afford them. In such cases, the cost of the pill depended on whether the doctor deemed the contraception to be necessary on medical or social grounds. Free provision was more likely if it was prescribed on the former rather than the latter criteria.[66] In 1967 local health authorities were allowed, if they so desired, to subsidize contraception in all cases without the need to consider health reasons or economic and marital status. However, this legislation was permissive, so free provision remained uneven. In 1974 the system was radically altered when the Conservative government agreed to make all contraception free under the National Health Service.[67]

This decision to allow free contraception followed years of debate. While some opposed the free provision of contraceptives on a universal basis because they feared it would promote promiscuity, others saw it as essential to population control. For the government, however, the major consideration was cost. In order to control the tax burden, the government initially explored possibilities of limiting free contraceptives to women with medical needs or those considered socially disadvantaged. The House of Lords, however, blocked this proposal in a spectacular rebellion in 1972, demanding that the government make the service comprehensive and free to all.[68] Interestingly, the call within the House of Lords for greater provision had come from representatives from across the political spectrum, reflecting wider pressures in society as a whole. Among those canvassing for such a service, for instance, was the Church of England's Board for Social Responsibility and the Women's Institutes, whose members were, on the whole, conservative.[69]

Much of the pressure for free contraception resulted from increasing concern over population growth and the need for government intervention. Indeed, many pointed to the disparity between funding population policies abroad while not attending to the issue at home.[70] Campaigners also highlighted the fact that abortion and vasectomies had recently been made freely available under the NHS. One of the reasons put forward for making all contraception free was that it would reduce abortion. Such arguments were based on the fact that in places like Aberdeen and in a number of London boroughs abortion rates had been reduced dramatically when contraception was made available without charge. At the heart of the debate was the fear that those who most needed contraception were not getting access to it. Immigrants were cited as well as the more socially deprived members of society.[71] Many saw such provision as the means of reducing the costs of other forms of social welfare. In 1972, for instance, the Conservative Secretary of State for Health, Sir Keith Joseph, pointed to the fact that unwanted children were a major cause of poverty and juvenile delinquency. Given that at least a quarter of all births in Britain each year were thought to be unwanted, this was a problem he felt the state could ill afford. While he and many others worried about the fact that the provision of free contraception would add at least £15 million to the annual NHS budget, all believed that its benefits far outweighed the social costs involved in unwanted pregnancies.[72]

Similar arguments continued in the following years. When the Labour government proposed to introduce fees for the pill in 1998 as part of its effort to cut £50 million off the £3.5 billion annual NHS drugs bill, it was opposed on the grounds that it would encourage unwanted pregnancies.

Hostility also stemmed from a belief that it would reduce women's choice and opportunities. Anger surfaced not only among Members of Parliament but also among the public. The proposal also raised protests from family planning experts. As Ann Furedi, director of the Birth Control Trust, put it: 'A charge for the Pill would be a tax on fertility. Society as a whole has an interest in preventing unwanted pregnancies and society should pay the price by providing free contraceptive services.'[73]

The increasing priority given to contraception by the British government over the years was not unique. Similar measures were also being taken in the Netherlands. In 1971 the Dutch government legislated for contraceptives to come under the medical benefits scheme, which provided for universal free contraception. Welcomed by all, this measure marked a significant change in public and official attitudes. During the 1960s the Netherlands had been primarily a conservative society with little public discussion of sexual matters or contraception. The display and sale of contraceptives was legally restricted, for example, and as had been the case in Britain the medical community was reluctant to become involved in anything to do with contraception. In addition, in 1966 the Dutch government had opposed making the pill free on the grounds of expense.[74]

The decision to make contraception free in the Netherlands in 1971 resulted in part, as in Britain, from a growing unease about population growth. The fact that the Netherlands was one of the most densely populated nations in the developed world made this a particularly intense debate. Free contraception was also seen as the best solution to the more politically difficult question of whether to legalize abortion. While abortion was seen as a woman's right, most saw it as something that should be considered only as the very last resort. As a result, effective contraceptives, such as the pill, were given the highest priority in terms of government funding. This provision was to have an important impact on the uptake of the pill. Within ten years of its first introduction into the Netherlands, it had become the most popular contraceptive method in the country, and its usage by far the largest reported internationally (see figure 8.2, p. 213 above). By 1972 at least 28 per cent of Dutch women aged 15–49 were taking the pill. Just four years later, in 1976, this figure had risen to 42 per cent. Overall this provision was thought to have helped the Netherlands experience one of the lowest rates of abortion in the world.[75] The high uptake of the pill may also be attributed to the good sex education that was instituted in the country's schools.

Table 10.5 Government policies concerning access to contraceptive methods, 1974–1993

Year	No. of countries	Access limited (% of countries)	Access not limited (% of countries)		
			No support	Indirect support	Direct support
1974	156	7	22	15	55
1983	168	4	19	17	60
1986	170	4	11	14	72
1989	170	4	12	12	72
1993	190	2	10	7	82

Source: UN, *Levels and Trends of Contraceptive Use as Assessed in 1994* (New York, 1996), 94, table 29

Government funding of contraceptive services was not confined to Europe. Table 10.5 indicates that between 1974 and 1993 the number of countries providing access to contraception increased substantially worldwide. This was achieved through a mixture of direct and indirect government sponsorship. During the 1980s access to family planning programmes expanded in all developing regions. Between 1982 and 1989 the percentage of developing countries that made contraception readily available to at least 50 per cent of their population increased from 39 to 60 per cent. By 1993, 89 per cent of national governments worldwide reported providing direct or indirect support to family planning services, and only 2 per cent had a policy of restricting access (notably Cambodia, the Holy See and Saudia Arabia.)[76]

This increased government sponsorship of contraception around the world has not extended to all methods of contraception, however. The pill became one of the most widely accessible contraceptive methods alongside the condom in the 1990s, with many governments allowing it to be distributed through non-medical personnel. By contrast sterilization and the IUD have tended to be provided only by physicians and are therefore less accessible, except where health services are highly developed or where special efforts have been made to provide these contraceptive methods through family planning programmes.[77]

AIDS and the pill

While government sponsorship of contraceptive services may have increased access to contraception over the years, worldwide usage of the pill continues to be uneven to this day. Its adoption has been conditioned by wider social, cultural and economic considerations, some of which have been outlined above. Since the mid-1980s, however, the uptake of the oral contraceptive has been affected by a new phenomenon: HIV and AIDS. The emergence of the HIV pathogen has had a major impact on the kinds of policies adopted by family planning programmes. While the prevention of pregnancy remains an important goal, attention is increasingly being focused on how to prevent the spread of sexually transmitted diseases, seen to be an important contributor to the transmission of HIV and AIDS. Within this context the pill has come to be seen as an increasingly inappropriate contraceptive method. Ironically the popularity of condoms, which the pill largely eclipsed during the 1960s,[78] is again rising in the more developed regions of the world. While the use of condoms initially increased most among homosexual couples, who were some of the first victims of AIDS, this contraceptive method has become increasingly important for heterosexuals, with implications for the use of the oral contraceptive. Figure 10.1 above (p. 239), for instance, indicates that the prevalence of the condom was just below that of the pill for more developed nations by the early 1990s.

The switch between the pill and the condom is best illustrated in the case of the United States. Here the percentage of women of reproductive age using the pill decreased from 31 to 27 per cent between 1988 and 1995. At the same time, use of the condom rose among American women from 15 to 20 per cent. Such a shift towards the condom came within two years of the General Surgeon of the United States publicly advising people to use this contraceptive to safeguard against HIV. The largest decrease in pill uptake and rise in condom use occurred among the 'never married' category of women. In this category use of the pill decreased from 59 to 44 per cent among teenagers and from 68 to 52 per cent among those aged between 20 and 24. Women in these categories showed an increasing propensity to use the condom in these years; the percentage of women aged 20 to 24 using it, for instance, grew from 20 to 30 per cent in the years between 1988 and 1995. Such shifts among teenagers and women in their early twenties is particularly striking given that it had been precisely these age-groups which had been most enthusiastic in embracing the oral con- traceptive in earlier decades. By contrast, married women showed much less of a switch from the pill to condom during the same years. It would therefore seem that the condom became the contraceptive of choice for those who were not in a stable relationship, unlike in the 1960s, when the pill became the method of choice for the free and single.[79]

It would be a mistake, however, to ascribe the shift away from the pill only to a rise in fears about HIV infection. In the United States use of the oral contraceptive had already begun to plummet in the mid-1970s when its associations with thrombosis and later possible links with breast and cervical cancer were announced.[80] Between 1973 and 1982, for instance, the percentage of currently married American women aged 15–44 using oral contraceptives fell from 25 to 13 per cent. This decline coincided with a dramatic increase in contraceptive sterilization. Between 1965 and 1975 the number of American couples resorting to voluntary sterilization tripled, and by 1988 sterilization had become the most common method of family planning, with over 10 million relying on it.[81] Such a switch from the pill to sterilization was not immediate, however. The vast majority of Americans who quit the pill between 1973 and 1982 initially turned to other non-permanent techniques. Not only did the condom regain its popularity, so did the diaphragm. Much of the decline in the use of the pill during these years was driven not by the attractiveness of other methods, but because of the perceived disadvantages of the oral contraceptive as a result of the publicized health reports. Significantly the number of pill users increased slightly in the United States during the late 1980s, when benefits of the pill began to be published, although it never regained the popularity it enjoyed in the 1960s.[82]

The patterns observed for the United States are not unique. In Britain the pill has also become a less popular method of contraception. Its decline in this country, however, has not been as dramatic as in the United States. Indeed the number of women taking the oral contraceptive in Britain remained high until the 1980s. Nonetheless, even here there was a significant decline in the wake of the news about its possible carcinogenic effects, most noticeably in 1977 and again in 1983.[83] Part of the trend away from pill use in Britain can be gauged from statistics collected from those attending family planning clinics in England. While the pill was one of the most common contraceptive methods from 1975, the proportion using it declined between 1965 to 1998 from 70 to 44 per cent.[84] By contrast the percentage using the condom rose from just 6 per cent in 1975 to 36 per cent in 1997–8. The shift towards the condom can be partly accounted for by government campaigns to promote safer sex after the mid-1980s.[85] Nonetheless, as in the United States the shift was also due to increasing disillusion with the pill, and the adoption of the condom was not immediate. Many British women initially turned towards other reversible methods such as the IUD, and began to choose sterilization on an unprecedented scale from the mid-1970s.[86]

In both the United States and Britain, it would therefore seem that the advent of HIV merely reinforced, rather than initiated, a decline in the use of the pill. Moreover it would be a mistake to argue that the issue had made oral contraceptives totally redundant. While HIV in the developed world has increasingly focused attention on the need to prevent sexually transmitted disease, the prevention of pregnancy remains a high priority for policy-makers. Part of this stems from the increasingly young age at which people are having sexual intercourse, and the rise in 'unwanted' births and abortions among teenage women in both Britain and the United States since the 1970s.[87] Within this context policy-makers have urged young unmarried people to use both the condom and the pill simultaneously.[88] What is important, however, is that the oral contraceptive is no longer seen as adequate protection. Illustration 17 captures the new message that family planning programmes in Canada promoted in the 1990s.

The current re-emergence of the condom is particularly interesting when viewed in relation to changes in the balance of power between women and men over contraception. One of the reasons that many women turned to the pill in its early days was because it represented a means of female control. This contrasted with previous methods of contraception, which had always necessitated some form of cooperation from the male partner. Adoption of the pill, however, has not always freed women. Indeed to some extent, it shifted the burden of the responsibility for contraception on to them. Moreover, it could be argued that the hidden nature of the oral contraceptive and the fact that it was taken at a time separate from intercourse meant that sexual intercourse could be pursued without any overt discussion of contraception between men and women. The AIDS epidemic, however, has transformed this situation. One of the important consequences of the disease is the way it can increase distrust between couples about their previous sexual liaisons and their HIV status. Yet while AIDS may have made some couples more distrustful of each other, it can also be argued that it has cultivated a greater awareness of the need to use a contraceptive such as the condom at the time of intercourse. The appearance of AIDS has therefore not only changed the types of contraceptive methods deployed, but has also necessitated much more explicit discussion about them than was the case in respect of the pill. This is apparent not only in the discussions taking place among individual couples, but also in the public arena, where politicians who were initially hesitant in talking about sex and contraception have been forced to debate such matters.[89]

Overall it can be argued that the public's increasing willingness to discuss sex and contraception since the AIDS epidemic is merely an extension of the sexual revolution of which the pill was a part. Nonetheless, this was not always a straightforwardly linear history. In some countries, such as Japan, public discussion about sexual matters did not occur when the pill began to be debated by the government in the 1960s, and only started in earnest with the arrival of HIV. Moreover, it cannot be assumed that the mere appearance of either the pill or AIDS has necessarily resulted in increasingly frank debates about sex and contraception everywhere. Nowhere is this more apparent than in parts of Africa, where governments were initially very reluctant to discuss AIDS or promote the condom.

Much depends on the power relationship between men and women, as well as overall cultural attitudes and the policies of individual governments over sexual matters and how to deal with disease and fertility control. While the AIDS epidemic may have rendered these issues more important than they were in the past, this has not resulted in the universal adoption of the condom. Like the pill the condom confronts major cultural barriers in its acceptance. This is most striking in Africa, where the spread of HIV and AIDS makes the question particularly acute. Here issues of male sexuality and reluctance to use condoms are major obstacles to safe sex and women are often powerless when negotiating sexual relations. Interestingly, women often resort to the pill and injectable hormones, which do not necessitate discussion with a partner and can be hidden more easily than other contraceptives. In sub-Saharan Africa, for instance, at least 27 per cent of those using any contraceptive method in 1994 used the pill, the most popular method, and 17 per cent used injectable hormones, the second most popular method. By contrast the condom was one of the least favoured contraceptives, accounting for only 4 per cent of all use.[90]

The prevalence of the pill in Africa, where HIV/AIDS is taking a very heavy toll on the population and the economy, raises important questions about whether it plays a part in the transmission of the disease. In 1987 a study of 115 sex workers in Nairobi showed that oral contraceptives could be helping to promote the spread of HIV. Some investigators feared that the contraceptive may have lowered the women's overall immunity to disease and thereby raised their susceptibility to HIV infection. Subsequent research in Rwanda, Zambia, Zaire and the United States did not endorse these conclusions, however. Much of the controversy over oral contraceptives and whether they contribute to the spread of HIV hinges on the fact that oral contraceptives can increase the size of the cervix, thus enlarging the area potentially susceptible to HIV infection. Others argue that the pill may in fact protect women because it can thicken cervical mucous, thus keeping the virus away from the upper reproductive tract. Concerns also focus on the fact that oral contraceptive use may increase the risk of sexually transmitted diseases, which are known to increase vulnerability to HIV infection. Women taking the pill, for instance, are more likely to get cervical infections than non-users. However, such infections are not known to be especially linked to HIV. Sexually transmitted diseases which are more closely associated with HIV are those which produce genital ulcers, such as syphilis and genital herpes, which are not usually linked with oral contraceptive use.[91]

Conclusion

While the debate continues as to whether oral contraceptives affect the spread of HIV, the rise of AIDS and the devastation it is causing around the globe will continue to raise questions about whether the pill remains an appropriate technique of contraception. The spread of HIV, however, will not be the only factor to influence the debate. As we have seen in this chapter, cultural attitudes towards contraception, as well as social, economic and religious factors, will continue to shape perceptions and access to oral contraceptives. Moreover, consumption of the pill will remain highly variable around the world. Much will depend on an individual woman's situation: where she lives, the types of health care and contraceptive services available, the nature of her sexual relationships, her age, whether or not she has children and how many, and how her body reacts to the medication. By 1990, for instance, there was a clear distinction between developed and developing nations in terms of the conjugal status of those taking the pill. While 95 per cent of all pill users in developing nations were either married or co-habiting, in the developing world such unions constituted only 61 per cent of the total.[92] Such a difference in conjugal status highlights the very different cultural issues surrounding sex and contraception in the developed and developing world and the intricate ways in which they determine the acceptance and use of the pill. Moreover, the history of the pill over the past four decades suggests that it will never be the universal panacea originally envisioned by its makers.

Bibliographical Abbreviations

AG-FCL	Alan Guttmacher's papers, Francis Countway Library, Boston
AJOG	*American Journal of Obstetrics and Gynecology*
AM	Archives and Manuscripts, Wellcome Library for the History and Understanding of Medicine, London
AMA	American Medical Association
AS-FCL	Abraham Stone's papers, Francis Countway Library, Boston
BMJ	*British Medical Journal*
CASH	Cancer and Steroid Hormone Study of the Centers for Disease Control
CG-FCL	Clarence Gamble's papers, Francis Countway Library, Boston
CIFC	Council for the Investigation of Fertility Control
CSD	Committee on Safety of Drugs (UK)
CSM	Committee on Safety of Medicines (UK)
FDA	Food and Drug Administration (US)
FPA	Family Planning Association (UK)
GP-LC	Gregory Pincus's papers, Library of Congress
IPPF	International Planned Parenthood Federation
JAMA	*Journal of the American Medical Association*
JDR III collection	John Rockefeller III's papers, Rockefeller Archive
JNCI	*Journal of the National Cancer Institute*
JR-FCL	John Rock's papers, Francis Countway Library, Boston
MRC	Medical Research Council (UK)
MS-LC	Margaret Sanger's papers, Library of Congress
MS-SS	Margaret Sanger's papers, Sophia Smith Collection, Smith College, Northampton, Mass.
Nelson hearings	US Congress, Senate, *Competitive Problems in the Drug Industry: Hearings before the Subcommittee on Monopoly of the Select Committee on Small Business, US Senate, 91st Congress, Second Session, on Present Status of Competition in the Pharmaceutical Industry*, parts 15–17, Jan.–Mar. 1970
NHS	National Health Service (UK)
OBT	Oliver Bird Trust
PPFA	Planned Parenthood Federation of America
PRO	Public Record Office (UK)

RCGP	Royal College of General Practitioners (UK)
SA/FPA	Papers of the Family Planning Association (UK) at the Archives and Manuscripts, Wellcome Library for the History and Understanding of Medicine, London
SIDA	Swedish International Development Authority
UN	United Nations
UNESCO	United Nations Educational, Scientific and Cultural Organization
UNICEF	United Nations Children's Fund
USAID	United States Agency for International Development
WHO	World Health Organization
WPEC	World Population Emergency Campaign

Notes

Introduction

1 'Oral contraceptives – 50 million users', *Population Report*, Series A, no. 1 (Apr. 1974), table 1, A-4.
2 Ibid., A-2, A-17; 'Lower-dose pills', *Population Report*, Series A, no. 7 (Nov. 1988), 8.
3 G. Guillebaud, 'Introduction', in J. Guillebaud, *The Pill* (Oxford, 1991), 3.
4 H. Lewin to A. Guttmacher, 22 July 1966, Population Council papers, Box 124, Rockefeller Archive.
5 Cited in L. McLaughlin, *The Pill, John Rock, and the Catholic Church* (Boston, 1982), 141.
6 F. D. Moore, 'Ethical boundaries in initial clinical trials', in P. A. Freund, ed., *Experimentation with Human Subjects* (New York, 1970), 363; Boston Women's Health Collective, *Our Bodies, Ourselves* (Boston, 1984); L. Grant, *Sexing the Millennium* (London, 1993), 54; B. Hartmann, *Reproductive Rights and Wrongs* (Boston, 1995), 190.
7 Letter from Irwin C. Winter, *JAMA*, 212/6 (11 May 1970), 1067–8. See also B. Asbell, *The Pill* (New York, 1995), 163–4; McLaughlin, *The Pill*, 139.
8 P. Galewitz, '"The pill" might prevent acne too', 30 Jan. 2000, Associated Press, Yahoo, http://biz.com.apf/000130/the_pill_3.html. The market advantage of expanding the medical conditions is not unique to the pill. The same was the case with aspirin, where pharmaceutical companies profited greatly from the discovery that it could be used to reduce heart problems. See C. C. Mann and M. L. Plummer, *The Aspirin Wars* (New York, 1991).
9 Galewitz, '"The pill" might prevent acne too'.
10 McLaughlin, *The Pill*, 136.
11 Mrs C. to G. Pincus, 31 Oct. 1957, GP-LC, cited in E. Watkins, *On the Pill* (Baltimore, 1998), 50.
12 Mr and Mrs H. to G. Pincus, 27 Oct. 1960, GP-LC, cited in Watkins, *On the Pill*, 50.
13 Mrs A. to G. Pincus, 28 June 1957, GP-LC, cited in Watkins, *On the Pill*, 147.
14 William L. Searle to US and Canadian Searlemen, divisional sales managers, and regional sales managers, 9 Aug. 1962, repr. in US Senate, *Hearings on Competitive Problems in the Drug Industry*, 6273, cited in Watkins, *On the Pill*, 51.

15 Watkins, *On the Pill*, 50–1.

16 Guillebaud, *The Pill*, 20.

17 E. Wilmsen, *Journeys with Flies* (Chicago, 1999), 127–8.

18 UN, *Levels and Trends of Contraceptive Use as Assessed in 1994* (New York, 1996), 56, 99, 100.

19 McLaughlin, *The Pill*, 140–4.

20 This attitude is captured in a statement by Oscar Hechter, who wrote shortly after the death of his friend Gregory Pincus:

> Pincus for me represents the prototype of a *new* scientist, whose life and achievements merit critical examination and analysis. On a planet rapidly being irreversibly transformed by science and technology in ways not clearly foreseen, we desperately need information about the mechanisms by which individual scientists change the world. Pincus and his life merit a critical case study, because if new Pincuses arise in the future, they will have a powerful impact upon the world. ... To oversimplify, some scientists become great by making important contributions to knowledge – discovery in the laboratory – and others become great as organizers and by making important applications of knowledge. Gregory Pincus, a scientist-statesman, was one of the latter. (O. Hechter, 'Homage to Gregory Pincus', *Perspectives in Biology and Medicine* (Spring 1968), cited in Asbell, *The Pill*, 319).

The importance of the use of 'father' is epitomized by the gravestone of Pincus's co-worker, Min Chueh Chang, which reads 'M.C. Chang, The Father of the Birth Control Pill' (Asbell, *The Pill*, 324). Engraved on the instructions of his wife, this inscription could be seen as making up for the fact that during his lifetime Chang had felt that his part in the pill had been underplayed. The idea of fathering the pill has been used in many ways to describe these scientists' role in the making of the pill. This is discussed in McLaughlin, *The Pill*, 93.

21 By using mother rather than father of the pill, Djerassi claims to be trying to challenge the patriarchal attitudes of society. C. Djerassi, 'The mother of the pill', *Recent Progress in Hormone Research*, 50 (1995), 1–18. Inside the dustjacket of one of his biographies he is described as the 'father of the pill'. See the dustcover of his *The Pill, Pygmy Chimps and Degas' Horse* (New York, 1992).

22 Subsequent scholars have adopted this approach. A survey undertaken by the National Science Foundation in 1967, for instance, summarizing the different scientific disciplines which went into the making of the pill, asserts the importance of individual scientists. One of the diagrams accompanying the survey highlights the part of individual scientists involved in the physiology of reproduction, hormone research and steroid chemistry, leading to the development of the pill. In this diagram the predominant names associated with the research are male. National Science Foundation, *Technology in Retrospect and Critical Events in Science*, vol.1 (15 Dec. 1968) and vol. 2 (30 Jan. 1969).

23 A. Biezanek, *All Things New* (New York, 1965). Anne Greene Biezanek, born into a Quaker family and educated in Aberdeen and at Oxford University, was an English medical doctor who converted to Catholicism when she married a Polish ex-army officer. After seven pregnancies, two of which had resulted in miscarriage, she was faced with the insurmountable difficulty of reconciling the teachings of her new-found church with the sexual demands of her husband and the financial needs of her family, and decided to take the pill. She is best known for her protest against the fact that women were unable to go to communion if they openly confessed to taking the pill. She also set up one of the first Catholic family planning clinics in

Britain in 1963, and published *All Things New* in 1965, a book which challenged the church's doctrine on contraception and provoked major debate within the Catholic establishment. For more information on Biezanek, see Asbell, *The Pill*, ch. 14.

24 For the ways journalists used this argument during the late 1960s, and how subsequent writers took the same line, see M. Mintz, 'The pill, press and public at the experts' mercy', *Columbia Journalism Review* (Winter 1968–9), 4–10; B. Seaman *The Doctors' Case against the Pill* (Alameda, Calif., 1995), 186; Statement by Washington Women's Liberation, cited in Nelson hearings, (vol. 3, part 16, 6470–1, and part 17, 7283–4; Boston Women's Health Collective, *Our Bodies, Ourselves* (Boston, 1984).

25 For the historical inaccuracy of such arguments, see S. W. Junod and L. V. Marks, 'Women on trial', forthcoming.

26 A. Clarke, 'Controversy and the development of reproductive sciences', *Social Problems*, 37 (1990), 18–37.

1 The Population Problem and the Pill

1 M. Sanger to K. McCormick, 27 Oct. 1950, MS-SS, cited in P. Vaughan, *The Pill on Trial* (Harmondsworth, 1972), 27.

2 *Planned Parenthood News*, no. 8 (Summer 1954), JR-FCL; J. Rock, *The Time has Come* (London, 1963), 18. Similar views were expressed by a number of other family planning activists. See for instance W. Vogt, *The Road to Survival* (New York, 1948), 280. In 1951, Robert Cook, who was later to become president of the Population Bureau, which was a major supplier of information to the US government economic aid programme, wrote that government funding of contraceptive research 'might cost no more than one destroyer; should it cost as much as an aircraft carrier, it would be one of the great research bargains of all time. It would offer mankind a good deal more promise of security than the atomic bomb or any worldwide agreement to "outlaw" war' (*Human Fertility* (New York, 1951), 296–7).

3 For the complexities of this issue, see D. Grigg, *The World Food Problem* (Oxford, 1993), ch. 4.

4 Mrs Harry Guthman to M. Sanger, 26 Jan. 1950, MS-SS, correspondence files.

5 Ibid. This theme continued in later years. Dr Edris Rice-Wray, for instance, who conduced the first large-scale clinical trials of the pill, argued in 1962, 'Unless population growth can be restrained, we may have to abandon for this generation, our hopes of economic progress in the crowded lands of Asia, Africa, and the Middle East' (E. Rice-Wray, 'Practical approach to the establishment of planned parenthood services in rural and urban areas', paper presented to the Joint Meeting of the Royal Swedish Endocrine Society and Swedish Gynecology Society, 9 Mar. 1962, 15, GP-LC, Box 55).

6 J. Rock, lecture to PPFA meeting, 1954, untitled MS, 5–6, JR-FCL. Similar sentiments are expressed in a letter from Mrs Raymond Ingersoll to Clara Higgins, 19 Oct. 1956, GP-LC, Box 23. The letter was aimed at obtaining support for the research just initiated for the development of an oral contraceptive.

7 T. Malthus, *An Essay on the Principle of Population* (London, 1798), 123–4, cited in A. Sen, 'Population and reasoned agency: food, fertility, and economic development', in K. Lindahl-Kiessling and H. Landberg, eds, *Population, Economic*

Development and the Environment (Oxford, 1994), 52–5. Malthus was Professor of Political Economy in the East India Company's college at Haileybury from 1805 to 1834, a place which inspired many British officials and scholars to study population issues in India within the context of Malthusian ideas. See J. Caldwell and P. Caldwell, *Limiting Population Growth and the Ford Foundation Contribution* (London, 1986), 4.

8 M. J. A. N. Condorcet, *Sketch for a Historical Picture of the Progress of the Human Mind* (1795), 187, cited in Sen, 'Population and reasoned agency'. Sen provides an important analysis of Malthus and Condorcet and their relevance for today's debates on population. See also A. Sen, 'Population', *New York Review of Books*, 22 Sept. 1992, 1–7.

9 For detail of the ways in which Malthus's ideas influenced later debates, particularly among demographers, see Caldwell and Caldwell, *Limiting Population Growth*, ch. 1.

10 Between 1800 and 1914 France changed from being one of the most densely populated countries in Europe to ranking the fifth. The birth-rate dropped from 26 per thousand in 1870 to 12 in 1918. For more information see A. Cova, 'French feminism and maternity', in G. Bock and P. Thane, eds, *Maternity and Gender Policies* (London, 1991), 119.

11 For the French preoccupation with depopulation see Cova, 'French feminism', and K. Offen, 'Body politics', in Bock and Thane, *Maternity and Gender Policies*, 138–59. For the British obsession with the question, see, A. Davin, 'Imperialism and motherhood', *History Workshop Journal*, 5 (1978), 9–66, and R. A. Soloway, *Demography and Degeneration* (London, 1995), xviii.

12 Soloway, *Demography and Degeneration*, 10–11; D. Kevles, *In the Name of Eugenics* (Los Angeles, 1985).

13 J. Macnicol, 'Eugenics and the campaign for voluntary sterilization in Britain between the wars', *Social History of Medicine*, 2/2 (Aug. 1989), 147–70.

14 Much has been written on the history of eugenics. For a general introduction to eugenics and the influence of evolutionary theory on scientific thought, see Kevles, *In the Name of Eugenics*, 85–112; S. J. Gould, *The Mismeasure of Man* (London, 1992), chs 3 and 4; N. Stepan, *The Hour of Eugenics* (Ithaca, 1991) . For the later application of eugenics in medical policy, see R. Proctor, *Racial Hygiene* (Cambridge, Mass., 1989), 177–222; S. Kuhl, *The Nazi Connection* (Oxford, 1994); and G. Bock, 'Antinatalism, maternity and paternity in National Socialist racism', in Bock and Thane, *Maternity and Gender Policies*, 233–55. See also C. Usbourne, *The Politics of the Body in Weimar Germany* (London, 1992), 4–5. For a detailed history of both the eugenic and neo-Malthusian movements in Britain, see Soloway, *Demography and Degeneration*.

15 Among the intellectuals strongly influenced by the eugenics movement were Julian Huxley, Lionel Penrose and C. P. Blacker in England, and Henry F. Osborn, Frederick Osborn, Robert Cook and Raymond Pearl in the United States. See Caldwell and Caldwell, *Limiting Population Growth*, 7.

16 Ann-Sofie Ohlander, 'The invisible child?', in Bock and Thane, *Maternity and Gender Policies*, 68–9; Offen, 'Body politics', 150.

17 For more on the ways in which this was pursued in various countries around Europe see further articles in Bock and Thane, *Maternity and Gender Policies*.

18 For the strengthening of punishment for abortion in France in the 1920s, see Offen, 'Body politics', 138.

19 Ibid., 139–40; J. Stepan and E. H. Kellogg, *The World's Laws on Contraceptives* (Medford, Mass., 1974), 16.

20 M. Nash, 'Pronatalism and motherhood in Franco's Spain', in Bock and Thane, *Maternity and Gender Policies*, 160–77. In a number of countries, notably Catholic countries such as Italy, France and Spain, the restrictions on contraception continued well into the 1970s.

21 Bock, 'Antinatalism, maternity and paternity', 240.

22 Kevles, *In the Name of Eugenics*, 100. Similar measures were also undertaken in Switzerland, see P. Ehrenstrom, 'Eugenics and the law in Switzerland', *Galton Institute Newsletter* (Sept. 1997), 4–5.

23 B. Hartmann, *Reproductive Rights and Wrongs* (Boston, 1995), 98–9; see also Kuhl, *The Nazi Connection*, and Kevles, *In the Name of Eugenics*.

24 M. Zaremba, 'A victim of the record-years', *Dagens Nyheter* (27 Sept. 1997); I. Blom, 'Voluntary motherhood 1900–1930', in Bock and Thane, *Maternity and Gender Policies*, 62.

25 Kevles, *In the Name of Eugenics*, 117, 118; Bock, 'Antinatalism, maternity and paternity'.

26 Kevles, *In the Name of Eugenics*, 118.

27 Gordon argues that the alliances between feminist advocates of birth control, such as Sanger, and the neo-Malthusians and eugenicists often resulted in the subordination of women's rights (L. Gordon, *Woman's Body, Woman's Right* (New York, 1976), 395–7). McCann, however, argues that such alliances were made with the explicit purpose of gaining scientific credibility for the cause of contraception in order to legitimate the social and economic justifications for using it, as well as to challenge medical authority and dissociate birth control from sexual controversy (C. R. McCann, *Birth Control Politics in the United States* (Ithaca, 1994), 19).

28 M. Sanger to K. McCormick, 27 Oct. 1950. Sanger is cited in B. Seaman and G. Seaman, *Women and the Crisis in Sex Hormones* (New York, 1977), 79; B. Asbell, *The Pill* (New York, 1995), 9; L. Gordon, 'Birth control and the eugenicists', cited in Hartmann, *Reproductive Rights and Wrongs*, 99. See also C. Usbourne, *The Politics of the Body in Weimar Germany* (London, 1992), 4–5; Kevles, *In the Name of Eugenics*, 12; E. Chesler, *Woman of Valor* (New York, 1992); Gordon, *Woman's Body, Woman's Right*; D. M. Kennedy, *Birth Control in America* (New Haven, 1970); L. Lader, *The Margaret Sanger Story and the Fight for Birth Control* (New York, 1955).

29 Gordon is highly critical of Sanger's alliance with eugenicists, seeing it as undermining her ability to increase women's powers (Gordon, *Woman's Body, Woman's Right*, 395–7). For a challenge to this argument see McCann, *Birth Control Politics*, 19. Women's support of eugenics was not confined to the United States. Some British women were also attracted to eugenic ideas, seeing its call for selective reproduction as a validation of motherhood and a means of raising the status of women. See L. Bland, *Banishing the Beast* (London, 1995), 230–5 and L. Hall, 'Women, feminism and eugenics', in R. Peel, ed., *Essays in the History of Eugenics* (London, 1998), 36–51.

30 Macnicol, 'Eugenics and the campaign for voluntary sterilization'.

31 Gordon, *Woman's Body, Woman's Right*, 345.

32 This is discussed in detail in ibid.

33 'The contribution of birth control to preparedness', draft statement by C. M. Smith,

11 June 1940, in PPFA archives, cited in Gordon, *Woman's Body, Woman's Right*, 350.

34 E. Tyler May, *Homeward Bound* (New York, 1988), ch. 4. Tyler points out that the nuclear family was built on an ideal family size and demanded traditional gender relations within marriage. See also N. Pfeffer, *The Stork and the Syringe* (Oxford, 1993), 20.

35 J. Rock, lecture to PPFA meeting, 1954.

36 Caldwell and Caldwell, *Limiting Population Growth*, 21–4.

37 Rock, lecture to PPFA meeting, 1954.

38 Articles from the *New York Times* and *Harpers* from 1954 onwards illustrate this fear. See also Caldwell and Caldwell, *Limiting Population Growth*, 20–1; and J. Reed, *The Birth Control Movement and American Society* (Princeton, 1984), ch. 21.

39 R. Coughlan, 'Control challenge', *Life*, 21 Nov. 1959, 159–76. A detailed account of the links between population growth and the threat of communism appears in R. Courey, 'Participants in the development, marketing and safety evaluation of the oral contraceptive, 1950–1965', Ph.D thesis, University of California, Berkeley, 1994, see esp. 124–35.

40 J. Rock, 'Keynote address to Symposium on Progestogen-Estrogen Compounds', *Applied Therapeutics*, 6/5 (May 1964), 406–9.

41 For more information on this issue see Gordon, *Woman's Body, Woman's Right*, 391–5; Reed, *The Birth Control Movement*, ch. 21.

42 Reed, *The Birth Control Movement*, 282–3.

43 From a letter from Lammont DuPont Copeland to G. Pincus, 3 Mar. 1960, 'C. 1960', GP-LC, Box 42. See also Courey, 'Participants', 136, 170–8.

44 Cited in *Lancet* (2 Feb. 1955); see also *Second Reading of Colonial Development and Welfare Bill Parliamentary Debates*, House of Commons, 2 Feb. 1955, 1151–8.

45 Renton's letter of 15 Nov. 1966, in *The Population Problem: Correspondence between the Prime Minister the Rt. Hon. Harold Wilson MP and Rt. Hon. Sir David Renton MP* (Huntington, 1967), 1. Such views continued into the following years. See 'Doctors concern re overpopulation', *Lancet* (8 Jan. 1972), 81–2, 89–90.

46 The Rockefeller family set up the foundation with the money they had accumulated from oil. The Scripps Foundation for Research in Population Problems was founded by Edward Scripps, the newspaper publisher, with help from the Laura Spelman Rockefeller Memorial, a branch of the Rockefeller Foundation. The Milbank Memorial Fund was one of the oldest foundations in the United States, dating back to 1905 when it began to sponsor work in public health. Early on it began to see birth control and the work carried out by Margaret Sanger as a key component of its public health policies. For more detailed information on these organizations and their sponsorship of research into population questions see O. Harkavy, *Curbing Population Growth* (New York, 1995), ch. 1. See also Reed, *The Birth Control Movement*, ch. 21 and Caldwell and Caldwell, *Limiting Population Growth*, 9–13.

47 This was funded by the Carnegie Corporation through the Milbank Memorial Fund.

48 S. Szreter, 'The ideas of demographic transition and the study of fertility change', *Population and Development Review*, 19/4 (Dec. 1993), 659–701, at 661–3, 668; Caldwell and Caldwell, *Limiting Population Growth*, 12.

49 Ibid.

50 E. Watkins, *On the Pill* (Baltimore, 1998), 17.

51 The explicit objective of the IPPF was to 'convert people and their governments to an acceptance of the need to persuade humanity to regulate its fertility in a fully responsible manner in the interests of individual families and mankind', see C. Deverell, 'The International Planned Parenthood Federation', *Demography*, 5/2 (1968), special issue, 574.

52 Gordon, *Woman's Body, Woman's Right*, 396; Reed, *The Birth Control Movement*, 282; Harkavy, *Curbing Population Growth*, chs 1 and 2.

53 Harkavy, *Curbing Population Growth*, 25.

54 *The Population Bomb*, pamphlet published by the Hugh Moore Fund, 20, kept in GP-LC, Box 28.

55 Cited in Reed, *The Birth Control Movement*, 426.

56 Hugh Moore had originally set up the Moore Fund in 1944 to promote world peace, see Reed, *The Birth Control Movement*, 303, and Harkavy, *Curbing Population Growth*, 35. For the antagonism of family planning activists to Moore's stand, see Chesler, *Woman of Valor*, 439. Moore was later instrumental in family planning legislation passed by the Nixon administration in 1970, which increased financial support for family planning, specifically making it freely available for the mentally ill, medically indigent, Cuban refugees, Native Americans, Alaskan natives and migrant workers and their families; see D. Critchlow, *Intended Consequences*, (Oxford, 1999) 93–4.

57 P. Piotrow, *World Population Crisis* (New York, 1973), 37–8.

58 Draper had been an economic adviser for the US occupation of Germany and had directed the European Recovery Program (Marshall Plan). Immediately prior to chairing the President's Committee, Draper was chairman of the Mexican Light and Power Company, which was seen as giving him expertise in the developing world. Others sitting on the committee included key military and industrial experts who had little interest in population questions. Harkavy, *Curbing Population Growth*, 34–5, and see also Courey, 'Participants', 137–40. Massive technical assistance was begun in Europe under the Marshall Plan of 1948–53. By the 1950s, however, similar strategies were being used in the provision of development to Third World countries. India played a major role in stimulating this policy. For more detail see Caldwell and Caldwell, *Limiting Population Growth*, 20–1.

59 Part of this was drawn from his experiences in Japan, which made Draper link Japan's economic recovery with its drastic reduction in fertility. He contrasted Japan's success with the impoverishment of other Asian countries, which continued to have rapid population growth; see Draper to F. W. Brown, 27 Dec. 1963, AG-FCL, Box 2.

60 The ultimate recommendation of the committee, however, was reworded to provide 'maternal and child welfare' aid. This wording was seen as less offensive to the Catholic church. Some committee members were themselves hostile towards American funding of birth control. General Gruenther, a prominent Catholic, refused to sign the committee's report if its recommendations were objectionable to the Catholic church. Testimony of W. H. Draper Jr before the Monopoly Subcommittee of the Senate Small Business Committee, 3 Mar. 1970, AG-FCL, Box 2; see also Harkavy, *Curbing Population Growth*, 36.

61 'An appeal to the President of the United States: Birth control must go with foreign aid', *Reader's Digest*, Sept. 1963, GP-LC, Box 62.

62 'Population profile', Population Reference Bureau, 22 July 1965, p.3, GP-LC, Box 89.

63 Up to 1968 the Ford Foundation was spending at least twice as much as the US government on population initiatives. For more information on spending patterns and Lyndon Johnson's support of population policies, see Harkavy, *Curbing Population Growth*, 34–7, 41, 53.

64 Critchlow, *Intended Consequences*, 51, 83–4.

65 For detailed information on the government's spending on fertility-related research in the 1960s and 1970s, see *Population and the American Future: The Report of The Commission on Population Growth and the American Future* (New York, 1972), 181–2; see also R. T. Ravenholt, 'The A.I.D. population and family planning program', *Demography*, 52 (1968), 561–73, special issue, ed. D. J. Bogue.

66 One of the reasons that Bird was interested in contraception stemmed from the sexual difficulties he had experienced when on honeymoon when he discovered his wife to have 'such a tough hymen' it 'was most difficult to penetrate'. During his life he had also faced the problem of premature ejaculation. Because of these experiences he felt it vital that people have access to good medical care and guidance on sexual matters, including contraception. See Oliver Bird to M. Pyke, 12 Mar. 1958, SA/FPA/A5/130, Box 246, AM).

67 Between 1900 and 1946 Oliver Bird was director of his family's company, the food firm Alfred Bird and Sons Ltd. He had been a Conservative MP for Wolverhampton West. Bird was able to finance the project by selling his oil shares in Trinidad. See obituaries in *Birmingham Post* (19 Apr. 1963); *Manchester Guardian* (12 June 1963); *Solihull, Warwick News*, n.d.; M. Pyke to OB, July 9 1956; all in SA/FPA/A5/130, Box 246; and Notes for Dr Parkes' visit to Captain Bird, 13 Feb. 1957, SA/FPA/127, Box 245, AM.

68 Deed of declaration of trust between Margaret Amy Pyke and Judith Anne Burrell and Dr Alan Stirling Parkes, 1957, SA/FPA/A5/126, AM.

69 CIFC material, SA/FPA/A5/126, Box 245, AM.

70 General Secretary to Oliver Bird, 31 Aug. 1959, SA/FPA/A5/130, Box 246, AM.

71 C. Deverell, Secretary-General to Regional Secretaries, IPPF, 4 Aug. 1964, GP-LC, Box 76.

72 Harkavy, *Curbing Population Growth*, 50-8.

73 S. L. Sayer and J. J. Bausch, *Towards Safe, Convenient and Effective Contraceptives*, Population Council (New York, 1978), 40.

74 Hartmann, *Reproductive Rights and Wrongs*, 175.

75 Critchlow, *Intended Consequences*, 79.

76 S. P. Johnson, *World Population and the United Nations* (Cambridge, 1987), 9–11; R. M. Salas, *International Population Assistance* (New York, 1979), xv–xvii.

77 Quoted in K. Sax, 'The world's exploding population', *Perspectives in Biology and Medicine*, 7 (1963), 326–7, cited in Courey, 'Participants', 58–9. See also E. Rice-Wray to G. Pincus, 10 Aug. 1958, GP-LC, Box 34; Stephen D. Mumford, 'The Vatican and world population policy', http://www.kzpg.com/Lib/Pages/Books/NSSM-200/29-APP3.html.

78 Courey, 'Participants', 58.

79 'Population profile', 1–2. Eisenhower, however, privately supported Draper's conclusions, see Eisenhower to Richard Nixon, President of the Senate, and Sam Rayburn, Speaker of the House, 24 June 1959, in *Composite Report of the President's Committee to Study the United States Military Assistance Program, Vol. 1* (Washington DC, 17 Aug 1959), 56.

80 Piotrow, *World Population Crisis*, 43.

81 *New York Times*, 13 Feb. 1950, 1. For the outcry against MacArthur's action, see in MS-SS: Mr and Mrs T. A. Styles to M. Sanger, 13 Feb. 1950; H. Bosworth to M. Sanger, 15 Feb. 1950; Mrs J. H. Edgar to M. Sanger, 15 Feb. 1950; H. Haken to M. Sanger, 17 Feb. 1950; H. C. Cooper to M. Sanger, 18 Feb. 1950; G. Bromley Oxnam to D. Loth, 28 Feb. 1950; M. Sanger to Bess, 28 Feb. 1950; F. Y. Amano to M. Sanger, 15 Mar. 1950.

82 General D. MacArthur to Bosworth, 6 Apr. 1950; M. Sanger to S. I. Kato, 26 Apr. 1950; in MS-SS.

83 Chesler, *Woman of Valor*, 422.

84 Reed, *The Birth Control Movement*, 286; see also Frederick Osborn to Fairfield Osborn, 14 Jan. 1953, JDR III collection, Box 44, Fo. Population-General, Rockefeller Archive.

85 *Lancet* (1 Jan. 1955) and (2 Feb. 1955).

86 Piotrow, *World Population Crisis*, 45.

87 Reed, *The Birth Control Movement*, 285.

88 Ibid., 286; Harkavy, *Curbing Population Growth*, 11, 33; Gordon, *Woman's Body, Woman's Right*, 360.

89 Reed, *The Birth Control Movement*, 286.

90 About a hundred academics lost their jobs, and several hundred more probably suffered discrimination as a result of the McCarthy crusade. For more information on McCarthyism and how it affected academics and others in the USA in the 1940s and 1950s see E. Schrecker, *The Age of McCarthyism* (Boston, 1994), 82–4.

91 The laws were called after Anthony Comstock, founder of the New York Society for the Suppression of Vice. Technically contraception was forbidden in Massachusetts, Wisconsin, Philadelphia and the Dakotas. For more information on Comstock and his legacy see V. L. Bullough, *Science in the Bedroom* (New York, 1994), 52–3, 102. See also Vaughan, *The Pill on Trial*, 25, 53; P. Fryer, *The Birth Controllers* (London, 1967), chs 18 and 19.

92 In 1966 the legal restrictions on contraception were amended, but even then only married people had a right to birth control advice. Those giving contraceptive help to single people risked fines or incarceration. See Vaughan, *The Pill on Trial*, 42–3.

93 *Population and the American Future*, 167–8.

94 Up to the 1970s such restrictions also limited the manufacture and importation of contraceptives in the former colonies of many of these countries. While contraception was allowed in many former British colonies in Africa and Asia, it was banned in Francophone African states, except Tunisia, and in certain Latin American countries. L. T. Lee, 'Law and family planning', *Studies in Family Planning*, 2/2 (Apr. 1971), 81–98, at 83–4; Stepan and Kellogg, *The World's Laws on Contraceptives*, 16.

95 For more on Pincus, see pp. 54–60. Reed, *The Birth Control Movement*, 322–3.

96 J. D. Ratcliff, 'No father to guide them', *Collier's Magazine*, (20 Mar. 1937), 19, cited in Reed, *The Birth Control Movement*, 323. Reed provides an excellent overview of the experiments Pincus conducted on rabbits and how they were received in the press.

97 Reed, *The Birth Control Movement*, 320–6; J. Turney, *Frankenstein's Footsteps* (New Haven, 1998), 117.

98 Interview with E. Caspi by L. Marks, 23 Mar. 1995, notes, 2.

99 Interview with John Pincus by D. Halberstam, in D. Halberstam *The Fifties* (New York, 1993), 292.

100 Halberstam, *The Fifties*, 292; Reed, *The Birth Control Movement*, 328–31.

101 Unposted letter from G. Pincus to Albert Raymond, Oct. 1951, GP-LC, cited in Reed, *The Birth Control Movement*, 332–3. From 1944 G. D. Searle had financed the salaries of five investigators and four technical assistants based at the Worcester Foundation. G. D. Searle also paid Pincus as a consultant. One of the most important early projects Pincus had carried out with G. D. Searle's aid was the development of a process (known as perfusion) for the commercial production of cortisone, a secretion of the adrenal cortex. See Reed, *The Birth Control Movement*, 331, 343–4.

102 Vaughan, *The Pill on Trial*, 52; L. McLaughlin, *The Pill, John Rock, and the Church* (Boston, 1982), 133–4.

103 McLaughlin, *The Pill*, 134.

104 Letter from Irwin C. Winter to *Journal of the American Medical Association*, 212/6 (11 May 1970), 1067.

105 This changed in 1959 when G. D. Searle realized the popularity of the pill and directed Pincus to reveal Searle's participation. See Raymond to Pincus, 28 July 1959, GP-LC, Box 111.

106 Cited in McLaughlin, *The Pill*, 136.

107 G. Pincus to D. Wolfle, 28 June 1967, GP-LC, Box 104.

108 Vaughan, *The Pill on Trial*, 54; C. Djerassi, *The Politics of Contraception* (New York, 1979), 249–52. In 1956 Parke-Davis refused to undertake any fertility research when approached by Warren Nelson from the Population Council on account of its fear of hostility from the Catholic community. While eventually contributing $5,000 to the Worcester Foundation, Parke-Davis continued to emphasize that its policy was to keep out of the contraceptive field. Reed, *The Birth Control Movement*, 362.

109 Vaughan, *The Pill on Trial*, 54; Djerassi, *The Politics of Contraception*, 249–52; Reed, *The Birth Control Movement*, 362; McLaughlin, *The Pill*, 136–7.

110 Vaughan, *The Pill on Trial*, 53; Courey, 'Participants', 60.

111 W. Dixon to G. Pincus, 23 Mar. 1959, GP-LC, Box 111.

112 D. Searle to G. Pincus, 31 July 1959 GP-LC, Box 111.

113 M. Sanger, *The Pivot of Civilzation'*, cited in Chesler, *Woman of Valor*, 209.

114 G. Swyer, OBT lecture, SA/FPA/A5/135, Box 246, AM.

115 Cited in Vaughan, *The Pill on Trial*, 6. Similar views were expressed by the philosopher Bertrand Russell, when he said that 'without science and the scientific approach to the problems of mankind there is no hope for his future', cited in Huber Speech, 'Man and his relation to natural resources', n.d., in Calderone papers, Box 4 file 50, Schlesinger Library.

116 A. S. Parkes lecture, *Lancet* (16 Jan. 1963), in SA/FPA/A5/126, Box 245, AM. In 1963 John Rock similarly argued, 'the major obligation of science [is] not to get to the Moon or Mars, or to solve any of the other scientific problems. It's up to the scientists to find the weak spots in the physiology of reproduction so that we may tackle them and break the connection between what is euphemistically called "the marriage act" and its all too likely result' (J. Rock, 'Science and charity to the rescue of humanity', *Pacific Medicine and Surgery (Ortho-Symposium)*, 73 (Feb. 1965), 1-A-25-27).

117 Hartmann, *Reproductive Rights and Wrongs*, 177–80; Courey, 'Participants', 323.

118 Report in *Science Newsletter*, cited in Turney, *Frankenstein's Footsteps*, 162.

119 Cited in Vaughan, *The Pill on Trial*, 54.

120 Vaughan, *The Pill on Trial*, 52–3.
121 Hartmann, *Reproductive Rights and Wrongs*, 177.

2 The Contraceptive Challenge

1 He based his hypothesis on experiments with mice and rabbits. H. H. Simmer, 'On the history of hormonal contraception I. Ludwig Haberlandt (1885–1932) and his concept of hormonal sterilization', *Contraception*, 1/1 (Jan. 1970), 3–27; H. H. Simmer, 'On the history of hormonal contraception II. Otfried Otto Fellner (1873–n.d.) and estrogens as antifertility hormones', *Contraception*, 3/1 (Jan. 1971), 1–21; E. Diczfalusy, 'Gregory Pincus and steroidal contraception', *Journal of Steroid Biochemistry*, 11 (1979), 3–11, at 3; N. Perone, 'The history of steroidal contraceptive development', *Perspectives in Biology and Medicine*, 36/3 (Spring 1993), 347–68, at 353.

2 For an overview of contraceptives in the eighteenth and nineteenth centuries, see A. McLaren, *A History of Contraception* (Oxford, 1994).

3 J. W. Goldzieher, 'Newer drugs in oral contraception', *Medical Clinics of North America*, 48/2 (Mar. 1964), 529–45, at 545; J. Riddle, *Contraception and Abortion from the Ancient World to the Renaissance* (London, 1992).

4 A. Huxley, *Brave New World* (London, 1994), 33–4: contraception is considered the norm for everyone who is not sterilized and is achieved by a 'Malthusian drill', which involves counting. How contraception works is not described in detail in the book. See 69, 108, 146.

5 M. Borell, 'Organotherapy, British physiology, and the discovery of internal secretions', *Journal of the History of Biology*, 9/2 (Fall 1976), 235–68; M. Borell, 'Brown-Sequard's organotherapy and its appearance in America at the end of the nineteenth century', *Bulletin of the History of Medicine*, 50/3 (Fall 1976), 309–20; W. Sneader, *Drug Discovery* (Chichester 1985), 192; N. Pfeffer, *The Stork and the Syringe* (Cambridge, 1993), 51, 68.

6 Starling was based at University College London. His work focused on pancreatic secretions, in particular insulin. Nowadays hormones are classified into three different groups: steroids, peptides and proteins. Peptidal hormones include the thyroid hormone. Proteins include insulin. Those in the steroidal group include sex hormones, which are vital to the process of reproduction, and adrenocortical hormones (also known as corticosteroids and corticoids), which regulate the body's metabolism. Cortisone is one of the adrenocortical hormones linked to stress responses. For more on Starling and on hormonal functions, see L. Crapo, *Hormones* (Stanford, 1985).

7 For more information on the discovery of insulin, thyroxine and their clinical applications see Sneader, *Drug Discovery*, 208–9, 213–17.

8 Sneader, *Drug Prototypes and their Exploitation* (Chichester, 1996); Pfeffer, *The Stork and the Syringe*, 68–71.

9 N. Pfeffer, 'Lessons from history', in P. Alderson, ed., *Consent to Health Treatment and Research*, Report of the Social Science Research Unit Consent Conference Series, no. 1, Dec. 1992, 31–7.

10 Hancock and Co. Ltd, *The Ravages of Time Defied* (London, 1934); see also Pfeffer, *The Stork and the Syringe*, 51, 68–71; Pfeffer, 'Lessons from history', 34.

11 Male hormones were first noted by the German zoologist A. A. Berthold

(1803–1861) as a result of his experiments with castrated roosters. Female hormones were discovered by the Viennese gynaecologist Emil Knauer (1867–1935), who noticed that immature female animals began to display mature sexual characteristics as a result of receiving ovary transplants from fully mature animals. V. N. Bullough, *Science in the Bedroom* (New York, 1994), 124; see also N. Oudshoorn, *Beyond the Natural Body* (London, 1994), 19.

12 Simmer, 'On the history of hormonal contraception I,' 5–9; Diczfalusy, 'Gregory Pincus and steroidal contraception', 3; Bullough, *Science in the Bedroom*, 129; S. Kostering, 'Etwas Besseres als das Kondom', in G. Staupe and L. Vieth, eds, *Die Pille* (Berlin, 1996), 115. The corpus luteum had first been described as early as the seventeenth century, but until the nineteenth century many presumed its function was to expel the egg rather than to suppress ovulation; see Perone, 'The history of steroidal contraceptive development', 353–4.

13 The hormone was called progesterone because of its ability to promote gestation. Sneader, *Drug Discovery*, 199–200; Bullough, *Science in the Bedroom*, 129.

14 Doisy and Allen were aided in their research by the development of a technique known as the vaginal smear. Developed in 1917, this method enabled scientists to study what was happening in the reproductive tract of female animals without resorting to sacrifice or operations. Bullough, *Science in the Bedroom*, 128.

15 In 1927 Leo Loeb also demonstrated that follicular extracts could render animals temporarily infertile. Simmer, 'On the history of hormonal contraception', I and II; Perone, 'The history of steroidal contraceptive development', 354.

16 Sneader, *Drug Prototypes and their Exploitation*, 306–7; J. W. Goldzieher, 'Estrogens in oral contraceptives', *Johns Hopkins Medical Journal*, 150 (1982), 165–9; Bullough, *Science in the Bedroom*, 128; Simmer, 'On the history of hormonal contraception II', 9.

17 See A. S. Parkes, 'The Biology of Fertility', in R. O. Greep, ed., *Human Fertility and Population Problems* (New York, 1963), 28. A useful guide to the different female hormones and their related synthesized compounds appears in Sneader, *Drug Prototypes and their Exploitation*, 304–34, and Sneader, *Drug Discovery*, 194.

18 Bullough, *Science in the Bedroom*, 131–2; Pfeffer, *The Stork and the Syringe*, 76–7.

19 For more information on this see the next chapter.

20 Oudshoorn, *Beyond the Natural Body*, 95–8.

21 Pfeffer, 'Lessons from history', 32–3; 'Experimental interruption of pregnancy', *BMJ* (10 Sept. 1938), 580; A. S. Parkes, E. C. Dodds and R. L. Noble, 'Interruption of early pregnancy by means of orally active oestrogens', *BMJ* (10 Sept. 1938), 557–8. The British research recognized that other compounds were also being found to be successful agents for temporary sterilization in Germany: Sneader, *Drug Discovery*, 195–6, 200.

22 For more information on the concern raised by abortion in these years and the number of official investigations that were set up to explore the question, see J. D. Thomas and S. Williams, 'Women and abortion in 1930s Britain', *Social History of Medicine*, 11/2 (1988), 283–310; see also B. Brookes, *Abortion in England, 1900–1967* (London, 1988).

23 E. Mellanby of the MRC to D. Veale, 13 Dec. 1938, MRC files 1523/60. I am grateful to Naomi Pfeffer for supplying this reference. Stilboestrol was subsequently used to treat menstrual disorders and recurrent miscarriage; Pfeffer, 'Lessons from history', 33.

24 Goldzieher, 'Estrogens in oral contraceptives', 165–9; J. W. Goldzieher, 'The

history of steroidal contraceptive development', *Perspectives in Biology and Medicine*, 36/3 (Spring 1993), 363–8, at 364.

25 For more on the shift in attitudes in Germany see C. Usborne, *The Politics of the Body in Weimar Germany* (London, 1992), ch. 3.

26 Kostering, 'Etwas Besseres als das Kondom', 118–19; see also Simmer, 'On the history of hormonal contraception I', 4–5, 20.

27 Perone, 'The history of steroidal contraceptive development', 353.

28 Ibid., 355.

29 Kostering, 'Etwas Besseres als das Kondom', 125; Diczfalusy, 'Gregory Pincus and steroidal contraception', 4. It is well known that Nazi doctors were carrying out experiments to bring about 'unnoticed' sterilization. A number of methods were tried, including drugs. For more information on this see T. Taylor, 'Opening statement of the prosecution, December 9, 1946', in G. J. Annas and M. A. Grodin, eds, *The Nazi Doctors and the Nuremburg Code* (Oxford, 1992), 79–80.

30 B. Zondek and S. Rozin, in *Lancet*, 236 (1939), 504.

31 Goldzieher, 'Estrogens in oral contraceptives'; Goldzieher, 'The history of steroidal contraceptive development'; Diczfalusy, 'Gregory Pincus and steroidal contraception', 4.

32 C. Gamble to M. Sanger, 21 Apr. 1954; 'Suggestions for procedure in testing oral contraceptive', 11 Apr. 1954, CG-FCL, Box 80/1276; S.N. Sanyal, 'Pisum sativum (linn). m-Xylohydroquinone as an oral contraceptive: a critical evaluation of the results of human trial and some biometric information', n.d., CG-FCL, Box 81/1286; S. Ghosh, Jyoti Sen and B. Mittra, 'Pisum sativum (linn). Contraceptive effects of m-Xylohydroquinone. A summary of two years trial results of human female subjects', CG-FCL, Box 81/1286; S. Ghosh and A. Gupta, 'The effectiveness as an oral contraceptive of synthetic metaxylohydroquinone, the active principle of the field pea (Pisum Sativum Linn): a preliminary report', *International Medical Abstracts and Reviews*, 16 (Nov. 1954), 89–90; and S. N. Sanyal, 'Ten years of research on an oral contraceptive from *Pisum Sativum Linn*', *Science and Culture*, 25 (June 1960), 661–5; S. N. Sanyal and S. Ghosh, 'Further clinical results with metaxylohydroquinone as an oral contraceptive', *International Medical Abstracts and Reviews*, 18/5 (Nov. 1955), 101–4; D. Williams and G. Williams, *Every Child a Wanted Child* (Boston, 1978), 316–7; H. Jackson, 'Antifertility substances', *Pharmacological Reviews*, 2 (1959), 135–72, at 157.

33 Sanyal, 'Ten years research on an oral contraceptive', 9. Companies involved in the manufacture of the drug included Distillation Products Industries, a subsidiary of the Eastman Kodak Company, and Merck Sharp and Dohme International, Railway, USA. Sanyal and Ghosh, 'Further clinical results with metaxylohydroquinone as an oral contraceptive'; S. N. Sanyal, 'Functional uterine bleeding', *Journal of Medicine and International Medical Abstract Review*, 24/5 (1960), 5–11.

34 *Sunday Dispatch*, 21 Sept. 1952, 3.

35 Ibid. Wiesner was a biologist of Austrian origin, married to Mary Barton, who ran her own infertility clinic. Together they established in 1946 the means for infertile couples to have artificial insemination in Britain. For more information see Pfeffer, *The Stork and the Syringe*, 59, 115, 118, 129.

36 Document, n.d., *c*.June 1953, verbatim, in MRC file FD1/4841, PRO: Outline of Research Project to Nuffield Foundation by Professor J. Yudkin. Experiments were also carried out with the plant elsewhere; see P. S. Henshaw, 'Physiologic control of fertility', *Science*, 117 (29 May 1953), 572–82, at 578.

37 See p. 46 above.

38 Green to J. Elliot Janney, 17 Nov. 1952; document, 21 Oct. 1952; Herald to MRC Secretary, memo, 24 Jan. 1952; Harrington to Himsworth, 11 Mar. 1952; Himsworth, 'Antifertility research', note, 10 Nov. 1952; all in MRC file FD1/1737, Substances producing temporary sterility, PRO. See also Jackson, 'Antifertility substances', 151–2.

39 Himsworth to A. S. Parkes, 20 July 1953, FD1/1737, MRC, PRO.

40 Himsworth, 'Antifertility research'.

41 B. F. Sieve, 'A new antifertility factor (a preliminary report)', *Science* (10 Oct. 1952), 373–85. See also M. C. Chang and G. Pincus, 'Does phosphorylated hesperidin affect fertility?', *Science*, 117 (13 Mar. 1953), 274–6; N. Millman and F. Rosen, 'Failure of phosphorylated hesperidin to influence fertility in rodents', *Science*, 118 (21 Aug. 1953), 212–13.

42 K. McCormick to M. Sanger 8 May 1956, MS-SS, correspondence files. For more information on the investment being put into basic research, see O. Harkavy, *Curbing Population Growth* (New York, 1995), ch. 1; see also J. Reed, *The Birth Control Movement in American Society* (Princeton, 1984), ch. 21; J. Caldwell and P. Caldwell, *Limiting Population Growth* (London, 1986), 9–13.

43 For more on Gamble see Williams and Williams, *Every Child a Wanted Child*; Reed, *The Birth Control Movement*, 225–38.

44 M. Sanger to Clarence J. Gamble, 1939, cited in G. Williams, 'Biography of Clarence Gamble', MS 20–1, research materials for James Reed's Family Planning Oral History Project, MC 223, Schlesinger Archives, cited in S. M. Berg, 'Gregory Goodwin Pincus', B.A. thesis, Harvard University, 1989, 81.

45 E. Chesler, *Woman of Valor* (New York, 1992), 22–3, 32–4, 39–43.

46 Ibid., 45–6, 48, 52–5, 62–6, 209–10, 213.

47 Cited in L. McLaughlin, *The Pill, John Rock and the Catholic Church* (Boston, 1982), 94.

48 Cited in Chesler, *Woman of Valor*, 96.

49 M. Sanger, 'The future of contraception', *Journal of Contraception*, 2 (Jan. 1937), 3–4, cited in Berg, 'Gregory Goodwin Pincus', 69–70.

50 Cited in M. Gray, *Margaret Sanger* (New York, 1979), 396. See also M. Sanger to R. L. Dickinson, 28 May 1946, MS-SS. Gray explains that part of Sanger's desire to find an oral contraceptive may have resulted from her repeated gall bladder attacks for which she had been prescribed pills. This had perhaps made her realize how easily a pill could be integrated into the routine of a person's daily life. Cited in Berg, 'Gregory Goodwin Pincus', 82–3.

51 The first woman to graduate from MIT was Ellen Swallow Richards: after she graduated in chemistry in 1873 her research into sanitary conditions resulted in the establishment of the first state water quality standards in the USA. Sherene ChenSee, *Women in Science* (Canadian Science Writers' Association, 1999).

52 See T. C. Boyle, *Riven Rock* (Viking, 1998), for a fictionalized account of Stanley McCormick's illness and life.

53 Reed, *The Birth Control Movement*, ch. 26.

54 Interview with James Dean, Harvard University, in Gray, *Margaret Sanger*, 413, 463, cited in Berg, 'Gregory Goodwin Pincus', 61–2.

55 K. McCormick to M. Sanger, 11 Apr. 1958, MS-SS.

56 K. McCormick to G. Pincus, 8 Aug. 1964, GP-LC, Box 73; see also interview with Celso Ramon Garcia by L. V. Marks, 16 Apr. 1995, transcript, 34–5.

57 K. McCormick to M. Sanger, 18 Oct. 1951 and 22 Jan. 1952, M. Sanger to K. McCormick, 26 Feb. 1952, MS-SS.

58 Cited in P. Vaughan, *The Pill on Trial* (Harmondsworth, 1972), 26.

59 In 1927, for instance, K. McCormick funded the establishment of a Neuroendocrine Research Foundation at Harvard University. This aimed to support the work of Roy G. Hoskins, an endocrinologist investigating the role of adrenal cortex malfunction in schizophrenia. Reed, *The Birth Control Movement*, 338.

60 Ibid., 339. Sanger suggested laboratories in England and Germany. Germany was a surprising recommendation given that the Second World War had only recently ended, but, as Vaughan argues, 'a cynic might suspect that Mrs Sanger had in mind that country's ill-gotten experience of sterilizing undesirables.' While Sanger was in favour of national sterilization, neither she nor McCormick pursued this as a serious option. Vaughan, *The Pill on Trial*, 27.

61 K. McCormick was not familiar with G. Pincus despite her contact with Hudson Hoagland, his co-director at the Worcester Foundation: see below. K. McCormick to M. Sanger, 13 Mar. 1952, MS-SS, correspondence files.

62 G. Pincus, *The Control of Fertility* (New York, 1965), 5–6.

63 Interview with G. Pincus in *Candide* (1966), cited in Reed, *The Birth Control Movement*, 309.

64 Reed, *The Birth Control Movement*, 317; McLaughlin, *The Pill*, 104.

65 McLaughlin, *The Pill*, 112.

66 Worcester Foundation, *Annual Report* (1949–50), 4.

67 For a more detailed description of G. Pincus's earlier work and the controversy it caused, see Reed, *The Birth Control Movement*, 320–1, 343–4; for more information on Pincus and the Worcester Foundation, see *Worcester Sunday Telegram*, 4 Mar. 1951, 14; see also Vaughan, *The Pill on Trial*.

68 Worcester Foundation, *Annual Report* (1949–50), 4.

69 Pincus had already received funds from the PPFA: between 1948 and 1949, the PPFA had awarded him $14,500 to investigate the early development of mammalian eggs. Reed, *The Birth Control Movement*, 340.

70 For some idea of the experiments being funded by the PPFA see P. S. Henshaw, 'Research activities 1952–3', 28 Apr. 1953, JDR III collection, Record Group 2, Box 45; see also A. Stone to M. Sanger, 1 Mar. 1952, MS-SS. One of these experiments concerned phosphorylated hesperidin, see G. Martin, 'Phosphorylated hesperidin', *Science*, 117 (3 Apr. 1953), 363.

71 J. Rock to G. Pincus, 26 June 1957, GP-LC, Box 29; G. Pincus to K. McCormick, 18 July 1959, GP-LC; P. Henshaw, 'Research needs in relation to family planning and fertility control', 10 Aug. 1953, MS-LC; PPFA Research Committee papers', Oct. 1951, MS-LC, cited in Berg, 'Gregory Goodwin G. Pincus', 77–8. See also J. Rock to K. McCormick, 26 Sept. 1958, JR-FCL, and K. McCormick to G. Pincus, 14 July 1959, GP-LC, Box 39; J. Rock to G. Pincus, 26 June 1957, JR-FCL; K. McCormick to M. Sanger, 17 Feb. 1954, MS-SS.

72 K. McCormick had originally met Hoagland when he was head of a small biology department at Clark University in Massachusetts; see Worcester Foundation, *Annual Report* (1945), 9; Reed, *The Birth Control Movement*, 338–9.

73 K. McCormick to M. Sanger, 4 June 1952, MS-SS, correspondence files.

74 K. McCormick to G. Pincus, 31 May 1954, GP-LC, cited in Berg, 'Gregory Goodwin Pincus', 86. See also K. McCormick to B. Crawford, 14 June 1956, GP-LC, Box 21; Minutes of a Special Meeting of the Trustees of the Worcester Foundation, 6 Dec.

1956, GP-LC, Box 23.

75 K. McCormick to M. Sanger, 1 Oct. 1952, 17 Feb. 1954 and 31 May 1955, MS-SS; K. McCormick to M. Sanger, 13 Nov. 1953, MS-LC. See also Reed, *The Birth Control Movement*, 433.

76 'Grantors' funds balances Jan. 31 1956', and 'Assets and principal accounts balances: grantors' funds March 31, 1957', GP-LC, cited in Berg, 'Gregory Goodwin Pincus', 87; R. C. Johnson, 'Feminism, philanthropy and science in the development of the oral contraceptive pill', *Pharmacy in History*, 19/2 (1977), 63–77, at 71. For a detailed breakdown of how K. McCormick's funds were spent on the pill project, see Mrs Stanley McCormick's grants, for the year ending December 31 1958', GP-LC, Box 39. A large proportion of the money went towards financing the salaries of the investigators.

77 National Science Foundation, *Interactions of Science and Technology in the Innovative Process* (19 Mar. 1973), 10–17; Reed, *The Birth Control Movement*, 340.

78 Interview with Celso Ramon Garcia by L. V. Marks, 41.

79 M. Sanger to K. McCormick, 5 Oct. 1953, MS-LC.

80 G. Pincus to D. Wolfle, 28 June 1967, GP-LC, Box 104; Vaughan, *The Pill on Trial*, 52; Reed, *Birth Control Movement*, 43–4, 331–3. See also K. McCormick to M. Sanger, 30 Nov. 1956, and Notes on McCormick's conversation with Dr Rock, 2 Apr. 1958, MS-SS. See also chapter 1 above.

81 P. S. Henshaw to G. Pincus, 27 Mar. 1953, GP-LC, Box 14.

82 G. Pincus to K. McCormick, 5 Mar. 1954, GP-LC, cited in Berg, 'Gregory Goodwin Pincus', 87; A. B. Ramirez de Arellano and C. Seipp, *Colonialism, Catholicism and Contraception* (London, 1983), 108–10.

83 B. Asbell, *The Pill* (New York, 1995), 134. In 1956 McCormick wrote, 'Everything is as slow as molasses, but both Rock and Pincus seem to be moving towards more extensive "field tests" and I am most anxious to get these going as fast as we can' (K. McCormick to M. Sanger, 30 June 1956, MS-SS).

84 Cited in Vaughan, *The Pill on Trial*, 26; interview with Celso Ramon Garcia by L. V. Marks, 34.

85 Memorandum from H. Hoagland to G. Pincus and B. Crawford, 14 Feb. 1957, GP-LC, Box 27; see also G. Pincus to K. McCormick, 15 Aug. 1960, GP-LC, Box 45.

86 Cited in Reed, *The Birth Control Movement*, 339.

87 G. Pincus to K. McCormick, 14 July 1956, GP-LC, Box 21. She was also asked to become a trustee of the Worcester Foundation in 1954. This request made it clear that she was regarded as more than just a sponsor. As Hudson Hoagland stated, 'We would value your advice and active participation in the affairs of the Foundation' (H. Hoagland to K. McCormick, 8 Apr. 1954, GP-LC, cited in Berg, 'Gregory Goodwin G. Pincus', 88).

88 K. McCormick to M. Sanger, 23 July 1954, 21 Oct. 1954, MS-SS; 'Procedure for progesterone tests', n.d., *c.*1954; and GP-LC, Box 17. See also documents 'Suitable experimental subjects', and 'Objectives for experimentation', Nov. 1954, JR-FCL. K. McCormick to M. Sanger 19, 21, 23 July 1954; 31 May 1955; 9 Jan 1956; 30 Jan. 1956; 11 Feb. 1956, 7 June 1956, MS-SS; K. McCormick to M. Sanger 6 Feb. 1956, GP-LC; K. McCormick to M. Sanger, 13 Nov. 1953, MS-LC; G. Pincus to K. McCormick, 5 Mar. 1954, MS-SS; G. Pincus to K. McCormick, 13 Dec. 1956, GP-LC, Box 21.

89 Pincus, *The Control of Fertility*.

90 K. McCormick to M. Sanger, 17 June 1954, 2 July 1954, 21 Oct. 1954, 1 Feb. 1955,

9 Jan. 1956, 13 Dec. 1957; M. Sanger to G. Pincus, 18 July 1957, MS-SS. M. Sanger to K. McCormick, 25 Sept. 1952 and 23 Mar. 1953, K. McCormick to M. Sanger, 13 Nov. 1953, MS-LC.

91 Cited in National Science Foundation, *Interactions of Science and Technology*, 10–15.

92 Pfeffer, 'Lessons from history', 32, 34–5. The fears about cancer proved well founded, because stilboestrol was later found to be carcinogenic.

93 F. B. Colton, 'Steroids and "the pill"', *Steroids*, 57 (Dec. 1992), 624–30, at 625.

94 National Science Foundation, *Interactions of Science and Technology*, 10–15.

95 M. Sanger to K. McCormick, 12 Dec. 1956, MS-SS, cited in Reed, *The Birth Control Movement*, 344, and Chesler, *Woman of Valor*, 435. Two years later, M. Sanger reiterated this line, stating 'I consider almost all, at least 90 % of his [G. Pincus's] recent scientific successes have been because of you, who have given him financial support as well as moral encouragement' (M. Sanger to K. McCormick, 19 Aug. 1958, MS-SS).

3 Sexual Chemistry

1 J. Reed, *The Birth Control Movement in American Society* (Princeton, 1984a), 313; N. Oudshoorn, *Beyond the Natural Body* (London, 1994), 69, 76.

2 D. Halberstam, *The Fifties* (New York, 1993), 283.

3 The term steroid comes from the fact that these substances are related to, and in most cases derived from, sterols (solid alcohols), which are abundant in nature.

4 Syntex Corporation, *A Corporation and a Molecule* (Palo Alto, 1966), 5–7; M. R. Henzl, letter to editor, *Lancet*, 347 (27 Jan. 1996), 257–8.

5 For a more detailed chemical description of steroids, see N. Applezweig, *Steroid Drugs* (New York, 1962), 9; C. Djerassi, 'The chemical history of the pill', in C. Djerassi, *The Politics of Contraception* (London, 1979), 228–31.

6 H. E. Dale, 'The chemistry of sex hormones', *Pharmaceutical Journal* (29 Apr. 1939), 432–41; Syntex Corporation, *A Corporation and a Molecule*, 13.

7 For more information on cholesterol and how it came to be used for the production of steroids see Applezweig, *Steroid Drugs*, 17.

8 Ibid., 10.

9 N. Perone, 'The history of steroidal contraceptive development', *Perspectives in Biology and Medicine*, 36/3 (Spring 1993), 347–68, at 348.

10 Applezweig, *Steroid Drugs*, 10, 23.

11 Interview with Alejandro Hernandez by L. V. Marks, 8 Apr. 1997, notes; Syntex Corporation, *A Corporation and a Molecule*, 22; Perone, 'The history of steroidal contraceptive development', 349.

12 A. Q. Maisel, *The Hormone Quest* (New York, 1965), 47.

13 Syntex Corporation, *A Corporation and a Molecule*, 23; Maisel, *The Hormone Quest*, 46; P. A. Lehmann, A. Bolivar and R. Quinteron, 'Russell E. Marker', *Journal of Chemical Education*, 50/3 (Mar. 1973), 195–9; Applezweig, *Steroid Drugs*, 23.

14 Maisel, *The Hormone Quest*, 47; interview with Hernandez, notes.

15 Maisel, *The Hormone Quest*, 47; Applezweig, *Steroid Drugs*; A. Pedro and F. Lehmann, 'Early history of steroid chemistry in Mexico', *Steroids*, 57 (Aug. 1992), 403–8. Lehmann et. al., 'Russell E. Marker', 198.

16 V. N. Bullough, *Science in the Bedroom* (New York, 1994), 128.

17 S. A. Szpilfogel and F. J. Zeelen, 'Steroid research at Organon in the golden 1950s and the following years', *Steroids*, 61 (1996), 483–91.

18 Bullough, *Science in the Bedroom*, 128. See also Syntex Corporation, *A Corporation and a Molecule*, 21; Szpilfogel and Zeelen, 'Steroid research at Organon'; W. Sneader, *Drug Prototypes and their Exploitation* (Chichester, N.Y., 1996).

19 Maisel, *The Hormone Quest*, 49; Applezweig, *Steroid Drugs*, 24–5.

20 Interview with Russell Marker, in C. Djerassi, *From the Lab into the World* (Washington DC, 1994), 26, 30.

21 This was collected between Cordova and Orizaba near Fortin; interview with Marker, in Djerassi, *From the Lab into the World*, 26.

22 Interview with Marker, in Djerassi, *From the Lab into the World*, 26.

23 Reed, *The Birth Control Movement*, 315; 'The early production of steroidal hormones', *CHOC News*, 4 (1987), 3–6; and 'Autobiography: Professor Russell Marker, transcribed from the facsimile of a manuscript of his handwriting', 15 May 1969, cited in R. M. Courey, 'Participants in the development, marketing and safety evaluation of the oral contraceptive, 1950–1965', Ph.D thesis, University of California, Berkeley, 1994, 32.

24 G. Rosenkrantz, 'From Ruzicka's terpenes in Zurich to Mexican steroids via Cuba', *Steroids*, 57 (Aug. 1992), 409–18, at 414; see also J. Fortes and L. Adler Lomnitz, *Becoming a Scientist in Mexico* (Philadelphia, 1994).

25 Dr Somlo had originally set himself up in 1928 as the Mexican commercial representative for Hungarian and German pharmaceutical drug houses, including Gedeon Richter; Rosenkrantz, 'From Ruzicka's terpenes', 414.

26 Lehmann had experience in pharmacology and endocrinology; Pedro and Lehmann, 'Early history of steroid chemistry in Mexico'.

27 Ibid.

28 Marker's rapid departure from Syntex was part of a long pattern. He had similarly abruptly left the University of Maryland when on the verge of receiving his Ph.D and also the Rockefeller Institute when he had what his colleagues thought to be a minor disagreement; see Reed, *The Birth Control Movement*, 314.

29 While at Syntex, Marker had not been paid a salary on the understanding that he would receive 40 per cent of Syntex's net profits at the end of the year. Pedro and Lehmann, 'Early history of steroid chemistry in Mexico'; Lehmann et al., 'Russell E. Marker', 198; Perone, 'The history of steroidal contraceptive development', 351.

30 Rosenkrantz, 'From Ruzicka's terpenes', 414; Oudshoorn, *Beyond the Natural Body*, 71; Syntex Corporation, *A Corporation and a Molecule*, 27.

31 Rosenkrantz, 'From Ruzicka's terpenes', 412.

32 Syntex Corporation, *A Corporation and a Molecule*, 28.

33 In addition to the recruitment of foreign-trained scientists, Rosenkrantz set up a Ph.D programme in organic chemistry in collaboration with the National University of Mexico (UNAM). A number of talented students who emerged from this programme subsequently worked for Syntex. Rosenkrantz, 'From Ruzicka's terpenes', 414. This article gives a detailed list of all the Mexican and international co-workers who were based at Syntex between 1945 and 1960 (at 418).

34 C. Djerassi, *The Pill, Pygmy Chimps, and Degas' Horse* (New York, 1992), 25–7.

35 Ibid., 26.

36 A. J. Birch, 'Steroid hormones and the Luftwaffe', *Steroids*, 57 (Aug. 1992), 363–77, at 364.

37 D. Cantor, 'Cortisone and the politics of empire', *Bulletin of the History of Medicine*

67/3 (1993), 463–93; H. M. Marks, 'Cortisone, 1949', *Bulletin of the History of Medicine* 6/3 (1992), 419–40. See also Reed, *The Birth Control Movement*, 331–2 for the relationship between the production of cortisone and the development of the pill.

38 *Harpers Magazine*, 1951, cited in C. Djerassi, 'Steroid Research at Syntex', *Steroids*, 57 (Dec. 1992), 631–41, at 638. Some idea of the importance attached to cortisone research in these years can be seen in M. E. Wall et al., 'Steroidal sapogenins. VII', *Journal of the American Pharmaceutical Association: Scientific Edition*, 13/1 (Jan. 1954), 1–7.

39 Syntex later sold its patent for its synthesis of cortisone to the pharmaceutical company Glaxo, whose production of cortisone remains reliant on this technique to this day. Djerassi, 'Steroid research at Syntex', 640; Rosenkrantz, 'From Ruzicka's terpenes', 416.

40 A. Zaffaroni, 'From paper chromatography to drug discovery', *Steroids*, 57 (Dec. 1992), 642–8, at 643. See also Maisel, *The Hormone Quest*, 44; Syntex Corporation, *A Corporation and a Molecule*, 35–6.

41 On the basis of this research, in November 1949 Marker, together with the chemist Norman Applezweig, predicted that plant sapogenins would provide the cheapest and most readily available starting material for the synthesis of corticoid hormones. Applezweig, *Steroid Drugs*, 25; interview with Hernandez, notes, 3; Perone, 'The history of steroidal contraceptive development', 351–2.

42 Zaffaroni, 'From paper chromatography to drug discovery', 644.

43 Rosenkrantz, 'From Ruzicka's terpenes', 413.

44 Ibid., 416.

45 Djerassi, 'Steroid research at Syntex', 632.

46 Interview with Hernandez, notes, 6–7.

47 Ehrenstein and Birch's research was influential in abolishing the idea that progesterone's biological activity was extremely specific and that almost any alteration of the molecule would diminish or abolish its activity. Djerassi, *The Pill*, 54–6.

48 W. M. Tullner and R. Hertz, 'High progestational activity of 19-norprogesterone', *Endocrinology*, 52 (1953), 359–60; W. Tullner and R. Hertz, 'Progestational activity of 19-norprogesterone and 19-norethisterone in the rhesus monkey', *Proceedings of the Society of Experimental Biology and Medicine*, 94 (1957), 298–300; R. Hertz, J. H. Waite and L. B. Thomas, 'Progestational effectiveness of 19-norethinyl-testosterone by oral route in women', *Proceedings of Experimental Biology and Medicine*, 91 (1956), 418–20. Interview with Celso Ramon Garcia by L. V. Marks, 16 Apr. 1995, transcript, 55; L. McLaughlin, *The Pill, John Rock and the Catholic Church* (Boston, 1982), 113.

49 Djerassi, 'Steroid research at Syntex'; Djerassi, *The Pill*, 58.

50 F. B. Colton, 'Steroids and "the pill"', *Steroids*, 57 (Dec. 1992), 624–30, at 625.

51 For more information on Pincus see the previous and following chapters.

52 Colton, 'Steroids and "the pill"', 626.

53 Ibid.; see also McLaughlin, *The Pill*, 114.

54 E. Diczfalusy, 'Gregory Pincus and steroidal contraception', *Journal of Steroid Biochemistry*, 11 (1979), 3–11, at 5.

55 Djerassi, *The Pill*, 59.

56 G. Pincus to D. Wolfle, 28 June 1967, GP-LC, Box 104.

57 McLaughlin, *The Pill*, 127, 136.

58 'Fertility and infertility', transcript of a panel meeting, *Bulletin of New York Academy of Medicine*, 37/10 (Oct. 1961), 689–712, at 699–700; Colton, 'Steroids and "the pill"', 627–8; R. A. Edgren, 'Early oral contraceptive history', letter to the editor, *Steroids*, 59 (Jan. 1994), 58.

59 G. Pincus to J. Boes, 4 Oct. 1957, GP-LC, Box 24.

60 Colton, 'Steroids and "the pill"', 628.

61 G. D. Searle and Co., *Proceedings of a Symposium on 19-Nor Progestational Steroids* (Chicago, 23 Jan. 1957), JR-FCL; G. Pincus to C. Gamble, 30 Jan. 1958, GP-LC, Box 31. Sneader, *Drug Prototypes and their Exploitation*, 331.

62 A. Zaffaroni (Syntex) to G. Pincus, 30 May 1956, and G. Pincus to A. Zaffaroni, 5 June 1956, GP-LC, Box 23; G. Pincus to Edris Rice-Wray, 6 Aug. 1956, GP-LC, Box 22; G. D. Searle and Co., *Proceedings of a Symposium on 19-Nor Progestational Steroids*, 22, 24.

63 CIFC Clinical Trial Committee, Minutes, 13 Oct. 1960, SA/FPA/A5/160, Box 250; E. Mears to the editor, *Guardian*, 6 Nov. 1961, SA/FPA/A5/161/2, Box 251, AM. For more information on these British trials see L. V. Marks, '"Public spirited and enterprising volunteers"', in M. Gijswijt-Hofstra and T. Tansey, eds, *Remedies and Healing Cultures in Britain and the Netherlands in the Twentieth Century*, (Amsterdam, 2001).

64 Some oestrogens are more potent than others. No trials, however, were ever conducted to see which type of oestrogen was most effective. Interview with Geoffrey Venning by L. V. Marks, 16 Oct. 1996 and 7 Nov. 1996, London, notes.

65 V. A. Drill, 'History of the first oral contraceptive', *Journal of Toxicology and Environmental Health*, 3 (1977), 133–8, at 137.

66 Djerassi, *The Pill*, 59–63.

67 Colton, 'Steroids and "the Pill"', 628.

68 Djerassi, *The Pill*, 122.

69 Memo from T. F. Gallagher to Sam R. Hall, 16 July 1954, GP-LC, Box 16. In 1958 the New York Academy of Science held a joint meeting with three drug companies to discuss the contraceptive potential of progestational compounds; these included Norlutin, Enovid and Delalutin, produced respectively by Parke-Davis, Searle and E. R. Squibb; copy of article for *Los Angeles Times* 18 Apr. 1958, MS-SS.

70 For a more detailed breakdown of the different steroid compounds available for contraception, see M. P. Vessey, 'Some epidemiological investigations into the safety of oral contraceptives', M.D. thesis, London University 1970, 12; I. Stockley, 'Drugs in use', *Pharmaceutical Journal*, 1 (1976), 140–3; Sneader, *Drug Prototypes and their Exploitation*. See also M. D. G. Gillmer, 'Metabolic effects of combined oral contraceptives', in M. Filshie and J. Guillebaud, *Contraception* (London, 1989), 11–38, at 12, 15.

71 Economist Intelligence Unit, 'Special report no. 1: contraceptives', *Retail Business Market Surveys*, no. 138 (Aug. 1969), 12–27, at 15; 'Oral contraceptives – 50 million users', *Population Reports*, Series A, no. 1 (Apr. 1974), A–4.

72 R. L. Kleinman, *Directory of Hormonal Contraceptives* (IPPF, 1992).

73 'Oral contraceptives – 50 million users', A–4.

74 FDA Advisory Committee on Obstretics and Gynaecology, *Report on the Oral Contraceptives* (1 Aug. 1966), appendix 1, 18.

75 B. Asbell, *The Pill* (New York, 1995), 168. In 1965 Searle was predicting that the pharmaceutical industry in the USA would sell $4 million worth of oral contraceptives to US state and local government birth control programmes; in 1964 the

sum had been $1.8 million. US Congress, Senate, *World Population and Food Crisis: Hearings before the Consultative Subcommittee on Economic and Social Affairs of the Committee on Foreign Relations* (29 June 1965), 123.

76 Syntex Corporation, *A Corporation and a Molecule*, viii.

77 *Pharmaceutical Journal* (11 June 1966), 619. In Britain oral contraceptives with norethynodrel had the largest share of the market in 1965; A. Klopper, 'Advertisement and classification of oral contraceptives', *BMJ* (16 Oct. 1965), 932–3, at 933.

78 Many of the shares had been sold to key employees of Syntex to avoid tax. Asbell, *The Pill*, 168.

79 Djerassi, *From the Lab into the World*, 21; Sneader, *Drug Prototypes and their Exploitation*, 327.

80 'Safety of drugs statement on oral contraceptives', *Pharmaceutical Journal*, 2 (20 Dec. 1969), 750–1. For more on thrombosis and the pill, see chapter 6 below.

81 Economist Intelligence Unit, 'Special report no. 1: contraceptives', 18.

82 Asbell, *The Pill*, 167.

83 As late as 1975 diosgenin remained an important source for steroidal compounds. At this time about 25 per cent of the world's annual production (600,000 kg) of diosgenin was being used to produce oestrogens and progestogens for oral contraceptives, the remainder being used to make other sex hormones, corticosteroids, diuretics and anabolic agents. See 'Advantages of orals outweigh disadvantages', *Population Reports*, Series A, no. 2 (Mar. 1975), A–32.

84 See interview with Hernandez, notes, 10. Djerassi's comment on this episode is as follows: 'The Mexican *Dioscorea* species was particularly rich in diosgenin, but even as early as the 1940s the Mexican government had had the foresight to make the exportation of diosgenin particularly expensive. This step resulted in the establishment of an advanced steroid manufacturing industry based on abundant and cheap, locally produced diosgenin in Mexico, initially started by Syntex but subsequently followed by local branches of foreign pharmaceutical firms' (*From the Lab into the World*, 34).

85 Maisel, *The Hormone Quest*.

86 Interview with Hernandez, notes, 12.

87 US Congress, Senate Subcommitte on Patents, Trademarks, and Copyrights of the Committee on the Judiciary, *Wonder Drugs, Hearings on S. Res. 167*, 84th Congress, 2nd Session (1956), 64–151; Reed, *The Birth Control Movement*, 357.

88 Syntex Corporation, *A Corporation and a Molecule*, 48.

89 Maisel, *The Hormone Quest*, 52–3; interview with Hernandez, notes.

90 A. Villar Borja, 'Productos Quimicos Vegetales Mexicanos, S.A. De C.V. (Proquivemex)', in X. Lozoya, *Estado Actual Del Conocimeiento en Plantas Medicanas* (Mexico City, 1976), 240–1.

91 Interview with Hernandez, notes, 15.

92 Villar Borja, 'Productos Quimicos Vegetales Mexicanos', 236.

93 Interview with Hernandez, notes, 12.

94 Villar Borga, 'Productos Quimicos Vegetales Mexicanos', 241; Djerassi, *From the Lab into the World*, 35.

95 Villar Borja, 'Productos Quimicos Vegetales Mexicanos'.

96 An *ejido* is a form of collective farming established after the Mexican Revolution in 1921. The land itself was owned by the state. Each farmer, *ejidatario*, was given a piece of the collective land to farm for himself. Land was distributed on the basis that farmers had a right to the land as long as they were farming it. No farmer,

however, could sell the land as if it was his own property. In 1994 the legislation regarding land and property changed, giving farmers the right to sell the land they had been working. The motivation for this transformation, was that the land could thus be consolidated into larger plots, allowing for more intensive farming as in the USA. Private investors were encouraged to buy up the land.

97 Villar Borja, 'Productos Quimicos Vegetales Mexicanos', 241.

98 Interview with Hernandez, notes, 14–16; Villar Borja, 'Productos Quimicos Vegetales Mexicanos'.

99 Interview with Hernandez, notes, 15; Djerassi, *From the Lab into the World*, 34–5.

100 Interview with Hernandez, notes, 15.

101 Villar Borja, 'Productos Quimicos Vegetales Mexicanos', 239–40.

102 'Is the pill too dependent on wild yams?', *New Scientist* (3 May 1973), 281; 'Microbes may replace yams for making the pill', *New Scientist* (5 Sept. 1974), 589. *Encyclopedia of Chemical Technology*, 3rd edn New York, (1978–84), vol. 6, 764.

103 'Microbes may replace yams', 589; Applezweig, *Steroid Drugs*; Djerassi, *From the Lab into the World*, 35.

104 N. Pfeffer, *The Stork and the Syringe* (Cambridge, 1993), 78.

105 Steroid hormones accounted for $140 million, and corticosteroids for $95 million. N. Applezweig, 'The big steroid treasure hunt', *Chemical Week*, 84 (21 Jan. 1959), 37–51, at 38.

106 Ibid., 41.

107 Other hormones had also fallen in price. The cost of a gram of testosterone in 1947 was $30; by 1957 a gram of testosterone was fetching just 35 cents; ibid.

108 'Birth control pills boom', *Business Week* (23 Feb. 1963), 62.

109 *Investors Chronicle*, 29 Apr. 1960.

110 *Pharmaceutical Journal* (22 Feb. 1964), 178. The main scientist involved in this development was the British scientist V. Petrow. For his work and the chemical composition of Volidan, see Sneader, *Drug Prototypes and their Exploitation*, 322, 326.

111 *Pharmaceutical Journal*, 2 (22 July 1967), 101.

112 Values estimated from theoretical consumer prices for 1964–8 and retail prices for 1970–4, based on Economist Intelligence Unit: 'Special report no. 1: contraceptives', 17; 'The UK contraceptive market', *Retail Business Market Surveys*, no. 210 (Aug. 1975), 22; 'Market survey 4: contraceptives', *Retail Business Market Surveys*, no. 444 (Feb. 1995), 110.

113 *Encyclopedia of Chemical Technology*, 4th edn (New York, 1991–8), vol. 7, 219–50, at 219.

4 Human Guinea Pigs?

1 Interview with Celso Ramon Garcia by L. V. Marks, 16 Apr. 1995, transcript, 29–32, 40–1. For more information on the history behind the establishment of strict controls in human experimentation, see P. M. McNeill, *The Ethics and Politics of Human Experimentation* (Cambridge, 1993). See also interview with A. Satterthwaite by L. V. Marks, 27 Apr. 1995, transcript, 23.

2 Originally developed in East Germany, thalidomide had been considered so safe a drug that it had been available without prescription in Germany. It had also been recommended for pregnant women both to combat severe morning sickness and

as a sedative. By 1962, however, the drug had been withdrawn from the European market because of the severe birth defects it caused. The outcry over the tragedy resulted in many new regulations being imposed on pharmaceutical manufacturers in Europe. Stricter rules governing the introduction of new drugs were also passed in the USA, where a licence for the drug had narrowly missed being granted. R. Harris, *The Real Voice* (New York, 1964); R. McFadyen, 'Thalidomide in America', *Clio Medica* 11/2 (1976), 79–93; H. Sjöström and R. Nilsson, *Thalidomide and the Power of the Drug Companies* (Harmondsworth, 1972), 23–8. While thalidomide prompted stricter testing procedures, debates continue to this day about how trials should be run to test the safety of drugs.

3 S. E. Lederer, *Subjected to Science* (Baltimore, 1995); R. Rupke, ed., *Vivisection in Historical Perspective* (London, 1987).

4 Cited in L. McLaughlin, *The Pill, John Rock and the Catholic Church* (Boston, 1982), 106.

5 M. C. Chang, 'On the study of animal reproduction', talk, GP-LC, cited in J. Reed, *The Birth Control Movement and American Society* (Princeton, 1978, 1983), 349.

6 McLaughlin, *The Pill*, 105–6.

7 P. Vaughan, *The Pill on Trial* (London, 1972), 28–9, 44; Reed, *The Birth Control Movement*, 349–51; interview with Garcia by Marks, transcript, 4; interview with Dot Hunt by L. V. Marks, Apr. 1995, transcript, 12.

8 The following publications were also listed as inspiration points for the experiments: E. B. Astwood, 'Progesterone inhibition of ovulation in the rat', *American Journal of Physiology*, 127 (1939), 127; R. H. Dutt and L. E. Casida, 'Alteration of estrual cycle in sheep by use of progesterone and its effects upon subsequent ovulation and fertility', *Endocrinology*, 43 (1943), 208–17; A. W. Makepeace, C. L. Weinstein and M. H. Friedman, 'The effect of progestin and progesterone on ovulation in the rabbit', *American Journal of Physiology*, 119 (1937), 512–16; G. Pincus and R. E. Kirsch, 'The sterility in rabbits produced by injections of oestrone and related compounds', *Journal of Experimental Physiology*, 115 (1936), 219–28; G. Pincus and N. T. Werthenssen, 'The comparative behaviour of mammalian eggs *in vivo* and *in vitro*. III. Factors controlling the growth of the rabbit blastocyst', *Journal of Experimental Zoology*, 78 (1938), 1–18; G. Pincus and N. T. Werthenssen, 'An analysis of the mechanism of oestrogenic activity', *Proceedings of the Royal Society*, 126 (1939), 506; G. Pincus, 'Factors controlling the growth of rabbit blastocysts', *American Journal of Physiology*, 133 (1941), 412–13; G. Pincus, 'The physiology of ovarian hormones', *The Hormones*, vol. 2 (New York, 1950), ch. 1; G. Pincus, 'Fertilization in mammals', *Scientific American*, 184/3 (1951).

9 See Worcester Foundation, 'Report of progress to Planned Parenthood Federation of America', 24 Jan. 1952, A. Stone's papers, FCL; also in GP-LC, Box 14.

10 Ibid.

11 K. McCormick to M. Sanger, 13 Nov. 1953, MS-LC.

12 Worcester Foundation, 'Report of progress to PPFA', 23 Jan. 1953, GP-LC, Box 14; Report to the Rockefeller Foundation on research on the physiology of mammalian eggs and sperm, 12 Mar. 1953, GP-LC, Box 23.

13 Interview with Anne Merrill and Mary Ellen Fitts Johnson by L. V. Marks, 8 Apr. 1995, transcript, 18; G. Pincus, *The Control of Fertility* (New York, 1965), 67–8.

14 Pincus, *The Control of Fertility*, 57, 67–8.

15 Interview with Hunt by Marks, transcript, 33.

16 Pincus, *The Control of Fertility*, acknowledgements.

17 Interview with Merrill and Fitts Johnson by Marks, transcript, 41.

18 Ibid.

19 Ibid., 38.

20 Ibid., 39.

21 Ibid., 47.

22 F. B. McCrea and G. E. Markle, 'The estrogen replacement controversy in the USA and UK', *Social Studies of Science*, 14 (1984), 1–26; N. Pfeffer, 'Lessons from history', in P. Alderson, ed., *Consent to Health Treatment and Research*, Report of the Social Science Research Unit Consent Conference Series, no. 1 (Dec. 1992), 31–7.

23 G. Pincus to P. S. Henshaw, 28 Jan. 1953, GP-LC, Box 14. By 1954 progesterone in oil was being sold in capsules on the American market to women for preventing abortion. M. Sanger to K. McCormick, 25 Mar. 1954, MS-SS. See also Vaughan, *The Pill on Trial*, 41–2.

24 G. Pincus to P. S. Henshaw, 28 Jan. 1958 and 19 Feb. 1953, GP-LC, Box 14; K. McCormick to M. Sanger, 13 Nov. 1953, MS-LC; Notes from McCormick's conversation with Dr Rock, 6 Oct. 1955, MS-SS.

25 Further biographical details for John Rock appear in chapters 4 and 9.

26 G. D. Searle, 'Clinical experience with and practical techniques for the use of Enovid in ovulation control', 18 Jan. 1961, 8, CG-FCL, file 214, fo. 3326; Vaughan, *The Pill on Trial*, 31; McLaughlin, *The Pill*, 109–10; Reed, *The Birth Control Movement*, 351–5. Other investigators found it difficult to duplicate the rebound effect achieved by Rock. Correspondence from Denise Pullen to L. V. Marks, 11 Sept. 2000.

27 McLaughlin, *The Pill*, 110.

28 Reed, *The Birth Control Movement*, 375; McLaughlan, *The Pill*, 110–11.

29 McLaughlin, *The Pill*, 111.

30 She had been classmates with Friedman, Weinstein and Makepeace at the University of Pennsylvania; interview with Garcia by Marks, transcript, 6.

31 McLaughlin, *The Pill*, 72–89; interview with Garcia by Marks, transcript, 6–8, 21.

32 Behind the scenes Menkin was also the 'reference researcher and manuscript editor for scientific articles that reported the stage of [the pill's] development'. In later years she helped Rock to write 'popular pieces on the pill and its role in curbing runaway birth rates'. McLaughlin, *The Pill*, 91.

33 G. D. Searle, 'Clinical Experience'; Vaughan, *The Pill on Trial*, 31. For more information on John Rock see McLaughlin, *The Pill*; Reed, *The Birth Control Movement*, 351–4.

34 Garcia had originally trained at Long Island College of Medicine, in Brooklyn, now New York State University Health Science Center.

35 Interview with Garcia by Marks, transcript, 8, 12.

36 Ibid., 13, 29–32, 40–1.

37 In the USA new pharmaceutical drugs were subject to formal regulatory review as early as 1938. This had been introduced after 109 people died from taking an untested new drug in 1937. Charles O. Jackson, *Food and Drug Legislation in the New Deal* (Princeton, 1970); James Harvey Young, *The Toadstool Millionaires* (Princeton, 1961). Senate Committee on Government Operations, *Interagency Co-ordination in Drug Research and Regulation Hearings*, part 3 (Mar. 1963), 987; T. Maeder, *Adverse Reactions* (New York, 1994), ch. 5.

38 For more information on the history of human experimentation, clinical trials and informed consent before the 1960s, see L. H. Glantz, 'The influence of the Nuremberg Code on U.S. statutes and regulations', in G. J. Annas and M. A. Grodin, eds, *The Nazi Doctors and the Nuremberg Code* (Oxford, 1992), 86; *The Human Radiation Experiments: Final Report of the President's Advisory Committee* (New York, 1996); Lederer, *Subjected to Science*; H. Marks, *The Progress of Experiment* (Cambridge, 1997), 89–97, 129; P. Temin, *Taking Your Medicine* (Cambridge, Mass., 1980), 125.

39 B. Zondek to G. Pincus, 27 June 1953, GP-LC, Box 15.

40 G. Pincus to J. Rock, 15 May 1953, JR-FCL.

41 'Procedure for progesterone tests', n.d., JR-FCL; K. McCormick to M. Sanger, 17 June 1954, MS-SS.

42 K. McCormick to M. Sanger, 17 June 1954, MS-SS.

43 G. Pincus to J. Rock, 15 May 1953, JR-FCL; Worcester Foundation, 'Report of progress to the Planned Parenthood Federation of America, Inc.', 4 Mar. 1954, MS-SS, and GP-LC, Box 17; Worcester Foundation, Application for a grant to the Robert L. Dickinson Memorial, PPFA, 6 Mar. 1954, G. Pincus to K. McCormick, 5 Mar. 1954, GP-LC, Box 17; L. Tsacona to G. Pincus, 10 Apr. 1954, GP-LC, Box 19.

44 Vaughan, *The Pill on Trial*, 42–3; McLaughlin, *The Pill*, 118–19.

45 G. Pincus to K. McCormick, 5 Mar. 1954, M. Sanger to G. Pincus, 29 May 1954, G. Pincus to K. McCormick, 28 Dec. 1955, GP-LC, Box 17; P. S. Henshaw to G. Pincus, 6 Aug. 1954, GP-LC, Box 16; G. Pincus to K. McCormick, 14 Mar. 1956, GP-LC, Box 21; K. McCormick to M. Sanger, 13 Nov. 1953, MS-LC; K. McCormick to M. Sanger, 17 June 1954, K. McCormick to M. Sanger, 21 June 1954, M. Sanger to N. Larsen, 10 Sept. 1954. Notes on conversation with Dr Rock, 9 Jan. 1956, MS-SS.

46 'Suitable experimental subjects' and 'Objectives for experimentation', Nov. 1954, JR-FCL.

47 K. McCormick to M. Sanger, 31 May 1955, MS-SS.

48 K. McCormick to M. Sanger, 13 Nov. 1953, MS-LC.

49 K. McCormick to M. Sanger, 21 July 1954, MS-SS.

50 K. McCormick to M. Sanger, 21 Oct. 1954, MS-SS.

51 K. McCormick to M. Sanger, 19 July 1954, MS-SS.

52 D. Tyler to G. Pincus, 20 Oct. 1954, M. F. Fuster to G. Pincus, 1 Nov. 1954, GP-LC, Box 17.

53 A. B. Ramirez de Arellano and C. Seipp, *Colonialism, Catholicism and Contraception* (London, 1983), 111.

54 C. R. Garcia to G. Pincus, 18 June 1955, J. Diaz Carazo to G. Pincus, 16 Sept. 1955, GP-LC, Box 18.

55 McLaughlin, *The Pill*, 119.

56 The fact that women could refuse to participate indicates that the investigators were following the guidelines laid down by the Nuremberg Code on medical experimentation. This stipulated that participants in trials should not be coerced and could leave a trial. For more on this, see Glantz, 'The Influence of the Nuremberg Code', 185–6.

57 J. Diaz Carazo to G. Pincus, 16 Sept. 1955 and G. Pincus to D. Tyler, 30 Sept. 1955, GP-LC, Box 18; J. Diaz Carazo to G. Pincus, 31 Jan. 1956, GP-LC, Box 22; K. McCormick's notes on conversation with G. Pincus, 5 Mar. 1956, MS-SS. See also McLaughlin, *The Pill*, 119.

58 'Protocol on progesterone therapy in psychotic women', n.d., GP-LC, Box 17; 'Progress report: studies of the effects of progestational compounds upon psychotic subjects', 22 July 1957, GP-LC, Box 30. See also Vaughan, *The Pill on Trial*, 39–40; McLaughlin, *The Pill*, 119–20.

59 Interview with Garcia by Marks, transcript, 8; Vaughan, *The Pill on Trial*, 39.

60 G. Pincus to W. Vogt, 30 Mar. 1954, GP-LC, Box 17; G. Pincus to M. Sanger, 31 Mar. 1954, MS-SS.

61 K. McCormick to M. Sanger, 21 July 1954, MS-SS.

62 K. McCormick's notes on talk with G. Pincus, 1 Feb. 1955, MS-SS.

63 K. McCormick to M. Sanger, 19 July 1954, MS-SS.

64 K. McCormick to M. Sanger, 11 Feb. 1956, MS-SS; letter from E. Rice-Wray to W. Vogt, 10 Dec. 1953, and 'A proposal to the PPFA for a program of action in fertility control in Puerto Rico', in GP-LC, Box 17; Ramirez de Arellano and Seipp, *Colonialism, Catholicism and Contraception*, 88, 109; N. Oudshoorn, *Beyond the Natural Body* (London, 1994), 127, 128; Vaughan, *The Pill on Trial*, 41.

65 Garcia, in 'Historical perspectives of the scientific study of fertility,' transcript from the Conference on Historical Perspectives of the Scientific Study of Fertility, Session III: The Development of Endocrinology, American Academy of Arts and Sciences, Boston, 5 May 1978, cited in Oudshoorn, *Beyond the Natural Body*, 126.

66 Edris Rice-Wray had graduated from Vassar College, and obtained her medical qualifications from the University of Michigan and Northwestern University. Before going to Puerto Rico, she had run her own private medical practice in Chicago and Evanston, Illinois and worked for Planned Parenthood clinics in these areas.

67 G. Pincus to M. Sanger, 31 Mar. 1954, K. McCormick to M. Sanger, 21 July 1954, MS-SS. Notes on talk with Dr Pincus, 1 Feb.1955, MS-SS. See also K. McCormick to M. Sanger, 21 July 1954, Notes on conversation with G. Pincus, 5 March 1956, K. McCormick to M. Sanger, 17 June 1954, M. Sanger to N. Larsen, 10 Sept. 1954, G. Pincus to G. J. Watumull, 3 Apr. 1956, Notes on conversation with Dr Rock, 9 Jan. 1956, MS-SS; K. McCormick to M. Sanger, 13 Nov. 1953, MS-LC: G. Pincus to K. McCormick, 5 Mar. 1954, M. Sanger to G. Pincus, 29 May 1954, G. Pincus to K. McCormick, 28 Dec. 1955, GP-LC, Box 17; P. S. Henshaw to G. Pincus, 6 Aug. 1954, GP-LC, Box 16; G. Pincus to K. McCormick, 14 Mar. 1956, GP-LC, Box 21.

68 'Report on Puerto Rico', n.d., 3, AS-FCL; Notes on conversation with G. Pincus, 5 Mar. 1956, MS-SS.

69 Reed, *The Birth Control Movement*, 359; Oudshoorn, *Beyond the Natural Body*, 128.

70 G. Pincus to M. Sanger, 23 Mar. 1956, MS-SS.

71 Ramirez de Arellano and Seipp, *Colonialism, Catholicism and Contraception*, 113.

72 The setting up of the trials in Rio Piedras also had the advantage that the superintendent of the housing project was enthusiastic to help with the contraceptive tests and made every possible effort to supply records of the families living in the new flats. E. Rice-Wray, 'Study project of SC-4642' (Jan. 1957), 1, CG-FCL, Box 50. See also Notes on conversation with Pincus, 5 Mar. 1956, MS-SS.

73 Cited in Vaughan, *The Pill on Trial*, 49.

74 E. Rice-Wray to G. Pincus, 11 June 1956, GP-LC, Box 23.

75 K. McCormick's notes on conversation with G. Pincus, 5 Mar. 1956, MS-SS; E. Rice-Wray, 'Study project of SC-4642'; interview with Merrill and Fitts Johnson, transcript, 20; G. Pincus et al., 'Fertility control with oral medication', *American*

Journal of Obstetrics and Gynecology, 75 (1958), 1335; Oudshoorn, *Beyond the Natural Body*, 128–9.

76 G. Pincus to A. Fishberg, 28 Feb. 1956, GP-LC, Box 22; Ramirez de Arellano and Seipp, *Colonialism, Catholicism and Contraception*, 114.

77 Rice-Wray, 'Study project of SC-4642'.

78 Satterthwaite had undertaken her medical training at the University of California, San Francisco. After graduating she had practised obstetrics and gynaecology in New Jersey and then went to work in surgery in Puerto Rico. At that time it was difficult for women physicians to get surgical placements. From Puerto Rico she went to work as a medical missionary in China. Widowed shortly after going to China, she was forced to return to Puerto Rico in 1952. Interview with Satterthwaite by Marks, transcript, 1, 4, 7.

79 G. Pincus to K. McCormick, 11 Mar. 1957, GP-LC, Box 27.

80 For more on Gamble, see p. 51 above.

81 Interview with A. Satterthwaite by J. Reed, 19 June 1974, transcript, 27, Oral History Project, Schlesinger Library. See also G. Pincus, J. Rock and C. R. Garcia, 'Field trials with norethynodrel as an oral contraceptive', *Report of the Proceedings of the Sixth International Conference on Planned Parenthood*, 14–21 Feb. 1959, New Dehli. See also G. Pincus et al., 'Fertility control with oral medication'.

82 Interview with Satterthwaite by Marks, transcript, 9, 11, 12, 15.

83 Letter to Dr H. J. Bhabha from G. Pincus, 28 June 1960, NDA 10976, vol. 21, FDA archives; G. D. Searle, pamphlet on 'Conovid E', Aug. 1963, Hetherington's papers, PP/RJH/A11/3, Box 5, AM. Little has been published on the trials conducted in Kentucky. These were conducted from 1958 among 100 women of Leslie County and were supervised by the nurse Mrs Mary Breckinridge, a personal friend of John Rock and his wife. Breckinridge established the trial under the auspices of the Frontier Nursing Service. One of the reasons for the trial was the fact that the women in this area had some of the highest fertility rates in the USA and also came from a deprived socioeconomic background with low levels of education and literacy. They were therefore considered important for understanding whether the pill would be acceptable in developing countries. The study was also designed to test whether the pill could be effectively provided and supervised by nurse-midwives rather than doctors. For more information on this trial, see H. Harris, 'Clinical trials of Enovid in Kentucky, 1958–1969', paper presented to American Association for the History of Medicine, Apr. 1998.

84 Rice-Wray, 'Study project of SC-4642'.

85 Pincus to A. Fishberg, 28 Feb. 1956, GP-LC, Box 22; McCormick's notes on conversation with Pincus, 5 Mar. 1956, MS-SS; Pincus et al., 'Fertility control with oral medication', 1335. The use of social workers to check the compliance of patients with medication had also been used in the trials conducted in India. S. Ghosh and A. Gupta, 'The effectiveness as an oral contraceptive of synthetic metaxylohydroquinone, the active principle of the field pea (Pisum Sativum Linn)', *International Medical Abstracts and Reviews*, 16 (Nov. 1954), 89–90.

86 Rice-Wray, 'Study project of SC-4642'; Pincus et al., 'Fertility control with oral medication', 1335; interview with Merrill and Fitts Johnson, 35.

87 Rice-Wray, 'Study project of SC-4642'; Pincus et al., 'Fertility control with oral medication', 1335.

88 F. Laraque to G. Pincus, 7 July 1958, GP-LC, Box 32; L. Honorat to R. Crosier, 27 Aug. 1958, GP-LC, Box 32.

89 Interview with Merrill and Fitts Johnson, 35.

90 'Study of the long-term administration of 17 Ethinyl-19 Nortestosterone in fertility control', Box 109, fo. 1789, and A. P. Satterthwaite and C. J. Gamble, 'Control of ovulation with norethynodrel', 1962, CG-FCL, Box 53 fo. 849.

91 Several patients also discovered that they were pregnant before taking the tablet. E. Rice-Wray to G. Pincus, 11 June 1956, GP-LC, Box 23.

92 Interview with Edris Rice-Wray by J. Reed, 14 Mar. 1974, Oral History Project, Schlesinger Library; McLaughlin, *The Pill*, 134; Vaughan, *The Pill on Trial*, 50. G. Pincus to K. McCormick, 11 Oct. 1956, JR-FCL. Modifications in the trials meant that by July the women seemed to stop complaining of side-reactions; D. Tyler to G. Pincus, 2 July 1956, GP-LC, Box 23.

93 Vaughan, *The Pill on Trial*, 54, 56.

94 McCormick's conversation with Dr Rock, 22 Feb. 1958, MS-SS. See also Oudshoorn, *Beyond the Natural Body*, 131. Critics of the pill trials have criticized the early investigators for assuming that the side-effects were psychosomatic and for not paying enough attention to the women's feelings. Yet, as we can see, it was not an easy issue to determine. For this criticism see B. Hartmann, *Reproductive Rights and Wrongs* (New York, 1987, 1995), 190.

95 Interview with Merrill and Fitts Johnson, 34.

96 Rice-Wray, 'Study project of SC-4642'; C. Tietze to M. Snyder, 15 Aug. 1957, GP-LC, Box 28; Satterthwaite and Gamble, 'Control of ovulation with norethynodrel'.

97 McCormick's notes on conversation with Pincus, 16 May 1957, MS-SS; Ramirez de Arellano and Seipp, *Colonialism, Catholicism and Contraception*, 116.

98 G. Pincus to K. McCormick, 11 Oct. 1956, GP-LC, Box 21; C. Tietze to M. Synder, 15 Aug. 1957, GP-LC, Box 28.

99 I. Rodriguez Pla to G. Pincus, May 1956 and E. Rice-Wray to G. Pincus, 10 May 1956, GP-LC, Box 22; K. McCormick to M. Sanger, 12 May 1956; E. Rice-Wray, 'Study project of SC-4642'.

100 Ibid.; interview with Satterthwaite by Reed, transcript, 21; interview with D. Pullen by L. V. Marks, Dec. 1996, transcript.

101 Translation from *El Imparcial*, 21 Apr. 1956, GP-LC, Box 22; G. Pincus to K. McCormick, 11 Oct. 1956, JR-FCL; I. Rodriguez Pla to G. Pincus, n.d., and E. Rice-Wray to G. Pincus, 10 May 1956, 11 June 1956, GP-LC, Box 22; K. McCormick to M. Sanger, 12 May 1956; E. Rice-Wray, 'Study project of SC-4642'.

102 Interview with Satterthwaite by Reed, transcript, 22.

103 E. Rice-Wray to G. Pincus, 20 Dec. 1956, GP-LC, Box 22; interview with Satterthwaite by Reed, transcript, 29.

104 E. Rice-Wray to G. Pincus,10 Aug. 1958, GP-LC, Box 26. Letter 'For our close friends and sympathisers' attached to Annual Report of the Associacion Mexicana Pro-Bienestar de la Familia', c.1959–60, GP-LC, Box 45. See also E. Rice-Wray to G. Pincus, 6 Apr. 1959, GP-LC, Box 40.

105 E. Rice-Wray to G. Pincus, 25 Jan. 1960, GP-LC, Box 45. Interview with Rice-Wray, n.d., transcript, 1. See also interview with Rice-Wray by Reed.

106 O. Mendoza to T. O. Griessemer, 25 June–16 July 1958, CG-FCL, Box 108, fo. 1786; E. Rice-Wray to C. J. Gamble, 2 July 1959, CG-FCL, Box 108, fo. 1787; E. Rice-Wray to G. Pincus, 6 Apr. 1959, GP-LC, Box 40.

107 E. Rice-Wray to G. Pincus, 25 Jan. 1960, GP-LC, Box 45.

108 In the end Rice-Wray directed her energies towards training health professionals in family planning; E. Rice-Wray to G. Venning, n.d., Venning's papers, personal collection. Letter was probably written c.1974. Interview with E. Rice-Wray, n.d., transcript, 13, 16.

109 'Progress report of the difficulties of the clinic of the Associacion Mexicana Pro-Bienestar de la Familia up to August 24th 1961', CG-FCL, Box 108, fo. 1791; interview with E. Rice-Wray, n.d., transcript, 2–5, 7–8. I am grateful to Dr Rice-Wray's daughter Lynne Carson for giving me a copy of this taped interview.

110 A. Satterthwaite to C. Gamble, 2 Dec. 1959, Gamble's papers, CG-FCL, Box 50, fo. 819; see also interview with Satterthwaite by Reed, transcript, 22.

111 Such accusations carried on into the 1970s; interview with Edris Rice-Wray, n.d., transcript, 10, 14–15.

112 An interesting article examining the long-term side-effects of the pill not only had as its title 'Women as guinea pigs, the continuing saga', but carried a drawing of women caged up like animals. The article argued that 'women have become oestrogen guinea-pigs' (*Critical List* (Summer 1977), 25–6).

113 Boston Women's Health Collective, *Our Bodies, Ourselves* (Boston, 1984); L. Grant, *Sexing the Millennium* (London, 1993), 54; Hartmann, *Reproductive Rights and Wrongs*, 190.

114 Satterthwaite and Gamble, 'Control of ovulation with norethynodrel'; interview with Satterthwaite by Reed, transcript, 24; interview with Satterthwaite by Marks, transcript, 15. Tensions emerged between Pincus and Satterthwaite when Pincus prematurely announced in 1961 that the pill suppressed cervical cancer. Satterthwaite felt the evidence collected at that point was not convincing. For more on this, see Ramirez de Arellano and Seipp, *Colonialism, Catholicism and Contraception*, 120–1.

115 C. Gamble to M. Sanger, 18 Nov. 1954, MS-SS; McCormick's notes on conversation with Rock, 10 Oct. 1956, MS-SS. Similar anxieties were expressed by Garcia; interview with Garcia by Marks. Rock was particularly cautious of the pill because he feared a negative backlash from the Catholic church. Moreover, he saw his reputation as on the line. See McLaughlin, *The Pill*, 121–3.

116 Vaughan, *The Pill on Trial*, 49; also see interview with Satterthwaite by Marks, transcript, 23–4. Since the 1890s biological and medical literature had discussed the possibility of hazardous effects of drugs on foetuses, and this was a continual matter of debate throughout the early twentieth century. For more information on this, see Sjöström and Nilsson, *Thalidomide and the Power of the Drug Companies*, 168–72. For more information on cancer, see chapter 7 below.

117 Hartmann, *Reproductive Rights and Wrongs*, 190.

118 For more information on this issue, see chapter 6 below.

119 M. Susser, 'Epidemiology in the United States after World War II', *Epidemiologic Reviews*, 7 (1985), 147–77; A. Lilienfeld 'Epidemiology of infectious and non-infectious disease', *American Journal of Epidemiology*, 97 (1973), 135–47.

120 Interview with Merrill and Fitts Johnson by Marks, transcript, 21.

121 Interview with Garcia by Marks, transcript, 32; G. Pincus to K. McCormick, 11 Oct. 1956, JR-CL.

122 Interview with Satterthwaite by Marks, transcript, 23.

123 Interview with Garcia by Marks, transcript, 29–32; interviews with Ellen Tyler May and Denise Pullen by L. V. Marks, 13 May 1996 and 16 Dec. 1996.

124 Interview with Garcia by Marks, transcript, 29–32, 40–1; interview with

Satterthwaite by Marks, transcript, 23. For more information on the history behind the establishment of strict controls in human experimentation, see McNeill, *The Ethics and Politics of Human Experimentation.*

125 Interview with Merrill and Fitts Johnson, transcript, 28, 43; interview with Satterthwaite by Marks, transcript, 23.

126 McLaughlin, *The Pill*, 131; Oudshoorn, *Beyond the Natural Body*, 130.

127 Pincus et al., 'Fertility control with oral medication'.

128 Interview with Merrill and Fitts Johnson, transcript, 20–31.

129 Interview with Satterthwaite by Marks, transcript, 23.

130 McLaughlin, *The Pill*, 117.

131 S. Perley et al., 'The Nuremberg Code', in Annas and Grodin, *The Nazi Doctors*, 156.

132 Interview with Satterthwaite by Reed, transcript, 27–8; interview with Satterthwaite by Marks, transcript, 20.

133 'Protocol on progesterone therapy in psychotic women'; 'Progress report: studies of the effects of progestational compounds upon psychotic subjects'; see also McLaughlin, *The Pill*, 119–20.

134 A. Hodges, *Alan Turing* (London, 1983), 467–71.

135 In Oregon doctors reported that the male prisoners liked taking it because their appetite improved and they felt better. Protocol by Pincus, 29 June 1956, GP-LC, Box 23; G. Pincus to K. McCormick, 13 Dec. 1956, GP-LC, Box 21; G. Pincus to K. McCormick, 27 July 1957, GP-LC, Box 27; Nelson in G. D. Searle and Co., *Proceedings of a Symposium on 19-Nor-Progestational Steroids* (Chicago, 23 Jan. 1957), 118, JR-FCL. McCormick's conversation with Rock, 22 Feb. 1958, MS-SS; W. Crosson to J. Rock, 29 July 1958, JR-FCL. Interestingly, however, the pill was never developed as a male contraceptive because it reduced the male libido. E. Mears to M. Smyth, 24 Apr. 1963, SA/FPA/A5/162.4, Box 252.

136 One of the first American litigation cases against Searle (*Meinert v. Searle*) in the wake of thrombotic complications in 1970 was premised on the idea that the pill had been insufficiently tested before marketing. This theory, however, was rejected by the court. See J. Barrett, 'Product liability and the pill', *Cleveland State Law Review*, 19 (1970), 468–78, reprinted in J. Katz, *Experimentation with Human Beings* (New York, 1972), 789–91. For a detailed critique of the argument that women were used as guinea pigs, see S. W. Junod and L. V. Marks, 'Women on trial', forthcoming.

137 W. J. Crosson from Searle to P. DeFelice, 9 Oct. 1959, and letter from DeFelice, 9 Dec. 1959, NDA 10976, vol. 15, FDA archives; and FDA Commissioner Larrick's statement to Senate Committee on Government Operations, *Interagency Coordination in Drug Research and Regulation, Hearings – 1962, Part 1*, 233–9; leaflet information submitted by Searle for Enovid, NDA 10976, vol. 16, FDA archives. J. Rock, 'Inhibition of ovulation in the human', reprint from *Control of Ovulation* (Oxford, 1961), 233, JR-FCL.

138 Oudshoorn, *Beyond the Natural Body*, 133.

139 Memo of meeting, 15 Apr. 1965, NDA 10976, AF20-787, FDA archives.

140 NDA 12249, Librium Hydrochloride Tablets, FDA archives.

141 Junod and Marks, 'Women on trial'.

142 Ibid.

143 Senate Committee on Government Operations, *Interagency Coordination*, 233–9. See also G. Pincus, 'Progestational agents and the control of fertility', *Vitamins and Hormones*, 169 (1959), 81.

144 Oudshoorn, *Beyond the Natural Body*, 132.

145 C. Tietze, 'The current status of fertility control', n.d., *c.*1960, GP-LC, Box 50. For a critique of this methodology, see M. Meldrum, '"Simple methods" and "determined contraceptors"', *Bulletin for the History of Medicine*, 70 (1996), 266–95, at 276.

146 W. J. Crosson from G. D. Searle to P. DeFelice, 9 Oct. 1959, NDA 10976, vol. 15, FDA archives.

147 E. T. Tyler and H. J. Olson, 'Fertility promoting and inhibiting effects of new steroid hormonal substances', *Journal of American Medical Association*, 169/16 (18 Apr. 1959), 1843–54, in FDA archives, NDA 10976, vol. 14; Crosson to DeFelice, 9 Oct. 1959. For a summary of the animal tests and clinical trials done with Enovid to measure its physiological effect, see V. A. Drill, 'The experimental control of fertility by steroidal substances', in *Report of the Proceedings of the Sixth International Conference on Planned Parenthood*, 14–21 Feb. 1959, New Dehli, 167–76, in NDA 10976, vol. 22. Drill was company director for G. D. Searle.

148 Council for the Investigation of Fertility Control, fact sheet, Nov. 1970, SA/FPA/15/160/3, Box 250, AM.

149 Tietze, 'The current status of fertility control', 436–7; H. H. Cook, A. P. Satterthwaite and C. J. Gamble, 'Oral contraception by norethynodrel: a three year field study', 7, submitted in NDA 10976, vol. 21, FDA archives.

150 Crosson to DeFelice, 9 Oct. 1959, 6.

151 American obstetrician-gynaecologist Edward Tyler reported a rate of '8.6% pregnancies (22 pregnancies in 3,082 woman-months)', but a number of the women on his Los Angeles trial were taking progestational agents other than Enovid. Memo from W. H. Kessenich to G. P. Larrick, 11 May 1960, 2, in NDA 10976, vol. 15, FDA archives.

152 E. Mears, 'The clinical application of oral contraceptives', paper read to Symposium on Agents Affecting Fertility, Middlesex Hospital, 24 Mar. 24 1964, SA/FPA/A5/158B, Box 249, AM.

153 'The pill', *Eugenics Review* (May 1960), SA/FPA/A5/161/1, Box 251; 'Oral contraceptives', *c.*1960, SA/FPA/A5/167, Box 254, AM.

154 A. E. Ledder, 24 Mar. 1960, NDA 10976, vol. 15, FDA archives.

155 'The pill', *Eugenics Review*, (May 1960); 'Oral contraceptives', *c.*1960.

156 P. DeFelice to W. H. Kessenich, 15 Feb. 1961, NDA 10976, vol. 21, FDA archives.

157 'Report of a medical conference of FPA medical officers and nurses', 19 Nov. 1960, SA/FPA/A5/167, Box 253, AM.

158 E. Mears, 'Future of the Council for the Investigation of Fertility Control', 6 May 1964, SA/FPA/A5/158B, Box 249; E. Mears to A. Herxheimer, 22 Mar. 1963, Medical Letter, RG891, Box 45, fo.2, Rockefeller Archive Center.

159 P. DeFelice to Searle, 25 Sept. 1959, NDA 10976, vol. 15, FDA archives; Third Meeting of Council for the Investigation of Fertility Control, Clinical Trials Committee, 12 Jan. 1961, SA/FPA/A5/157/1, Box 249, AM.

160 These time limits seem not to have been observed in the rush to allow physicians to provide oral contraceptives, but evidence on this is admittedly scarce; Beth Bailey 'Prescribing the pill', *Journal of Social History* (Summer 1997), 827–56.

161 Crosson to P. DeFelice, 9 Oct. 1959, letter from DeFelice, 9 Dec. 1959, Ralph W. Weilerstein memo to Dr Granger, 2 Feb. 1960, all in NDA 10976, vol. 15, FDA archives.

162 Memo from Kessenich to Larrick, 11 May 1960.

163 In 1965 the FDA Advisory Committee on Obstetrics and Gynecology pointed out that 'Oral contraceptives were probably unique in that they were one of a very few and possibly [the] only class of drugs where these time restrictions had been inserted in their labelling' (First meeting, 22 and 23 Nov. 1965, 9–10, 16–17).
164 M. Jackson at IPPF press conference, 30 Mar. 1960, SA/FPA/A5/161/4, AM.
165 Interview with Roger Short by L. V. Marks, 13 Nov. 1995, notes.

5 Doctors and the Pill

1 T. Stuttaford, 'Political barriers to population control', *Spectrum*, no. 1 (1973), Hetherington's papers, PP/RJH/A6/1, Box 2, AM.
2 *BMJ*, 1 (1962), 878.
3 *BMJ*, 2 (1962), 52.
4 H. Curtis Wood, 'Unplanned children', *Medical Opinion and Review* (Mar. 1966), 28–35, cited in US Congress, Senate, *Hearings before the Subcommittee on Foreign Expenditures of the Committee on Government Operations*, 89th Congress, 2nd session, June 1966, 1153–6.
5 Stuttaford, 'Political barriers to population control'.
6 A. Leathard, *The Fight for Family Planning* (London, 1980), 108, 223.
7 Ridgeley C. Bennett, 'Remarks to the Fertility and Maternal Health Drugs Advisory Committee', 15 Jan. 1988, paper; Sharon Snider, 'The pill', *FDA Consumer*, 24/10 (1990), 8–11.
8 O. Moscucci, *The Science of Woman* (Cambridge, 1990); L. Jordanova, *Sexual Visions* (London, 1989).
9 C. McCann, *Birth Control Politics in the United States, 1916–1945* (Ithaca, 1994), ch. 3; J. Ray and F. G. Gosling, 'American physicians and birth control, 1936–47', *Journal of Social History*, 18 (1985), 399–411; E. Chesler, *Woman of Valor* (New York 1992), 270–1; J. Peel and M. Potts, *Textbook of Contraceptive Practice* (Cambridge, 1969), 14.
10 Peel and Potts, *Textbook of Contraceptive Practice*, 14; M. S. Calderone, 'Family planning and sexuality: retrospect 1953–74', MS, 2, Worcester Foundation archives; Ray and Gosling, 'American physicians and birth control', 40; Leathard, *The Fight for Family Planning*; see also interview with Denise Pullen by L. V. Marks, 16 Dec. 1996, transcript, 2.
11 McCann, *Birth Control Politics in the United States*, 97; Ray and Gosling, 'American physicians and birth control', 403–5. By 1962, two years after the pill had been put on the American market, 35,320 women were getting their pill from 83 Planned Parenthood Federation Association centres; M. S. Calderone, 'Survey of Enovid use in Planned Parenthood centers', 20 Aug. 1962, MS-SS.
12 E. Draper, *Birth Control in the Modern World* (Harmondsworth, 1972), 238; Leathard, *The Fight for Family Planning*, 118–19; Peel and Potts, *Textbook of Contraceptive Practice*, 17.
13 NHS Act 9 and 10 Geo. 6, c. 81 (1945–46), sec. 22; Government Act 1948, 11 and 12 Geo. 6, c. 26 (1947–48). See also Draper, *Birth Control in the Modern World*, 237. See also L. Hall, 'Malthusian mutations', in B. Dolan, ed., *Malthus, Medicine and Morality* (Amsterdam, 2000), 141–63 and L. Hall, '"A suitable job for a woman"?', in L. Conrad and A. Hardy, eds, *Women and Modern Medicine* (Amsterdam, 2001).
14 Draper, *Birth Control in the Modern World*, 238.

15 Leathard, *The Fight for Family Planning*, 86.

16 Draper, *Birth Control in the Modern World*, 238; Leathard, *The Fight for Family Planning*, 1–8; see also I. Kelt, 'The medical profession and the pill', B.Sc. dissertation, Wellcome Institute, June 1998, 33–4.

17 Correspondence from Dr Irvine Loudon to L. V. Marks, 1 and 2 Sept. 1998.

18 Draper, *Birth Control in the Modern World*, 147.

19 One of the first countries where physicians were actively encouraged to give women advice on contraception was Iceland, which in 1935 made it a duty for physicians. In 1966 Denmark also enacted a law which required contraceptive advice to be given to all women within six weeks of giving birth. For some idea of the variations in medical attitudes to contraception worldwide, see Draper, *Birth Control in the Modern World*, ch. 8.

20 Ray and Gosling, 'American physicians and birth control', 407; see also M. Calderone to E. V. Blasingame, American Medical Association, Chicago, 27 Dec. 1962, Calderone's papers, Box 9, fo. 154, Schlesinger Library; on the Comstock Laws, see p. 33 above.

21 McCann, *Birth Control Politics in the United States*, 95; Ray and Gosling, 'American physicians and birth control', 402–5.

22 McCann, *Birth Control Politics in the United States*, 75.

23 Ray and Gosling, 'American physicians and birth control'; Draper, *Birth Control in the Modern World*, 237–8.

24 A. Stone, 'The teaching of contraception in medical schools', *Human Fertility*, 7 (Aug. 1942), 108.

25 McCann, *Birth Control Politics in the United States*, ch. 3. See also M. Calderone to J. Rock, 14 Aug. 1963, Calderone's papers, Box 9, fo. 154, Schlesinger Library.

26 Report of Medical Director to Medical Committee meeting, 4 June 1958, JR-FCL.

27 Curtis Wood, 'Unplanned children', and S. M. Spencer, 'The birth control revolution', *Saturday Evening Post*, (15 Jan. 1966), in US Congress, Senate, *Hearings before the Subcommittee on Foreign Expenditures*, June 1966, 1153–6, 1274.

28 I. Loudon, 'Some international features of maternal mortality, 1880–1950', in V. Fildes, L. Marks and H. Marland, eds, *Women and Children First* (London, 1992), 21. See also US Congress, House of Representatives, Select Commitee on Population, *Report: Fertility and Contraception in the United States*, Dec. 1978, 24–5. McCann, *Birth Control Politics in the United States*, 93.

29 *Obstetrics and Gynecology*, 23 (Apr. 1964), cited in E. Watkins, *On the Pill* (Baltimore, 1999), ch. 2.

30 Ibid.

31 Watkins, *On the Pill*, 36.

32 Ibid., 34, 36–7.

33 US Congress, House of Representatives, *Fertility and Contraception in the United States*, 24–5.

34 Correspondence from Loudon to Marks, 1 and 2 Sept. 1998.

35 R. D. T. Farmer and T. D. Preston, 'The risk of venous thromboembolism associated with low oestrogen oral contraceptives', *Journal of Obstetrics and Gynaecology*, 15 (1995), 195–200, at 199.

36 Leathard, *The Fight for Family Planning*, 109; interview with Pullen, transcript, 32–3.

37 *BMJ*, 1 (1964), 267 of supplement, cited in Kelt, 'The medical profession and the pill'. See Kelt also for a summary of the medical profession's attitude towards government bearing the cost of contraceptive prescriptions.

38 J. Silverman and E. F. Jones, 'The delivery of family planning and health services in Great Britain', *Family Planning Perspectives*, 20/2 (Mar./Apr. 1988), 68–79, at 69.

39 C. M. Langford, *Birth Control Practice and Marital Fertility in Great Britain* (Oxford, 1976), 55. The rise in demand was also affecting family planning clinics. By 1967 the FPA was opening two or three new clinics a week to cope with the demand, and patients were reaching the half million mark. Leathard, *The Fight for Family Planning*, 123.

40 Correspondence from Loudon to Marks, 1 and 2 Sept. 1998.

41 The same was true in the USA; see Watkins, *On the Pill*, 49–52.

42 A. Cartwright, *Parents and Family Planning Services* (London, 1970), 223.

43 Peel and Potts, *Textbook of Contraceptive Practice*, 249.

44 Cartwright, *Parents and Family Planning Services*, 40, 48–9, 59–60, 62.

45 Ibid., 42–3, 48–9, 75, 223, 224, 239; M. Bone, *Family Planning Services in England and Wales* (London, 1973), 14.

46 Silverman and Jones, 'The delivery of family planning', 69.

47 Women doctors were more likely than their male counterparts to raise the issue of family planning with their patients; Cartwright, *Parents and Family Planning*, 81–5.

48 Ibid., 25, 64.

49 WHO, *Technology of Reproduction Series* (1966), no. 326.

50 Peel and Potts, *Textbook of Contraceptive Practice*, 230.

51 Ibid.

52 For more information on this, see E. Vayena, 'Cancer detectors', Ph.D thesis, University of Minnesota, Nov. 1999, chs. 4 and 5.

53 'What do consultants think of the pill?', *World Medicine* (27 Feb. 1968), 82–3.

54 Interview with Ellen Tyler May by L. V. Marks, 13 May 1996, notes.

55 This, however, did not include treatment if problems were detected. For this clinics had to refer the patients elsewhere.

56 Cartwright, *Parents and Family Planning Services*, 63; A. Wiseman, 'Family planning policies and practice in population control', Symposium on Population, n.d., 109, Wiseman's personal papers; interview with D. Pullen by L. V. Marks, 16 Dec. 1996, transcript, 32–3; interview with J. Infield by L. V. Marks, 29 Jan 1996, transcript, 24–5.

57 Cartwright, *Parents and Family Planning Services*, 56–8, 63.

58 Ibid., 239.

59 'What do consultants think of the pill?', 82–3.

60 Silverman and Jones, 'The delivery of family planning', 70.

61 For more information on national differences in medical practice, see L. Payer, *Medicine and Culture* (London, 1989).

62 In some instances doctors in the USA can be more cautious about prescribing drugs than those in Britain. For more on this issue, see F. B. McCrea and G. E. Markle, 'The estrogen replacement controversy in the USA and UK', *Social Studies of Science*, 14 (1984), 1–26.

63 Dr David B. Clark, professor of neurology at the Kentucky University Medical Centre, evidence; US Congress, Senate, *Competitive Problems in the Drug Industry: Hearings before the Subcommittee on Monopoly of the Select Committee on Small Business, US Senate, 91st Congress, Second Session, on Present Status of Competition in the Pharmaceutical Industry* (henceforth Nelson hearings), part 15 (Jan. 1970), 6136.

64 J. Guillebaud, *The Pill* (Oxford, 1991), 6, 165–7; see also Hilary Hill, 'Risks of the pill', FPA release c.1960s, SA/FPA/A5/160/2, Box 250.

65 Goldzieher was the director of the clinical sciences division of the South West Foundation for Research and Education in San Antonio.

66 Nelson hearings, part 15, 6353–4. A similar argument is made in C. Wood, *Birth Control Now and Tomorrow* (Gateshead, 1969), 156–8.

67 Nelson hearings, part 15, 6354; see also D. F. Hawkins, 'Thromboembolic risks in contraception', *Spectrum*, no. 1 (1973).

68 I. Loudon, *Deaths in Childbirth* (Oxford, 1992), 352–4; J. Leavitt, 'Joseph DeLee and the practice of preventive obstetrics', *American Journal of Public Health*, 78/10 (1988), 1353–9.

69 G. J. Engelmann, *Labour among Primitive Peoples* (St. Louis, Ind., 1882); J. DeLee, 'The prophylactic forceps operation', *AJOG*, 1 (1920–1), 34–44, 77–84. See also Loudon, *Deaths in Childbirth*, 340–3, 354–7; Leavitt, 'Joseph DeLee'.

70 *BMJ*, 1 (1961), 432. In earlier controversies over whether pregnancy was pathological, William Whitridge and Grantley Dick-Read both argued similarly that pregnancy should be seen as natural and medical intervention should be used sparingly; see Loudon, *Deaths in Childbirth*, 349–50 and 356–8.

71 Nelson hearings, part 15, 5933. See also L. Grant, *Sexing the Millennium* (London, 1993), 184–5. Davis had a vested interest in promoting intrauterine devices in place of oral contraceptives. During the 1960s he had been among the many physicians who had begun to experiment with new models of intrauterine devices. He was involved in the development of the Dalkon Shield, which he had begun to test at Johns Hopkins. The Dalkon Shield later proved hazardous to women's health. Davis's publications were used to market the IUD. For more on Davis and the Dalkon Shield, see N. J. Grant, *The Selling of Contraception* (Columbus, Ohio, 1992), 31–2, 37, 43–51.

72 *Lancet* (11 Oct. 1970), cited in Nelson Hearings, part 15, 5927.

73 Letter from Mrs G. M. Bonser to Dr E. Mears, Apr. 1960, SA/FPA/A5/161/1, Box 251, AM.

74 W. H. W. Inman, 'Role of drug-reaction monitoring in the investigation of thrombosis and "the pill"', *British Medical Bulletin*, 26/3 (1970), 248–56, at 252–3.

75 Department of Health and Social Security, *Report on Confidential Enquiries into Maternal Deaths in England and Wales: 1964–1966* (1969), cited in Inman, 'Role of drug-reaction monitoring'.

76 This was based at the Rockefeller University. Hertz also worked in various capacities for the National Institute of Health.

77 Ironically when speaking about the idea of survival, Hertz was referring to the debate taking place over the need to curb the population. The need for the prevention of births for the world population to survive contrasted with the background discussions occurring at the time of Engelman and De Lee, who saw their medical interventions as helping mothers to have more and healthier children so as to ensure the survival of the race. For more discussion on the twists and turns in the population debate, see N. Pfeffer, *The Stork and the Syringe* (Cambridge, 1993).

78 Nelson hearings, part 15, 6041.

79 Peel and Potts, *Textbook of Contraceptive Practice*, 255; see also Guillebaud, *The Pill*, 6, 165–7.

80 Dr Gabriel V. Jaffe, letter in *BMJ*, 1 (1961), 1043. WHO also promoted oral contra-

ceptives for this reason. See letter from G. G. Robertson to G. J. W. Hunter, 25 Mar. 1966, Searle archives, High Wycombe.

81 J. Rock, *The Time has Come* (New York, 1963), 167.

82 Physicians booklet, *Conovid*, Searle, July 1960, SA/FPA/A5/161/3, Box 251; see also transcript from the broadcast by Margaret Pyke on the Overseas Service of the BBC, 21 May 1962, SA/FPA/A5/161/4, Box 251, and pamphlet put out for doctors advertising Lyndiol, SA/FPA/A7/90, Box 284; information for volunteers, n.d., SA/FPA/A5/162/3, Box 252 and similarly SA/FPA/A5/157/1, Box 249, AM.

83 G. Venning, letter to editor, *BMJ* (8 Aug. 1962); 'Meet the Press', July 1962, transcript from a programme on Australian television, 7, SA/FPA/A7/109, Box 284; letter from G. Venning to V. Wynn, 1 Oct 1962, SA/FPA/A5/155, Box 248, AM.

84 A. S. Parkes, in the *Lancet* (16 Jan. 1963), SA/FPA/A5/126, Box 245, AM.

85 Nelson hearings, part 15, 6382.

86 Ibid., 5925. Interview with Victor Wynn by L. V. Marks, 6 Apr. 1994, transcript.

87 Advertisement in *Enovid Bulletin*, no. 20 (May 1964), cited in Nelson hearings, part 15, 6222.

88 The story of Andromeda is more complex than the advertisement implies. One of the reasons Andromeda had been chained to the rock was because her mother had incensed the gods by boasting about the beauty of her daughter and herself. Once freed, Andromeda's marriage to Perseus did not go smoothly. During the wedding festivities Agenor claimed Andromeda was originally betrothed to him. This made Andromeda's parents turn on Perseus, who then turned them into stone. Perseus then fled with Andromeda back to Seriphos. See R. Graves, *Greek Myths* (Wakefield, R.I., 1988); Ovid, *Metamorphoses, Book IV* (Cambridge, Mass., 1985).

89 See, for instance 'Female reproductive physiology', abridged proceedings of a symposium organized in Sept. 1964, in Birmingham, Alabama, by the Birmingham Medical Society with a grant from G. D. Searle and Co., Hetherington's papers, PP/RJH/B4/1, Box 8, AM.

90 Payer, *Medicine and Culture*, 130–1.

91 Jordanova, *Sexual Visions*; E. Martin, *The Woman in the Body* (Milton Keynes, 1987), 27–31.

92 Some examples of this are the use of forceps in childbirth, caesareans and hysterectomies. One obstetrician argued that oral contraceptives were the closest thing to surgical sterilization that had ever been devised. Nelson hearings, Part 15, 5938.

93 Ibid., 6354. See also advertisement for Ortho-Novin in *Practitioner*, Oct. 1964, in Hetherington Papers, PP/RJH/A6/2 Box 2; E. Mears, 'The clinical application of oral contraceptives', 7, paper read to Symposium of Agents Affecting Fertility, Middlesex Hospital Medical School, 24 Mar. 1964, SA/FPA/A5/158b, Box 249, AM.

94 Mears, 'Clinical application of oral contraceptives', 7.

95 G. Pincus, 'Field trials with norethynodrel as an oral contraceptive', n.d., SA/FPA/A5/161/3, Box 251, AM, also in MS-SS.

96 Dr Wiseman to E. Mears, 15 Dec. 1963, SA/FPA/158b, Box 249; E. T. Tyler, 'Eight years' experience with oral contraceptives and an analysis of use of low-dosage norethisterone', *BMJ* (3 Oct. 1964), 843–7, at 844.

97 See Dr G. Swyer's comments on Australian television, transcript 'Meet the press', July 1962, 14, SA/FPA/A7/109, Box 284, AM.

98 Dr J. Goldzieher reporting on a study by Dr Moos, Nelson hearings, part 15,

6347–8; see also Notes from Mrs Clifford Smith to Dr Pyke, 4 Mar. 1960, SA/FPA/A5/161/1, Box 251, AM.

99 Dr F. J. Kane (associate professor of psychiatry, University of North Carolina School of Medicine), Nelson hearings, part 16, 6448.

100 Some studies in the late 1960s showed that those women who had a predisposition to psychiatric disorders had a greater tendency towards depression when on the pill than those with no such previous history. Ibid..

101 Ibid.

102 Ibid., 6457.

103 Fourth meeting of doctors conducting CIFC trials, in CIFC Minutes, 10 Aug. 1964, SA/FPA/A5/155, Box 248, AM. Interestingly, those who had a history of mental problems experienced an enhanced sexual desire and capacity of orgasm when on the pill.

104 E. Mears to Dr Margaret Smyth, 24 Apr. 1963, , SA/FPA/A5/162.4, Box 252, AM.

105 T. Laqueur, *Making Sex* (Cambridge, Mass. 1990); see also G. Greer, *The Change* (London, 1993) for a critique of the treatment of women by the medical profession and the pharmaceutical industry.

106 Dr Guttmacher's comments in 'Clinical experience with and practical techniques for the use of Enovid in ovulation control', 8, transcript from a closed circuit TV symposium sponsored by Searle, 18 Jan. 1969, New York, SA/FPA/A7/110.1, Box 284, AM; see also Kane, in Nelson hearings, part 16, 6457; P. Vaughan, *The Pill on Trial* (London, 1970).

107 One such study was carried out in West Park Hospital, Surrey. See Brenda Herzberg to Christine Butler, 28 Oct. 1970, SA/FPA/A5/160/3, Box 250, AM.

108 E. Chesler, *Woman of Valor* (New York, 1992), ch. 13; McCann, *Birth Control Politics in the United States*, ch. 3.

6 Handling Health Concerns of the Pill

1 W. M. Jordan (Suffolk), letter to editor, *Lancet*, (18 Nov. 1961), 1146–7.

2 Memo from G. D. Searle to shareowners, 9 Aug. 1962, Smithsonian Collection; *New York Times*, 9 Aug. 1962; Memo to PPFA affiliates from M. S. Calderone, 6 Aug. 1962, Calderone's papers, Box 12, fo.216, Schlesinger Library, Cambridge, Mass.; *BMJ* (11 Aug. 1962), 426; J. Davey, 'How safe are the birth control pills', *Redbook*, Feb. 1963, GP-LC, Box 60.

3 *BMJ* (4 Aug. 1962), 236, 315–16, and (11 Aug. 1962), 426; *New York Times*, 9 Aug. 1962; Evidence from E. Mears in G. D. Searle, *Proceedings of a Conference: Thromboembolic Phenomena in Women* (Chicago, 1962), 42, in Calderone's papers, Box 6 fo.86; see also Memo to PPFA affiliates from M.S. Calderone, 6 Aug. 1962. In 1967 the USSR also decided to ban the pill, see B. Asbell, *The Pill* (New York, 1995), 305.

4 M. P. Vessey and J. I. Mann, 'Female sex hormones and thrombosis', *British Medical Bulletin*, 34/2 (1978), 157–62; M. P. Vessey and W. H. W. Inman, 'Speculations about mortality trends from venous thromboembolic disease in England and Wales and their relation to the pattern of oral contraceptive usage', *Journal of Obstetrics and Gynaecology of the British Commonwealth*, 80 (June 1973), 562–6, fig. 1.

5 Testimony of Richard Dickey before the FDA Advisory Committee on Oral Contraceptives, *Minutes*, 12 Oct. 1973, 5–6, table 1. For a detailed breakdown on the

kinds of dosages of pills available in the USA, see J. M. Piper and D. L. Kennedy, 'Oral contraceptives in the United States', *International Journal of Epidemiology*, 16/2 (1987), 215–21.

6 In 1980 it was calculated that preparations containing 5 mg of oestrogen were still the most widely prescribed product on the market, although lower preparations were steadily increasing. FDA Fertility and Maternity Drugs Advisory Committee, *Minutes*, 10 Apr. 1980, 66, and 23 Oct. 1980, 32.

7 R. C. Bennett, 'Impact of FDA regulation of oral contraceptives on public health', Remarks to the Society of Alumni, Johns Hopkins University School of Hygiene and Public Health Annual Meeting and Recognition Banquet, 14 Nov. 1988; R. C. Bennett, 'High dose estrogen oral contraceptives', unpublished remarks to the FDA, Fertility and Maternal Health Drugs Advisory Committee, 15 Jan. 1988; see also R. C. Bennett, 'It's effective, but is it safe: the pill', paper, n.d., Bennett's personal papers. In 1988 75 per cent of oral contraceptives on the US market contained less than 5 mg of oestrogen; B. Seaman, *The Doctors' Case against the Pill* (New York, Alameda, Calif., 1995), 222, 226. See also R. Schwarz, 'FDA panel recommends limiting estrogen dose in contraceptives', *Medical World News* (14 Mar. 1988), 13; B. Burt Gerstman et al., 'Trends in the content and use of oral contraceptives in the United States, 1964–88', *American Public Health Journal*, 81/1 (Jan. 1991), 89–96.

8 Similar arguments have been made about the different approaches the American and British have taken towards hormonal replacement therapy. In the case of HRT, however, it has been the Americans who have tended to show more caution in prescribing than the British. For more information, see F. B. McCrea and G. E. Markle, 'The estrogen replacement controversy in the USA and UK', *Social Studies of Science*, 14 (1984), 1–26.

9 Much of the information on thrombosis in this paragraph and the next is drawn from W. Inman, 'Memoirs' (unpublished), ch. 11. Inman's experiences are particularly useful for this chapter because he was the key medical officer at the Committee on Safety of Drugs (CSD) who uncovered the earliest connections between thrombotic problems and the pill. For the distress of those who witnessed the dramatic death of women suffering pulmonary embolism, see Seaman, *The Doctors' Case against the Pill*, chs 5 and 6; B. Surface, 'Controversy over "the pill"', *Good Housekeeping*, Jan. 1970, 64–5, 123–7.

10 Inman, 'Memoirs', ch. 11.

11 Ibid.

12 Searle, *Proceedings of a Conference*, 9, 74, 87; editorial in *JAMA*, 185/2 (13 July 1963), 131–2; memo from M. S. Calderone to all Planned Parenthood–World Population affiliates, Aug. 1963, PPFA papers, Sophia Smith Collection, Northampton, Mass. In order to assess the natural incidence of thrombotic disease, Searle had contacted 250,000 physicians, hospitals and pharmacists in 1962. See FDA Advisory Committee on Obstetrics and Gynecology, *Minutes*, First Meeting, 22 and 25 Nov. 1965, 26.

13 CSD, *Annual Report for the Year ending December 1966* (London, 1967), 6. For a more detailed history of the evolution of drug regulation in both the USA and Britain, see J. Abraham, *Science, Politics, and the Pharmaceutical Industry* (New York, 1995), ch. 2. See also H. Sjöström and R. Nilsson, *Thalidomide and the Power of the Drug Companies* (Harmondsworth, 1972), 23–8.

14 Today the British mechanism for monitoring adverse reactions has been severely

criticized because it relies heavily on general practitioners filling in cards, which they often fail to do.

15 Dr Carr, in Nelson hearings, Part 15 (Jan. 1970), 6002–5, 6113; US Congress, Senate, *Interagency Coordination in Drug Research and Regulation, Hearings before the Subcommittee on Reorganization and International Organizations of the Committee on Government Operations*, part 3 (Mar. 1963), 1105–7, 1168–9; CSD, *Annual Report for the Year ending December 1966*, 6.

16 I am grateful to an anonymous referee for pointing this out.

17 A. F. Guttmacher to T. Fox, 16 Mar. 1965, AG-FCL, Box 2; see also Tietze's remarks in Searle, *Proceedings of a Conference*, 12.

18 B. Seaman and G. Seaman, *Women and the Crisis in Sex Hormones* (New York, 1977), 101.

19 Interview with W. Inman by L. V. Marks, 13 Oct. 1994, transcript, 74–5; W. H. W. Inman and M.P. Vessey, 'Investigation of deaths from pulmonary, coronary, and cerebral thrombosis and embolism in women of childbearing age', *BMJ*, 2 (27 Apr. 1968), 193–211, at 194.

20 Some states, such as Pittsburgh, had better prescription monitoring than others; see FDA Advisory Committee on Obstetrics and Gynecology, *Minutes*, Second Meeting, 20 and 21 Jan. 1966, 6.

21 FDA Advisory Committee on Obstetrics and Gynecology, *Report on Oral Contraceptives* (1 Aug. 1966), 19, 61, 63–4.

22 FDA Advisory Committee on Obstetrics and Gynecology, *Second Report on Oral Contraceptives* (1 Aug. 1969), 2–3.

23 W. H. W. Inman, 'Role of drug-reaction monitoring in the investigation of thrombosis and "the pill"', *BMJ*, 26/3 (1970), 248–56, at 248. The CSD compared the number of spontaneous reports it received with the number of death certificates sent to the Registrar General.

24 Interview with Inman by Marks, 74–6. From the mid-1980s a number of computer-based general practice clinical and administrative record systems were established in Britain, which made monitoring the effects of the pill even simpler. See R. D. T. Farmer and T. D. Preston, 'The risk of venous thromboembolism associated with low oestrogen oral contraceptives', *Journal of Obstetrics and Gynaecology*, 15 (1995), 195–200.

25 Until 1963 the FPA sought the written consent of general practitioners when putting a patient on a clinical trial for the oral contraceptive pill. See CIFC Minutes, 23 Mar. 1960, 103; letter to GPs, 14 July 1960; letter to GPs, 8 June 1961, 145, SA/FPA/A5/154; see also letter from E. Mears to Hadfield, 21 Sept. 1961; letter from E. Mears to Baxter, 18 Oct. 1963, SA/FPA/A5/161/2, 51; memo from E. Mears to C. Smith, n.d., c.1965, SA/FPA/A5/161/3. All in FPA papers, AM, Box 251.

26 R. C. Elston to the editor of the *Daily Herald*, 6 Mar. 1962, SA/FPA/A5/161/2; Second Meeting of the Medical Advisory Council, Minutes, 4 Oct. 1961, 3, SA/FPA/A5/161/4. Both files in FPA papers, AM, Box 251. Interview with J. Nabarro by L. V. Marks, 9 Dec. 1996, notes; interview with D. Pullen by L. V. Marks, 16 Dec. 1996, notes.

27 Searle, *Proceedings of a Conference*.

28 Editorial in *JAMA*, 185/2 (13 July 1963), 131–2.

29 Searle, *Proceedings of a Conference*, 27–8.

30 Letter from Dr R. L. Day (medical director of the PPFA) to Mrs T. M. Evans, 12 Jan. 1966, MS-SS; see also Nelson hearings, part 15 (Jan. 1970), evidence from

D. Siegel, 6415. The sample size needed varies according to the disease studied. Myocardial infarction and strokes, for instance, which are less common events than deep vein thrombosis, would need larger sample sizes for the problem to be detected.

31 In the USA, for instance, investigators found that couples rarely stuck to a contraceptive method they were randomly assigned. Pincus pointed out that in countries where there were few other resources available to women, such as in Puerto Rico, couples were more likely to accept the method allocated to them. Searle, *Proceedings of a Conference*, 54, 58.

32 D. Seigel and P. Corfman, 'Epidemiological problems associated with studies of the safety of oral contraceptives', *JAMA*, 203/11 (11 Mar. 1963), 950–4.

33 For a more detailed breakdown of the various epidemiological studies that were undertaken between 1960 and 1970, see tables 1–4 in Vessey and Mann, 'Female sex hormones and thrombosis', 157–62. See also M. P. Vessey, 'Female hormones and vascular disease', *British Journal of Family Planning, Supplement*, 6/1 (Oct. 1980), 1–12.

34 Ad Hoc Advisory Committee, 'FDA report on Enovid', *JAMA*, 185 (1963), 776.

35 'Report from the ad hoc committee for the evaluation of a possible etiologic relation with thromboembolic conditions', Aug. 1963, 7, circulated with memo from M. Calderone to all Planned Parenthood–World Population affiliates, PPFA papers, Sophia Smith Collection; and the final report of the same committee, 14, submitted to the Commissioner of the FDA of the Department of Health, Education and Welfare, 12 Sept. 1963, Medical Letter Collection RG891, Box 56, fo.10, Rockefeller Archive.

36 FDA Advisory Committee on Obstetrics and Gynecology, *Minutes*, First Meeting, 22 and 23 Nov. 1965, 27. See also the committee's *Report on Oral Contraceptives* (1 Aug. 1966), 6.

37 P. Sartwell et al., 'Thromboembolism and oral contraceptives: an epidemiological case-control study', in FDA Advisory Committee on Obstetrics and Gynecology, *Second Report on Oral Contraceptives* (1 Aug. 1969), 21–36.

38 By March 1965 the number of reports had risen dramatically, to 38 cases of pulmonary embolism with 7 deaths, 31 cases of stroke with 2 deaths and 3 coronary thrombotic deaths. Three women had also suffered blockages to arteries in their limbs, leading to limb amputations in two of the cases. Inman, 'Memoirs', ch. 11, p. 3.

39 'Risk of thromboembolic disease in women taking oral contraceptives', *BMJ*, 2 (6 May 1967), 355–9, at 356.

40 Inman, 'Memoirs', ch. 11, p. 4.

41 FDA Advisory Committee on Obstetrics and Gynecology, *Report on Oral Contraceptives*; G. I. M. Swyer, letter to the editor *BMJ*, 1 (1966), 355; and WHO, *Technology of Reproduction Series. World Health Organization*, (1966), no. 326. Not everyone who had been present at the WHO task-force meeting on the pill agreed that there was no association between the pill and thrombotic problems. Seaman, *The Doctors' Case against the Pill*, 193. Metabolic studies conducted in Britain indicated that oral contraceptive users developed abnormalities of carbohydrate and lipid metabolism similar to steroid diabetes. This was disturbing to a number of practitioners because of the strong link between diabetes mellitis and coronary thrombosis. See V. Wynn and J. W. H. Doar, 'Some effects of oral contraceptives on carbohydrate metabolism', *Lancet*, 2 (1 Oct. 1966), 715–19; V. Wynn,

J. W. H. Doar and G. L. Mills, 'Some effects of oral contraceptives on serum-lipid and lipoprotein levels', *Lancet*, 2 (1 Oct. 1966), 720–3.

42 Inman, because of his position as a civil servant on the CSD, was initially prohibited from officially publishing his own findings. Inman, 'Memoirs', ch. 11, pp. 4, 6; interview with Inman by Marks, transcript, 26, 29; and Inman, 'Role of drug-reaction monitoring', 250.

43 MRC, 'Risk of thromboembolic disease in women taking oral contraceptives', *BMJ*, 2 (6 May 1967), 355–9; see also Inman, 'Role of drug-reaction monitoring', 251.

44 MRC, 'Risk of thromboembolic disease'.

45 Inman and Vessey, 'Investigation of deaths', M. P. Vessey and R. Doll, 'Investigation of relations between use of oral contraceptives and thromboembolic disease', *BMJ*, 2 (14 June 1969), 651–7; W. H. W. Inman et al., 'Thromboembolic disease and the steroidal content of oral contraceptives', *BMJ*, 2 (25 Apr. 1970), 203–9; M. P. Vessey et al., 'Postoperative thromboembolism and the use of oral contraceptives', *BMJ*, 3 (1970), 123–6.

46 Inman et al., 'Thromboembolic disease'.

47 P. D. Stolley et al., 'Cardiovascular effects of oral contraceptives', *Southern Medical Journal*, 71/7, (July 1978), 82–4, table 3.

48 Vessey and Mann, 'Female sex hormones and thrombosis', R. C. Bennett, 'The safety and utility of oral contraceptives containing 50 micrograms of estrogen', paper prepared for FDA Fertility and Maternal Health Drugs Advisory Committee meetings, 28 Oct. 1993.

49 Inman and Vessey, 'Investigation of deaths', p. 209.

50 M. P. Vessey and R. Doll, 'Evaluation of existing techniques', *Proceedings of the Royal Society of London*, 195 (1976), 69–80, at 73–7. In 1989 a British prospective cohort study of 17,032 women over 20 years indicated that 'mortality from ischaemic heart disease was over three times higher in the pill entry cohort than in the diaphragm and intrauterine device entry cohort (relative risk 3.3)'. Oral contraceptives were also more likely than other contraceptives to cause cerebrovascular disease. M. P. Vessey et al., 'Mortality among contraceptive users', *BMJ*, 299 (16 Dec. 1989), 1487–91, at 1488.

51 *Parliamentary Debates*, House of Commons, vol. 685, 2 Dec. 1963, written answers; vol. 711, 26 Apr. 1965, written answers, 17; vol 721, 29 Nov. 1965, oral answers, 983; vol. 729, 17 June 1966, written answers, 340; vol. 744, 4 Apr. 1967, written answers, 28–9; vol. 763, 30 Apr. 1968, oral answers, 987; vol. 783, 12 May 1969, 958; House of Lords, 5 June 1967, 163–4, 172–3, 176–7. See also *Lancet* (8 Dec. 1962), 1231; (4 Dec. 1965), 1181; (4 Feb. 1967), 284; and (11 Feb. 1967), 337.

52 US Congress, Senate, *Interagency Coordination in Drug Research and Regulation*, parts 1–5; US Congress, House of Representatives, *Hearings of the Subcommittee on Government Operations, Drug Safety*, 1964, part 1; US Congress, Senate, *Hearings before the Subcommittee on Foreign Expenditures of the Committee on Government Operations*, 89th Congress, 2nd Session, June 1966; US Congress, Senate, *Hearings before the Subcommittee on Small Business*, 90th Congress, 2nd Session, 1968, part 8.

53 *Lancet* (28 Aug. 1965), 438, and (11 Sept. 1965), 548.

54 *BMJ* cited in 'Impasse on birth control pill', *The Times*, 29 Aug. 1969.

55 See, for instance, 'Birth pill killed wife', *The Times*, 16 Oct. 1969; 'Death risk from birth control pill "inevitable"', *Daily Telegraph*, 17 Nov. 1969.

56 'The sun says a million women wait', the *Sun*, 29 Nov. 1969. Wynn's work had highlighted the detrimental effects of the pill on carbohydrate metabolism in women. See Wynn and Doar, 'Some effects of oral contraceptives on carbohydrate metabolism'; Wynn, Doar and Mills, 'Some effects of oral contraceptives on serum-lipid and lipoprotein levels'.

57 Interview with V. Wynn by L. V. Marks, 2 July 1994, transcript, 26–9.

58 Inman, 'Memoirs', chapter 11.

59 E. F. Scowen (chairman of the CSD), letter to the editor, *Lancet* (20 Dec. 1969), 1369; and *BMJ* (1969), 759.

60 R. Crossman, *The Diaries of a Cabinet Minister*, vol. 3: Secretary of State for Social Services, 1968–70 (London, 1977), 761–7.

61 Inman, 'Memoirs', ch. 11; interview with Inman by Marks, transcript, 30–2, 34, 39–40, 48–9; *Parliamentary Debates*, House of Commons, vol. 793, 15 Dec. 1969, 919; Crossman, *Diaries of a Cabinet Minister*, vol. 3, 877. The importance of the media in pushing for stronger action on the issue can be seen from the fact that the previous May, when asked about the possible withdrawal of the pill, Crossman had declared in Parliament that 'despite the evidence of adverse reactions' found among oral contraceptives, they were still to be sold; *Parliamentary Debates*, House of Commons, vol. 783, 12 May 1969, 959.

62 Seaman, *The Doctors' Case against the Pill*.

63 B. Yuncker, 'A reporter finds a cause', *New York Post*, 24 Jan. 1970, 21.

64 Seaman, *The Doctors' Case against the Pill*, 223–5; interview with B. Seaman by L. V. Marks, 12 May 1996, notes. Seaman's public profile was also raised by her appearance with Wynn on the American version of the Frost Programme on 29 Dec. 1969; transcript from Frost Programme (I am grateful to Professor Wynn for giving me a copy of this transcript). See also B. Yuncker, 'Researcher predicts ban on the pill', *New York Post*, 22 Dec. 1969, 3. One irony of Seaman's book is the fact that the preface was written by Dr Hugh Davis, who was later to become infamous for his promotion of the Dalkon Shield which was responsible for the injury of many women across the world. Seaman's role in the hearings and her appearance on television did not occur without some personal cost; see her chapter in C. Looper Baker and C. Baker Kline, eds, *The Conversation Begins* (New York, 1996), 124.

65 These hearings took place over a decade, leading to 30 volumes of published material.

66 The aim of the hearings coincided with Gaylord Nelson's main interest, which was to weaken the monopoly of businesses in providing information to the consumer. See Seaman, *Doctors' Case against the Pill*, 224; Nelson hearings; Yuncker, 'Researcher predicts ban on the pill', 3.

67 Reported in *Newsweek*, cited in 'Pill pariah', *In These Times* (7 Aug. 1995), 10–11.

68 While women had protested at the hearings themselves at not being allowed a voice, they later disrupted a closed meeting at the FDA that had been convened to talk about policy on the pill. Initiated by Alice Wolfson, this disruption set a precedent in making FDA meetings open to the public. See FDA Obstetrics and Gynecology Advisory Committee, *Minutes*, 1 Apr. 1970, 2–3; testimony of B. Seaman to FDA Fertility and Maternal Health Drugs Advisory Committee, *Minutes*, 11 Feb 1982, 1.

69 Lord Beswick (Parliamentary Under-Secretary of State for Commonwealth Affairs). Similar views were also expressed by Lord Newton. All quoted in *Lancet* (4 Feb. 1967), 284.

70 Testimony of Seaman to FDA, 11 Feb. 1982, 1. 'The book that brought consumer advocacy to the medical system', *Health Facts: Center for Medical Consumers*, 20/196 (Sept. 1995), 3–4. Paradoxically, in later years, doctors and pharmaceutical companies were able to defend themselves from lawsuits from patients over the pill on the pretext of the patient package insert, for it was difficult for patients to prove that they had not read the insert. Interview with Inman by Marks, trancript, 68.

71 'The book that brought consumer advocacy', 3–4. Women health campaigners also took up a similar cause in the context of childbirth in the 1970s.

72 B. Seaman's and Dr Easterling's evidence to FDA Fertility and Maternal Health Drugs Advisory Committee meeting, *Minutes*, 11 Feb. 1982, 1, 101. Problems with patient package inserts are discussed in greater length in chapter 10 below.

73 The high dose of the first pill stands in marked contrast to other drugs in that every other drug that has been introduced on the market has been arrived at by titrating the dose upwards from a low dose to the minimum necessary to achieve the effect required.

74 A. E. Ledder, 24 Mar. 1960, NDA 10976, vol. 15, FDA archives.

75 For more information on the difference in the original policy over the dose of the pill, see S. W. Junod and L. V. Marks, 'Women on trial', forthcoming.

76 'Oral contraceptives – 50 million users', *Population Report*, Series A, no. 1 (Apr. 1974), A–12

77 Interview with Inman by Marks, transcript, 51; *Report of the Committee of Enquiry into the Relationship of the Pharmaceutical Industry with the National Health Service, 1965–7*, Cmnd. 3410 (London, 1967).

78 Inman, 'Memoirs', chapter 11.

79 Congress, House of Representatives, *Intergovernmental Relations Subcommittee of the Committee of Government Operations, FDA Regulation of Oral Contraceptives*, 15 July 1970, 27, 87. The problem of introducing new lower dose oral contraceptives had been under discussion since 1966. See FDA Obstetrics and Gynecology Advisory Committee, *Minutes*, 17 May 1968, 3.

80 Memo from the conference held between pharmaceutical companies and the FDA, 7 Apr. 1970, in US Congress, House of Representatives *Intergovernmental Relations Subcommittee*, 15 July 1970, 30, 32–7, 41–2, 81.

81 FDA Obstetrics and Gynecology Advisory Committee, *Minutes*, 6 Jan. 1977, open session.

82 Interview with P. Corfman by L. V. Marks, May 1996, notes. See also Dr Preston, director of clinical investigations from Parke-Davis and Co., FDA Obstetrics and Gynecology Advisory Committee, *Minutes*, 12 Oct. 1973, 40; FDA Fertility and Maternal Health Advisory Committee, *Minutes*, 11 Feb. 1982, 75–6, 81–6, 101–2. See also R. C. Bennett, 'High dose estrogen oral contraceptives', unpublished remarks to the FDA Fertility and Maternal Health Drugs Advisory Committee, 15 Jan. 1988 and Bennett, 'The safety and utility of oral contraceptives'.

83 Seaman, *The Doctors' Case against the Pill*, ch. 5.

84 The total number of cases screened by the FDA for pre-marketing amounted to a total of 897 cases; 500,000 additional women, however, had taken the pill for gynaecological treatment. W. J. Crosson from Searle to P. DeFelice, 9 Oct. 1959, NDA 10976, vol. 15, FDA archives; see also letter from DeFelice, 9 Dec. 1959, NDA 10976, vol. 15, FDA archives; and FDA Commissioner Larrick's statement, in US Congress, Senate, *Interagency Coordination in Drug Research and Regulation*,

Hearings, part 1, 233–9. Precise numbers tested are hard to determine. See a discussion of this in Junod and Marks, 'Women on trial'.

85 As late as 1990 an Institute of Medicine publication made the point that women's health would be better served if less money were spent on preclinical trials and some way was found of using money from the sale of the pill to fund post-marketing surveillance. Nonetheless, despite the fact that it was largely government-funded case-control and cohort studies that unravelled the risks of thrombotic problems associated with the pill, such research continues to be underfunded to this day. This is paradoxical given that such studies cost less than the 'less useful' preclinical trials. I am grateful to an anonymous referee for this information.

86 M. P. Vessey, 'Epidemiologic studies of oral contraception', *International Journal of Fertility, Supplement*, 34 (1989), 64–70.

87 At this time 6 per cent of the American users of oral contraceptives were taking such doses. Of this group 15 per cent were women aged 45 and over, those who were considered to be at higher risk of thrombotic problems when taking the pill; Bennett, 'The safety and utility of oral contraceptives'.

88 Committee on Safety of Medicines, *Combined Oral Contraceptives and thromboembolism* (London, 1995); WHO (collaborative study of cardiovascular disease and steroid hormone contraception), 'Effect of different progestogens in low oestrogen oral contraceptives on venous thromboembolic disease', *Lancet*, 364 (1995), 1582–8; V. Gurewich et al., 'Risk of idiopathic cardiovascular death and non-fatal venous thromboembolism in women using oral contraceptives with different progestagen components', *Lancet*, 346 (1995), 1589–93; J. Guillebaud, 'Advising women on which pill to take', *BMJ*, 311 (28 Oct. 1995), 1111–12; D. Garnall, 'Controversy rages over new contraceptive data', *BMJ*, 311, (28 Oct. 1995), 1117–18; WHO, 'WHO publishes research findings on oral contraceptives and risk of venous thromboembolism', press release, WHO/92, 15 Dec. 1995, 'Row as women are warned of blood clot risk', *Daily Express*, 20, Oct. 1995, 1–2; 'Blood clot alert on the pill', *Guardian*, 20, Oct. 1995, 1–3; 'Danger pill', *Daily Mail*, 20 Oct. 1995, 1–2; 'Outrage at pill warning', *Evening Standard*, 20 Oct. 1995, 1–2.

89 *BMJ*, 311 (28 Oct. 1995), 1111–12; Summary Proceedings: Task Force on Third Generation Oral Contraceptives and the Health of Young Women, Montreal, 19–20 Oct. 1995; letter from Committee on Safety of Medicines, to doctors and pharmacists, 18 Oct. 1995, Lock's personal papers.

90 D. Williams et al., 'Effect of the British warning on contraceptive use in the General Medical Service in Ireland', *Irish Medical Journal*, 91/6 (Dec. 1999).

91 In Europe the brands accounted for between 10 and 25 per cent of the user market. Fax from W. O. Spitzer to S. Lock, 15 Oct. 1995, Lock's personal papers.

92 J. Ferguson and M. Jenkins, 'General practitioners in England prescribe second generation pills instead', letter, *BMJ*, 313 (1996) 363; S. Suissa et al. 'First-time use of newer oral contraceptives and the risk of venous thromboembolism', *Contraception*, 56/3 (Sept. 1997) 114–6.

93 D. Williams et al., 'Effect of the British warning', O. Iverson and S. Nilsen, 'Abortions increased by nearly 8 per cent in Norway', letter, *BMJ*, 313 (1996), 363–4; J. Murty and S. Firth, 'Contraceptive effectiveness may be being sacrificed for safety', letter, *BMJ*, 313 (1996), 363; E. Ketting 'CSM's advice will harm women's health world-wide', letter, *BMJ*, 312 (1996), 576; S. Hope '12 per cent of women stopped taking their pill immediately they heard CSM's warning', letter, *BMJ*, 312 (1996), 576.

94 *BMJ*, 311 (28 Oct. 1995), 1111–12, 1117–18, 1162, 1172; 'Row as women are warned of blood clot risk', *Daily Express*, 20 Oct. 1995, 1–2; 'Blood clot alert on the pill', *Guardian*, 20 Oct. 1995, 1–3; H. Katz, 'British jump gun on pill data', *Montreal Gazette*, 21 Oct. 1995, 1; 'Outrage at pill warning', *Evening Standard*, 20 Oct. 1995, 1–2; 'Whipping up panic about the pill', *Nature* 377 (26 Oct. 1995), 663.

95 Fax from Spitzer to Lock, 15 Oct. 1995.

96 K. McPherson, 'Third generation oral contraception and venous thromboembolism', *BMJ*, 312 (13 Jan. 1996), 68–9. W. O. Spitzer et al., 'Third generation oral contraceptives and risks of venous thromboembolic disorders', *BMJ*, 312 (13 Jan. 1996), 83–8; W.O. Spitzer et al., 'Third generation oral contraceptives and risk of myocardial infarction', *BMJ*, 312 (13 Jan. 1996), 88–90.

97 M. A. Lewis 'The epidemiology of oral contraceptive use', *AJOG*, 179/4 (Oct. 1998), 1086–97; S. O. Skouby, 'Oral contraceptives and venous thrombosis', *European Journal of Contraception and Reproductive Health Care*, 3/2 (June 1998), 59–64; W. O. Spitzer, 'The 1995 pill scare revisited', *Human Reproduction*, 12/11 (Nov. 1997), 2347–57; A. Szarewski, 'New evidence of risk of VTE and combined oral contraceptives', *Clinical Pulse* (2 Sept. 2000), 53, 57, 61.

98 P. M. Ridker et al., 'Ethnic distribution of factor V Leiden in 4047 men and women', *JAMA*, 277/16 (23–30 Apr. 1997), 1305–7; B. Dahlback, 'Factor V and protein S as cofactors to activated protein C', *Haemotologica*, 82/1 (Jan.–Feb. 1997), 91–5; L. Shen and B. Dahlback, 'Factor V and protein S as synergistic cofactors to activated protein C in degradation of factor VIIIa', *Journal of Biological Chemistry*, 269/29 (22 July 1994), 18735–8.

99 R. M. Bertina et al., 'Mutation in blood coagulation factor V associated with resistance to activated protein C', *Nature* 369/6475 (5 May 1994), 64–7.

100 I am grateful to Deborah Scopes for this information.

7 The Pill and the Riddle of Cancer

1 Written questions by Miss Joan Vickers, House of Commons, 7 Apr. 1960; letter to A. J. Bradshaw, from Chairman of National Marriage Guidance Council, 5 Apr. 1960; letter to Margaret Howard, from General Secretary of National Marriage Guidance Council, 31 Mar. 1960; CIFC General Secretary to Mrs A. K. Court, 28 Apr. 1960, SA/FPA/A5/161/1, Box 251, AM.

2 Evidence from Roy Hertz, in Nelson hearings, part 15, Jan. 1970, 6023.

3 G. M. Bonser to E. Mears, Apr. 1960, SA/FPA/A5/161/1, Box 251; CIFC Minutes, 21 Apr. 1960, 110, SA/FPA/A5/154, AM.

4 'How safe are the birth control pills?', *Redbook*, Feb. 1963.

5 *Time*, 84 (3 July 1964), 46. See also E. Watkins, *On the Pill* (Baltimore, 1998), 43–4, 83.

6 *BMJ* (31 Jan. 1970), 252. See also *Pharmaceutical Journal* (13 Dec. 1975), 597; E. Horvath, et al., 'Ultrastructural findings in a well differentiated hepatoma', *Digestion*, 7 (1972), 74; J. F. Baum et al., 'Possible association between benign hepatomas and oral contraceptives', *Lancet*, 2 (1973), 926–8; E. T. Mays et al., 'Hepatic changes in young women ingesting contraceptive steroids', *JAMA*, 235 (1976), 730–2; H. A. Edmonsen et al., 'Liver-cell adenomas associated with the use of oral contraceptives', *New England Journal of Medicine*, 294 (1976), 470–2; P. Vaughan, 'The pill turns twenty', *New York Times Magazine*, 13 June 1976.

See also G. R. Huggins and R. L. Giuntoli, 'Oral contraceptives and neoplasia', *Fertility and Sterility*, 32/1 (July 1979), 1–23, at 8–11; R. L. Prentice and D. B. Thomas, 'On the epidemiology of oral contraceptives and disease', *Advances in Cancer Research*, 19 (1987), 359. See *PDR* (Physician's Desk Reference) (1979), product information for Ovcon-35, warnings, 1122.

7 *Pharmaeutical Journal* (18 Sept. 1976), 257; Prentice and Thomas, 'On the epidemiology of oral contraceptives', 335–6.

8 Between 1943 and 1959 nearly 6 million American women had been prescribed stilboestrol. Nearly 3 million children had therefore been exposed to the drug. For more information on the stilboestrol episode, see B. Seaman and G. Seaman, *Women and the Crisis in Sex Hormones* (New York, 1977), 13–24, 40–2; A. Direcks and E. Hoen, 'DES: the crime continues', in K. Donnell, ed., *Adverse Effects* (Toronto, 1986), 41–50; D. B. Dutton, *Worse than the Disease* (Cambridge, 1988), ch. 3.

9 E. R. Greenblatt et al., 'Breast cancer in mothers given diethylstilboestrol in pregnancy', *New England Journal of Medicine*, 311 (1984), 1393–7.

10 Seaman and Seaman, *Women and the Crisis in Sex Hormones*, 116.

11 G. Pincus to D. Norman, 7 June 1960, GP-LC, Box 45; see also G. Pincus and C. R. Garcia, 'Studies in vaginal, cervical and uterine histology', *Metabolism*, 3 (1965), 344–7; 'How safe are the birth control pills?', *Vogue*, 8 Jan. 1961, 90–1, 128.

12 WHO, 'Fifty facts from the World Health Report 1998', Geneva, 1998.

13 General Register Office, *Registrar General's Statistical Review of England and Wales*, part 1 (London, 1969); *Newsweek*, 19 May 1969, 118; A. Kalache et al., 'Oral contraceptives and breast cancer', *British Journal of Hospital Medicine* (23 Oct. 1983), 278–84; R. Lincoln, 'The pill, breast and cervical cancer, and the role of progestogens in arterial disease', *Family Planning Perspectives*, 16/2 (Mar./Apr. 1984), 55–63, at 56, 58; C. H. Hennekens et al., 'A case-control study of oral contraceptive use and breast cancer', *JNCI*, 72/1 (Jan. 1984), 39–42; J. J. Schlesselman, 'Oral contraceptives and breast cancer', *AJOG*, 163/4, part 2 (Oct. 1990), 1379–87; WHO, 'The dimensions of reproductive ill-health, 1990–1995', Geneva, 1995.

14 S. S. Devesa et al., 'Cancer incidence and mortality trends among whites in the United States, 1947–84', *JNCI*, 79 (1987), 701–70; General Register Office, *Registrar General's Statistical Review*, part 1; *Newsweek*, 19 May 1969, 118; Lincoln, 'The pill, breast and cervical cancer', 56, 58; Schlesselman, 'Oral contraceptives and breast cancer'. By the 1990s developing countries had an incidence of cervical cancer almost four times greater than more industrialized ones; WHO, 'Fifty facts from the World Health Report 1998'. Between 1990 and 1995 the World Health Organization calculated that the number of women worldwide living with invasive cervical cancers was 2 million, and that 450,000 new cases were being diagnosed annually; WHO, 'The dimensions of reproductive ill-health'. See also R. D. Mann, 'Breast cancer risk and the administration of human hormones: Part 1. Hormone replacement therapy', *Adverse Drug Reaction Toxicology Review*, 11/3 (1992), 149–72; C. J. L. Murray and A. D. Lopez, eds, *Global Health statistics*, Harvard School of Public Health on behalf of WHO and the World Bank, Boston, 1996; J. D. Sherris, 'Cervical cancer prevention', *Family Planning Perspectives*, 25 (Jan. 1999), supplement; R. M. Richart, 'Cervical cancer in developing countries', in *Special Challenges in Third World Women's Health*, presentations at

the 1989 annual meeting of the American Public Health Association, at http://www.iwhc.org/sc_cc.html; J. Elkas and R. Farias-Eisner 'Cancer of the uterine cervix', *Current Opinion, Obstetrics and Gynecology*, 10 (1998), 47–50.

15 W. U. Gardner, 'Tumors in experimental animals receiving steroid hormones', *Surgery*, 16 (1944), 8–32, and 'Studies on steroid hormones in experimental carcinogenesis', *Recent Progress in Hormone Research*, 1 (1946), 217–60; F. Bielschowsky and E. S. Horning, 'Aspects of endocrine carcinogenesis', *British Medical Bulletin*, 14/2 (1958), 106–15, at 107; L. S. Goodman and A. Gilman, *The Pharmacological Basis of Therapeutics*, 2nd edn (New York, 1960), 1594; W. Sneader, *Drug Prototypes and their Exploitation* (Chichester, 1996), 315. See also N. Oudshoorn, *Beyond the Natural Body* (Routledge, 1994), 107.

16 Gardner, 'Tumors in experimental animals' and 'Studies on steroid hormones'; Bielschowsky and Horning, 'Aspects of endocrine carcinogenesis', 107; Goodman and Gilman, *The Pharmacological Basis of Therapeutics*, 1594; Sneader, *Drug Prototypes and their Exploitation*, 315.

17 J. P. Lippincott and Co., *New and Nonofficial Remedies* (Philadelphia, 1951), 330; Goodman and Gilman, *The Pharmacological Basis of Therapeutics*, ch. 61; R. Hertz et al., 'Observations on the effect of progesterone on carcinoma of the cervix', *JNCI*, 11 (Apr. 1951), 867–75. C. Djerassi, *The Pill, Pygmy Chimps and Degas' Horse* (New York, 1992), 56.

18 Interview with Celso Ramon Garcia by L. V. Marks, 16 Apr. 1995, transcript, 8, 12.

19 *Newsweek*, 30 Jan. 1961, 71; *Business Newsweek*, 21 Jan. 1961, 32; 'How safe are the birth control pills?', *Vogue*.

20 G. Pincus, 'Control of contraception by hormonal steroids', *Science*, 153 (19 July 1966), 493–500, at 497; E. T. Tyler, 'Oral Contraceptives', *JAMA*, 175 (1961), 225; E. T. Tyler, *JAMA*, 187 (1964), 562; J. W. Goldzieher, L. E. Moses and L. T. Ellis, *JAMA*, 180 (1962), 352; E. Rice-Wray et al., 'Clinical trials of a combination of lynestrenol and menstranol (lyndiol) as an oral contraceptive agent', *Canadian Medical Association Journal*, 9 (12 Nov. 1966), 1024–30. See also Watkins, *On the Pill*, 82.

21 Gynaecologists tended to be more nervous about the risks than endocrinologists who were a younger and more pioneering profession. 'How safe are the birth control pills?', *Vogue*.

22 J. Rock to G. Pincus, 29 Sept. 1961 and G. Pincus to J. Rock, 7 Oct. 1961, GP-LC, Box 50.

23 R. Hertz to G. Pincus, 30 Mar. 1964, GP-LC, Box 72; R. Hertz and J. C. Bailar, 'An appraisal of some unresolved problems involved in the use of estrogen-progestogen combinations for contraception', National Institutes of Health staff paper, Apr. 1964.

24 R. Hertz to J. Rock, 14 May 1964, GP-LC, Box 72. Hertz and Bailar, 'An appraisal'.

25 G. Pincus to R. Hertz, 29 Apr. 1964, GP-LC, Box 72.

26 J. Goldzieher to R. Hertz, 7 Apr. 1964 and R. Greenblatt to R. Hertz, 20 Apr. 1964, GP-LC, Box 72.

27 R. Hertz to G. Pincus, 4 May 1964, GP-LC, Box 72.

28 *Time*, 84 (3 July 1964), 46; see also Watkins, *On the Pill*, 43–4, 83.

29 National Advisory Cancer Council, Subcommittee on Carcinogenesis and Prevention, 'Report of meeting on oral contraceptives', 23 July 1964, 2–3, Rockefeller Archive, National Committee on Maternal Health, Box 94, fo. 1752, record group IV3B4.4. I am grateful to Effy Vayena for this report.

30 Ibid.

31 Ibid., 7. Until the end of the 1970s scientists lacked a consensus on the relevance of animals for testing oral contraceptives in relation to cancer. G. C. Buehring, 'Oral contraceptives and breast cancer', *Biomedicine and Pharmacotherapy*, 42 (1988), 525–30.

32 National Advisory Cancer Council, 'Report of meeting on oral contraceptives', 7–8. For more information on the complex number of methods used by epidemiologists to explore the connection between the pill and cancer, see Huggins and Giuntoli, 'Oral contraceptives and neoplasia'.

33 FDA Advisory Committee on Obstetrics and Gynecology, *Report on Oral Contraceptives* (1 Aug. 1966), appendix 5; R. Hertz and J. C. Bailar, 'Estrogen-progestogen combinations for contraception', *JAMA*, 198 (Nov. 1966), 136–42; R. Hertz, 'Experimental and clinical aspects of the carcinogenic potential of steroid contraceptives', *International Journal of Fertility*, 13 (Oct.–Dec. 1968), 273–86. See also Watkins, *On the Pill*, 87.

34 FDA Advisory Committee, *Report on Oral Contraceptives*, Appendix 5, 51; see also Watkins, *On the Pill*, 87.

35 Watkins, *On the Pill*, 87.

36 FDA Advisory Committee, *Report on Oral Contraceptives*; FDA Advisory Committee on Obstetrics and Gynecology, *Second Report on Oral Contraceptives* (1 Aug. 1969), 3, 6.

37 FDA Advisory Committee, *Second Report on Oral Contraceptives*, 6–7.

38 M. R. Melamed et al.,'Prevalence rates of uterine cervical carcinoma in situ for women using the diaphragm or contraceptive oral steroids', *BMJ*, 3 (1969), 195–200; FDA Advisory Committee, *Report on Oral Contraceptives*, 6–8, 21–31; FDA Advisory Committee, *Second Report on Oral Contraceptives*, 6–7, 63–4.

39 Melamed et al., 'Prevalence rates'; see also Watkins, *On the Pill*, 93–4.

40 *Newsweek*, 11 Aug. 1969, 59.

41 FDA Advisory Committee, *Report on Oral Contraceptives*, 6–8, 21–31; FDA Advisory Committee, *Second Report on Oral Contraceptives*, 6–7, 63–4.

42 FDA Advisory Committee, *Second Report on Oral Contraceptives*, 7; see also P. Vaughan, 'The pill on trial', *Observer Review*, 1 Mar. 1970, 29.

43 FDA Advisory Committee, *Second Report on Oral Contraceptives*, 65.

44 Vaughan, 'The pill turns twenty'.

45 Royal College of General Practitioners (RCGP), *Oral Contraceptives and Health* (Oxford, 1974), 78–9; M. P. Vessey and R. Doll, 'Evaluation of existing techniques', *Proceedings of the Royal Society of London*, 195 (1976), 69–80, 71; M. Vessey, 'Contraceptive methods: risks and benefits', *BMJ* (9 Sept. 1978).

46 Interview with Valerie Beral by L. V. Marks, 17 and 26 Dec. 1998, notes and tape.

47 M. P. Vessey et al., 'Investigations of the possible relationship between oral contraceptives and benign and malignant breast disease', *Cancer*, 28 (1971), 1395; M. Vessey et al., 'Oral contraceptives and breast neoplasia', *BMJ*, 3 (1972), 719–34. RCGP, *Oral Contraceptives and Health*, 84, fig. 13.1; P. E Sartwell et al., 'Epidemiology of benign breast lesions', *New England Journal of Medicine*, 288 (1973), 551; Boston Collaborative Drug Surveillance Programme, 'Oral contraceptives and venous thromboembolic disease, surgically confirmed gallbladder disease, and breast tumours', *Lancet* (23 June 1973), 1399–404, at 1403. See also L. A. Brinton et al., 'Risk factors for benign breast disease', *American Journal of Epidemiology*, 113/3 (Mar. 1981), 203–14; Huggins and Giuntoli, 'Oral contraceptives and neoplasia', 6–7.

48 B. MacMahon et al., 'Etiology of human breast cancer', *JNCI*, 50 (1973), 21–42; for more discussion of this issue, see Huggins and Giuntoli, 'Oral contraceptives and neoplasia', 4–5, 6–7. One of the difficulties with benign breast disease is the considerable lack of agreement about what constitutes a pathological and what a normal lesion in the breast; V. L. Ernster, 'The epidemiology of benign breast disease', *Epidemiological Reviews*, 3 (1981), 184–202.

49 RCGP, *Oral Contraceptives and Health*, fig. 13.1; M. Vessey et al., 'A long term follow-up study of women using different methods of contraception', *Journal of Biosocial Science*, 8 (1976), 373.

50 Vessey and Doll, 'Evaluation of existing techniques', 69; see also R. W. Shaw, 'Adverse long-term effects of oral contraceptives', *British Journal of Obstetrics and Gynaecology*, 94 (Aug. 1987), 734–30, at 728.

51 D. M. Parkin et al., 'Estimates of worldwide frequency of sixteen major cancers in 1980', *International Journal of Cancer*, 41 (1988), 184–97. V. Beral et al., 'Does pregnancy protect against ovarian cancer?', *Lancet* (20 May 1978), 1083–6, at 1083.

52 M. L. Newhouse et al., 'A case-control study of carcinoma of the ovary', *British Journal of Preventive Social Medicine*, 31 (1977), 148–9, 152–3.

53 Ibid., 152–3.

54 Beral et al., 'Does pregnancy protect against ovarian cancer?'

55 J. T. Cassagrande et al., '"Incessant ovulation" and ovarian cancer', *Lancet* (28 July 1979), 170–3.

56 Prentice and Thomas, 'On the epidemiology of oral contraceptives and disease', 343–7.

57 J. L. Stanford, 'Oral contraceptives and neoplasia of the ovary', *Contraception*, 43/6 (1991), 543–56.

58 WHO, 'Epithelial ovarian cancer and combined oral contraceptives', *International Journal of Epidemiology*, 18 (1989), 538–45.

59 Cancer and Steroid Hormone Study of the Centers for Disease Control (CASH), 'Oral contraceptive use and the risk of ovarian cancer', *JAMA*, 249 (1983), 1596–9, cited in Stanford, 'Oral contraceptives and neoplasia of the ovary'.

60 B. S. Cutler, 'Endometrial carcinoma after stilboestrol therapy in gonadal dysgenesis', *New England Journal of Medicine*, 287 (1972), 628, cited in Seaman and Seaman, *Women and the Crisis in Sex Hormones*, 60–1, see also 402–6, 418–19; Prentice and Thomas, 'On the epidemiology of oral contraceptives and disease', 335.

61 *Pharmaceutical Journal* (18 Sept. 1976), 257; see also Seaman and Seaman, *Women and the Crisis in Sex Hormones*, 96–7; Prentice and Thomas, 'On the epidemiology of oral contraceptives and disease', 335; Huggins and Giuntoli, 'Oral contraceptives and neoplasia', 12–13. As early as 1963, the year that the first sequential preparation was marketed in the USA, one British investigator involved with clinical trials of the sequential pills had expressed concern that because of their high oestrogen component, sequential pills might be potentially carcinogenic. CIFC Minutes, 20 June 1963, 99, SA/FPA/A5/155, AM.

62 Prentice and Thomas, 'On the epidemiology of oral contraceptives and disease', 336–7. This article provides a good summary of the investigations during the 1980s. See also also Huggins and Giuntoli, 'Oral contraceptives and neoplasia', 12–13; J. A. Fortney et al., 'Oral contraceptives and life expectancy', *Studies in Family Planning*, 17/3 (May/June 1986), 117–25, at 118–19.

63 M. C. Pike et al., 'Breast cancer in young women and use of oral contraceptives',

Lancet, 2 (1983), 926–30; K. McPherson et al., 'Oral contraceptives and breast cancer', *Lancet*, 2 (1983), 1414–15. The same month the pill's link with liver cancer was further confirmed by a new study; *Medical News* (27 Oct. 1983). For a medical discussion on the results in 1983 see *Lancet* (22 Oct. 1983), 947–8.

64 Vessey and Doll, 'Evaluation of existing techniques', 71. Preliminary research from the RCGP also indicated that the results of Vessey's study might have exaggerated the extent of the risk of the pill causing cervical cancer. See C. R. Kay, letter to the editor, 'Oral contraceptives and cancer', *Lancet* (29 Oct. 1983), 1018.

65 *Evening Chronicle*, 28 Oct. 1983.

66 K. Dunnell, *Family Formation* (London, 1976), M. Bone, *The Family Planning Services* (London, 1978) and C. A. Bachrach, 'Contraceptive practice among young American women, 1973–1982', *Family Planning Perspectives*, 16/6 (1984), 253–9, all cited in K. McPherson, 'Modelling latent effects in any association between oral contraceptives and breast cancer', in H. Morgenstern et al., eds, *Models of Non-Communicable Diseases: Health Status and Health Service Requirements* (Heidelberg, 1992), 74–5. K. McPherson and J. Owen, letters to the editor, *BMJ*, (20 Sept. 1986), 710. See also M. Thorogood and M. Vessey, 'Trends in use of oral contraceptives in Britain', *British Journal of Family Planning*, 16 (1990), 46, table 4. By 1987 over 80 per cent of all British general practitioners' prescriptions of the pill were for women under the age of thirty. M. Thorogood and L. Villard-Mackintosh, 'Combined oral contraceptives', *British Medical Bulletin*, 49/1 (1993), 124–39, at 125; R. Russel-Briefel et al., 'Prevalence and trends in oral contraceptive use in pre-menopausal females, ages 12–54, United States, 1971–1980', *American Journal of Public Health*, 75 (1985), 1173–6.

67 *Sunday Telegraph*, 23 Oct. 1983; *Guardian*, 25 Oct. 1983; 'More worries about the pill', *Nature*, 305 (27 Oct. 1983), 749–50; *Mid-Sussex Times*, 28 Oct. 1983; *Windsor, Slough and Eton Express*, 28 Oct. 1983. Lincoln, 'The pill, breast and cervical cancer', 55–63.

68 Letters to the editor, *Lancet* (29 Oct. 1983), 1019; (5 Nov. 1983), 1081; (17 Dec. 1983), 1414–15. For a critique of the progestogen potency issue by a representative of a pharmaceutical company, see F. M. Sturtevant, 'Breast cancer and oral contraceptives', *Biomedicine and Pharmacotherapy*, 38 (1984), 371–9. See also C. R. Kay, 'Latest views on pill prescribing', *Journal of the Royal College of General Practitioners* (Nov. 1984), 611–14, at 612.

69 Lincoln, 'The pill, breast and cervical cancer'.

70 J. Laurence, 'More bad news for the pill', *New Society* 22/29 (Dec. 1983), 50; see also *Hospital Doctor* (19 Jan. 1984), 9.

71 Ibid. According to WHO, breast cancer posed one of the most serious challenges in the prevention of cancer field; D. Parkin et al., 'Estimates of worldwide frequency of twelve major cancers', *WHO Bulletin*, 2 (1984), 163–82.

72 'Breast cancer and the pill – a muted reassurance', *BMJ*, 282/6282 (27 June 1981), 2075–6; see also 'Another look at the pill and breast cancer', *Lancet* (2 Nov. 1985), 985–7.

73 Editorial, 'Oral contraceptives', *JAMA*, 249/12 (25 Mar. 1983), 1624–5; Hennekens et al., 'A case-control study of oral contraceptive use', 41.

74 Interview with Beral by Marks.

75 E. Fasal and R. S. Paffenberger, 'Oral contraceptives as related to cancer and benign lesions of the breast', *JNCI*, 55/4 (Oct. 1975), 767–73.

76 RCGP, *Oral Contraceptives and Health*; S. Ramcharan, ed., *The Walnut Creek*

Contraceptive Drug Study, vol. 1 (Washington DC, 1974). For a summary of the investigations in the 1980s, see M. P. Vessey, 'Epidemiologic studies of oral contraception', *International Journal of Fertility, Supplement*, 34 (1989), 64–70; Schlesselman, 'Oral contraceptives and breast cancer', 1379; and D. C. G. Skegg, 'Risks and benefits of oral contraceptives', in Institute of Medicine, *Oral Contraceptives and Breast Cancer* (Washington, 1991).

77 Men given oestrogen, for instance, had an increased risk of getting breast cancer. 'Breast cancer and the pill – a muted reassurance'.

78 H. Leis, 'Endocrine prophylaxis of breast cancer with cyclic estrogen and progesterone', *International Surgery*, 45/5 (May 1966), 496–503, at 497–8. L. A. Brinton et al., 'Oral contraceptives and breast cancer', *International Journal of Epidemiology*, 11/4 (1982), 316–22; Kalache et al., 'Oral contraceptives and breast cancer', 278–84; D. B. Thomas, 'Do hormones cause breast cancer?', *Cancer*, 53 (1 Feb. 1984), Supplement, 595–601; Huggins and Giuntoli, 'Oral contraceptives and neoplasia', 4; Prentice and Thomas, 'On the epidemiology of oral contraceptives', *Advances in Cancer Research*, 19 (1987), 342; M. Vessey, 'Oral contraceptives and breast cancer', *IPPF Medical Bulletin*, 21/6 (Dec. 1987), 1–2, at 1.

79 The first hypothesis that the pill in early life could lead to breast cancer was presented in R. S. Paffenberger et al., 'Cancer risk as related to use of oral contraceptives during fertile years', *Cancer*, 39 (1977), 1887–91.

80 M. C. Pike et al., 'Oral contraceptive use and early abortion as risk factors for breast cancer in young women', *British Journal of Cancer*, 43 (1981), 72–6; M. C. Pike et al., 'Breast cancer in young women'; McPherson et al., 'Oral contraceptives and breast cancer'; all cited in Skegg, 'Risks and benefits of oral contraceptives', 169. See also Prentice and Thomas, 'On the epidemiology of oral contraceptives', 342. Another case-control investigation carried out in Sweden and Norway, which had appeared in 1986, confirmed earlier findings that young women taking the pill for long periods of time might increase their risk of breast cancer. The risk, however, seemed unrelated to age at the time of first oral contraceptive use. O. Meirik et al., 'Oral contraceptive use and breast cancer in young women', *Lancet* (20 Sept. 1986), 650–3.

81 UK National Case-Control Study Group, 'Oral contraceptive use and breast cancer risk in young women', *Lancet*, 1 (1989), 973–82; M. P. Vessey et al., 'Oral contraceptives and breast cancer: Latest findings in a large cohort study', *British Journal of Cancer*, 59 (1989), 613–17; M. P. Vessey et al., 'Mortality among oral contraceptive users.', *BMJ*, 299 (16 Dec. 1989), 1487–91. The results of this national investigation to some extent confirmed the results of other research carried out by Vessey, McPherson and other colleagues in 1982. See M. P. Vessey et al., 'Oral contraceptive use and abortion before first term pregnancy in relation to breast cancer risk', *British Journal of Cancer*, 45 (1982), 327–31.

82 B. V. Stadel et al., 'Oral contraceptives and breast cancer in young women', *Lancet* (2 Nov. 1985), 970–3, at 970; CASH, 'Oral contraceptive use and the risk of breast cancer', *New England Journal of Medicine*, 315/7 (1986), 405–11. Preliminary findings of this study had been released as early as 1982. See CASH, 'Long-term oral contraceptive use and risk of breast cancer', *JAMA*, 249 (1983), 1591–5. See also 'Another look at the pill and breast cancer', *Lancet* (2 Nov. 1985), 985–7. Such results were reconfirmed on re-analysing the data according to methods used by McPherson. FPA, 'Joint statment on oral contraception and breast cancer', 20 Nov. 1987.

83 L. Rosenberg et al., 'Breast cancer and oral contraceptive use', *American Journal of Epidemiology*, 119 (1984), 167; Lincoln, 'The pill, breast and cervical cancer', 56–8; Hennekens et al., 'A case-control study of oral contraceptive use', 39–42; D. R. Miller et al., 'Breast cancer risk in relation to early oral contraceptive use', *Obstetrics and Gynecology*, 68/6 (Dec. 1986), 863–8; R. J. Lipnick, 'Oral contraceptives and breast cancer', *JAMA*, 255/1 (3 Jan. 1986), 58–61.

84 J. J. Schlesselman et al., 'Breast cancer in relation to type of estrogen contained in oral contraceptives', *Contraception*, 36 (1987), 595.

85 J Peto, 'Oral contraceptives and breast cancer', *Lancet*, 1 (1989), 552; B. V. Stadel et al., 'Oral contraceptives and breast cancer', *Lancet*, 1 (1989), 1257.

86 Lincoln, 'The pill, breast and cervical cancer', 56.

87 See, for instance, letters from K. McPherson and J. O. Drife in *BMJ* (20 Sept. 1986), 710 and J. M. Kaldor et al., *BMJ*, 293 (29 Nov. 1986), 1433.

88 FPA, 'Joint statement on oral contraception and breast cancer', 20 Nov. 1987.

89 J. J. Schlesselman et al., 'Breast cancer in relation to early use of oral contraceptives', *JAMA*, 259/12 (25 Mar. 1988), 1828–33; C. Paul et al., 'The pill and breast cancer', letter to the editor, *BMJ*, 293 (29 Nov. 1986), 1433; O. Meirik et al., 'Oral contraceptive use and breast cancer in young women', 650; 'Another look at the pill and breast cancer', *Lancet* (2 Nov. 1985), 985–7; C. Paul et al., 'Oral contraception and breast cancer in New Zealand', in R. D. Mann, ed., *Oral Contraceptives and Breast Cancer* (Carnforth, Lancs, 1990), 85–94.

90 Skegg, 'Risks and benefits of oral contraceptives', 170.

91 K. McPherson et al., 'Early oral contraceptive use and breast cancer', *British Journal of Cancer*, 56 (1987), 653; S. S. Jick et al., 'Oral contraceptives and breast cancer', *British Journal of Cancer*, 59 (1989), 618; UK National Case-Control Study, 'Oral contraceptives and breast cancer risk in young women'.

92 C. E. D. Chivers and J. M. Deacon, 'Oral contraceptives and breast cancer', *British Journal of Cancer* 61/1 (1990), 3; Schlesselman, 'Oral contraceptives and breast cancer'.

93 Buehring, 'Oral contraceptives and breast cancer', 526.

94 Chivers and Deacon, 'Oral contraceptives and breast cancer'.

95 J. M. Kaldor et al., letter to the editor, *BMJ*, 293 (29 Nov. 1986), 1433.

96 Interview with Beral by Marks.

97 Ibid. See also P. A. Wingo, et al., 'Age specific differences in the relationship between oral contraceptive use and breast cancer', *Obstetrics and Gynecology*, 78/2 (1991), 161–70.

98 UK National Case-Control Study Group, 'Oral contraceptive use and breast cancer risk in young women', 982.

99 V. Beral, 'Parity and susceptibility to cancer', in *Fetal Antigens and Cancer*, Ciba Foundation Symposium 96 (London, 1983), 182–203.

100 This research was summarized in V. Beral, 'Childbearing, oral contraceptives and breast cancer', *Lancet*, 3/41 (1993), 110–12.

101 CASH, 'Breast cancer and hormonal contraceptives', *Lancet*, 347 (22 June 1996), 1713–27; CASH, 'Breast cancer and hormonal contraceptives: Further results', *Contraception*, 53/3s (1996), 1s–106s; see also *Lancet*, 348 (7 Sept. 1996), 683. The data collected together came not only from studies conducted in Britain, the United States, Australia and New Zealand, but also Chile, China, Colombia, Kenya, Mexico, Nigeria, the Philippines and Thailand. Interview with Beral by Marks.

102 CASH, 'Breast cancer and hormonal contraceptives'.

103 Ibid.

104 'Pill scares and public responsibility', *Lancet*, 347/9017 (22 June 1996), 1707.

105 V. Beral et al., 'Mortality associated with oral contraceptive use', *BMJ*, 318 (9 Jan. 1999), 96–100.

106 Skegg, 'Risks and benefits of oral contraceptives', 166.

107 Beral et al., 'Mortality associated with oral contraceptive use'.

108 Ibid.

109 *IPPF Medical Bulletin*, 32/6 (Dec. 1998), 2; D. Grimes, 'The safety of oral contraceptives', AJOG, 166/6 (June 1992), part 2, 1950–4, at 1952.

110 Interview with Beral by Marks, notes.

111 Grimes, 'The safety of oral contraceptives', 1951.

112 J. W. Goldzieher, 'Are low-dose oral contraceptives safer and better?', *AJOG*, 171/3 (Sept. 1994), 587–90, at 590.

113 Grimes, 'The safety of oral contraceptives', 1951. Oral contraceptives are also known to help protect against pelvic inflammatory disease and ectopic pregnancy.

114 Meta-analysis is the combining of results of separate studies carried out to answer the same question. The foundations of this approach were laid in the 1970s by epidemiologists such as Richard Peto in the UK and Thomas Chalmers in the USA. Their aim was to find a method for understanding the confusing amount of data thrown up by the growing number of clinical trials. Instead of setting up a new trial, the aim was to collect and reanalyse all the data available from previous trials. See C. Cookson, 'The nature of things', *Financial Times*, 26–27 Nov. 1994, 3.

8 'A Dream Come True'

1 M. Sanger, *The New Motherhood* (London, 1922), 120, 11.

2 M. Stopes, *Enduring Passion* (London, 1928), 28, cited in A. McLaren, *A History of Contraception* (Oxford, 1990), 224.

3 Interview with Mrs A. C. by Ros O'Brien, Autumn 1997, transcript, 1.

4 Claire Boothe Luce cited in B. Seaman, *The Doctors' Case against the Pill* (Alameda, Calif., 1995), 5, 56.

5 A. F. Guttmacher, 'The pill around the world', Sept. 1966, paper for *IPPF Medical Bulletin*, AG-FCL, Box 18.

6 E. Draper, *Birth Control in the Modern World* (Harmondsworth, 1965, 2nd edn 1972), 74. The figures are approximate and apply only to the married female population. Statistics collected in later years show the percentages to be much lower when measured against the total female population (married and single) of childbearing age. See 'Oral contraceptives in the 1980s', *Population Reports*, Series A, 10/3 (May–June 1982), A-192, fig. 2.

7 See chapter 1 and R. M. Courey, 'Participants in the development, marketing and safety evaluation of the oral contraceptive, 1950–1965', Ph.D thesis, University of California, Berkeley, 1994.

8 Letter to G. Pincus, cited in L. Grant, *Sexing the Millennium* (New York, 1994), 53.

9 Draper, *Birth Control*, 288–93, 312; K. Fisher, 'An oral history of birth control practice *c*.1925–50', D.Phil. thesis, Oxford, 1997, 203–4.

10 Draper, *Birth Control*, 90, 93–4, 339.

11 McLaren, *A History of Contraception*, 235.

12 A. Tone, 'Contraceptive consumers', *Journal of Social History*, 29/3 (1996), 485–506.

13 McLaren, *A History of Contraception*, 236.

14 This is not to suggest that there was not a substantial market for such contraceptives in Britain. By the early 1960s there were approximately 7,000 retail outlets for contraceptives in England and Wales. Over 80 per cent of the sales were handled by pharmacies. Contraceptives were also supplied through barbers' shops, clinics, surgical stores, general practitioners' surgeries and mail order firms. J. Peel, *Manufacture and Retailing of Contraceptives in England* (1963), cited in Draper, *Birth Control*, 340.

15 The extensive use of withdrawal was not unique to Britain, but had a very long historical tradition across cultures; see Draper, *Birth Control*, 81–2. The use of coitus interruptus disappeared sooner in the United States. This was initially most noticeable among the college-educated middle-class whites, but was observable in other classes by the late 1920s. See J. Reed, *The Birth Control Movement and American Society* (Princeton, 1984), 124–6.

16 Draper, *Birth Control*, 82–3.

17 J. Peel and M. Potts, *Textbook of Contraceptive Practice* (Cambridge, 1969), 25–6; McLaren, *A History of Contraception*, 235; A. Wiseman, 'Oral contraceptives in family planning', *Journal of the College of General Practice of Canada* (June 1966), 18–21; Fisher, 'An oral history', 99.

18 Draper, *Birth Control*, 82–3.

19 Differences in health-care structures and the ways the medical profession viewed contraception and the pill also had an important influence on the uptake of the pill; for more on this see chapter 5 above.

20 L. A. Westoff and C. F. Westoff, *From Now to Zero* (Boston, 1971), 21; US Congress, House of Representatives, Select Committee on Population, *Report: Fertility and Contraception in the United States* (Dec. 1978), 22–3; H. W. Ory, *Making Choices* (New York, 1983), 10.

21 W. F. Pratt and C. A. Bachrach, 'What do women use when they stop using the pill?', *Family Planning Perspectives*, 19/6 (1987), 257–66, at 259.

22 Peel and Potts, *Textbook of Contraceptive Practice*, 26

23 Confirmed by figures from the US Bureau of the Census, International Database.

24 A. Cartwright, *How Many Children?* (London, 1976), 50–1.

25 C. M. Langford, *Birth Control Practice and Marital Fertility in Great Britain* (London, 1976), 26–7, 34; see also Draper, *Birth Control*, 309.

26 See also M. Woolf, *Family Intentions* (London, 1971), 86.

27 This is also confirmed by figures from the US Bureau of the Census, International Database.

28 *General Household Survey* (London, 1983), 47; A. Cartwright, 'Family size, contraceptive practice and fertility intentions in England and Wales, 1967–1975', *Family Planning Perspectives*, 11/2 (1979), 128–37, at 129.

29 This was not always the case. In some cases men, most working class, were unwilling for their wives to be on the pill for years after their family size had been completed.

30 Fisher 'An oral history', 30, 158, 161, 201, 208, 219–20, 226, 235, 244, 273, 275, 297.

31 A Scottish study undertaken in the 1980s showed that the efficacy of the pill continued to be a powerful component in people's choice of contraceptives in general in later years; see K. Hunt, 'The first pill-taking generation', *British Journal of Family Planning*, 16 (1990), 3–15, at 13.

32 Cartwright, *How Many Children?*, 168–9; Woolf, *Family Intentions*, 86.

33 E. F. Jones, J. R. Beninger and C. F. Westoff, 'Pill and IUD discontinuation in the United States, 1970–1975', *Family Planning Perspectives*, 12/6 (1980), 293–300, at 294; M. N. Bhrolcháin, 'The contraceptive confidence idea', *Population Studies*, 42 (1988), 205–25, at 225.

34 A. Cartwright, *Parents and Family Planning Services* (London, 1970), 30–3, table 15.

35 Interview with Denise Pullen by L. Marks, 16 Dec. 1996, transcript, 51.

36 Interview with Mrs M. B. by Ros O'Brien, 15 Mar. 1997, transcript, 14.

37 Cartwright, *Parents and Family Planning Services*, 32.

38 Interview with Mrs P. C. by Wendy Neil, 13 Nov. 1997, transcript, 2. Mrs P. C. had worked in the heartland of Sheffield's heavy steel industry. See also interview with Mrs J. S. by O'Brien, 25 Mar. 1997, transcript, 2, 8; interview with Mrs R. T. by O'Brien, Winter 1997, transcript, 1.

39 Betty Vincent comment in *Timewatch* TV programme: 'The pill: prescription for revolution', National Sound Archive.

40 See, for instance, interview with Mrs S. S. by O'Brien, Winter 1997, transcript 1.

41 Interview with Mrs J. F. by O'Brien, 25 Mar. 1997, transcript, 7. See also interview with Mrs R. T. by O'Brien, 1.

42 Interview with Mrs M. B. by O'Brien, Winter 1997, transcript, 3. Similar feelings were expressed by American women. See E. Watkins, *On the Pill* (Baltimore, 1998), 54.

43 Interview with Jean Infield by L. V. Marks, 29 Jan. 1996, transcript, 21–2.

44 A. Wiseman, 'Oral contraceptives in family planning', 21. See also interview with Pullen by Marks, 41; Seaman, *The Doctors' Case against the Pill*, 108.

45 This was not uncommon and a phenomenon recognized by psychologists in the 1970s; see K. Luker, *Taking Chances* (Berkeley, 1975), 25.

46 See for instance interview with Maureen Delenian, *Timewatch* tape, C612/02/C612/03, transcript, 34.

47 Interview with Mrs J. F. by O'Brien, transcript, 7; see also interview with Mrs R. T. by O'Brien, transcript, 1.

48 Interview with Helen Gurley Brown for *Timewatch*, tape C612, transcript, 22.

49 Interview with Mrs A. C. by O'Brien, transcript, 2; letter from Mrs A. C. to Lara Marks, n.d.

50 Interview with Denise Pullen, *Timewatch*, tape C612/07/08, transcript, 13; see also interview with Heather Bailey, *Timewatch*, tape C612/05/C612/06, transcript, 13.

51 Interview with Mrs R. W. by O'Brien, transcript, 6. See also Woolf, *Family Intentions*, 61–2 for more discussion of the ways in which the effectiveness of contraception shaped people's expectations about the ideal family size.

52 Fisher, 'An oral history', 253, 275.

53 Draper, *Birth Control*, 311; see also Woolf, *Family Intentions*, 76, 83.

54 Interview with Mrs R. T. by O'Brien, transcript, 4.

55 Interview with Pullen by Marks, 3–4, 20–1.

56 Interview with Maureen Delenian, *Timewatch*, transcript, 31, 41, 45.

57 S. M. Scrimshaw, 'Women and the pill', *Family Planning Perspectives*, 13/6 (Nov./Dec. 1981), 254–62, at 260.

58 Antoinette, cited in Seaman, *The Doctors' Case against the Pill*, 52.

59 Interview with Mrs C. H. by O'Brien, transcript, 3; correspondence between Mrs C. H. and L. Marks, 30 Aug. 2000 and 1 Sept. 2000.

60 Ibid.

61 Interview with Maureen Delenian, *Timewatch*, transcript, 31, 41, 45.

62 Interview with Mrs C. H. by O'Brien, transcript, 6; see also interview with R.W. by O'Brien, transcript, 6.

63 Interview with Mrs R. T. by O'Brien, transcript, 4.

64 Interview with Pullen by Marks, 26–7.

65 Ibid., 28.

66 Ibid. See also Seaman, *The Doctors' Case against the Pill*, 107; Luker, *Taking Chances*, 116.

67 Cartwright, *Parents and Family Planning Services*, 151.

68 Interview with Mrs S. S. by O'Brien, transcript, 4; interview with Mrs J. A. S. by O'Brien, transcript, 4; interview with Helen Gurley Brown for *Timewatch*, transcript, 14; see also Luker, *Taking Chances*, 127–8.

69 Andy, cited in Seaman, *The Doctors' Case against the Pill*, 54.

70 Woolf, *Family Intentions*, 75–6, 120.

71 Luker, *Taking Chances*, 123, 127–8.

72 Westoff and Westoff, *From Now to Zero*, 104, 106, 111.

73 Ibid., 103.

74 Cartwright, 'Family size', 130.

75 Westoff and Westoff, *From Now to Zero*, 61–4.

76 Ibid., 104; Luker, *Taking Chances*, 7, 102.

77 W. Mosher, 'Fertility and family planning in the 1970s', *Family Planning Perspectives*, 14/6 (1982), 314–20, at 315, 316.

78 Cartwright, *Parents and Family Planning Services*, 202–6, table 82.

79 Cartwright, 'Family size', 130; A. Cartwright, 'Trends in family intentions and the use of contraception among recent mothers, 1967–84', *Population Trends*, 49 (1987), 31–4, 33.

80 'Proposed trial of Searle contraceptive tablet', 2 May 1960, CMAC, SA/FPA/A5/157/1, Box 249; 'Proposed trial of Searle contraceptive pill', 23 Mar. 1960, in CIFC Minutes, AM, SA/FPA/A5/154.

81 Interview with Infield by Marks, 27–8.

82 Watkins, *On the Pill*, 64, 67; Office of Health Economics, *Family Planning in Britain* (London, 1972), 19; A. Leathard, *The Fight for Family Planning* (London, 1980), 16.

83 Interview with Mrs M. B. by O'Brien, transcript, 2, 4; interview with Pullen by Marks, transcript, 31; interview with Infield by Marks, transcript, 22.

84 CIFC Minutes, 81, AM file A5/154; memo from Dr Bond, CIFC Minutes, 10 Mar. 1960, 77–8, AM file A5/154; interview with Pullen by Marks, transcript, 25, 29.

85 J. Davey, 'How safe are the birth control pills?', *Redbook*, Feb. 1963; see also S. M. Spencer, 'The birth control revolution', *Saturday Evening Post*, 15 Jan. 1966, 21–5, 64, 67–90, in US Congress, Senate, *Hearings before the Subcommittee on Foreign Expenditures of the Committee on Government Operations*, 89th Congress, 2nd session, June 1966, 1264–5.

86 Interview with Mrs M. B. by O'Brien, 15 Mar. 1997, transcript, 2, 4; interview with

Pullen by Marks, transcript, 31; interview with Infield by Marks, transcript, 22.

87 Leathard, *The Fight for Family Planning*, 139–41.

88 L. Grant, *Sexing the Millennium* (London, 1993), 99–106, 115.

89 K. Kiernan, H. Land and J. Lewis, *Lone Motherhood in Twentieth-Century Britain* (Oxford, 1998), 25–9.

90 Ibid., 31; see also K. Dunnell, *Family Formation* (London, 1976), 7, 11–12.

91 B. Asbell, *The Pill* (New York, 1995), 200; Spencer, 'The birth control revolution', 21–5, 64, 67–90.

92 Kiernan, Land and Lewis, *Lone Motherhood*, 56, table 2.17.

93 S. Humphries, *A Secret World of Sex* (London, 1991), ch. 3.

94 Interview with Helen Gurley Brown for *Timewatch*, transcript, 2–4, 9–10.

95 Interview with Jan Williams for *Timewatch*, Tape C612/04, transcript, 15–16.

96 Ibid., 19.

97 Ibid., 9.

98 Kiernan, Land and Lewis, *Lone Motherhood*, 85, 113, 114.

99 Ibid., 85.

100 Ibid., 31.

101 Wiseman, 'The pill', MS., n.d., *c.*1966, ch. 2, 15.

102 Kiernan, Land and Lewis, *Lone Motherhood*, 114.

103 A. Wiseman, 'Should you tell your daughter?' *Evening Standard*, 4 Nov. 1966.

104 Spencer, 'The birth control revolution', 21–5, 64, 67–90.

105 Ibid., see also Watkins, *On the Pill*, 74.

106 Watkins, *On the Pill*, 64.

107 US Congress, House of Representatives, Select Committee on Population, *Fertility and Contraception in the United States*, 68–9.

108 Dunnell, *Family Formation*; M. Bone, *The Family Planning Services* (London, 1978) and C. A. Bachrach, 'Contraceptive practice among young American women, 1973–1982', *Family Planning Perspectives*, 16/6 (1984), 253–9, all cited in K. McPherson, 'Modelling latent effects in any association between oral contraceptives and breast cancer', in H. Morgenstern et al., eds, *Models of Non-Communicable Diseases: Health Status and Health Service Requirements* (Heidelberg, 1992), 74–5. K. McPherson and J. Owen, letters to the editor, *BMJ* (20 Sept. 1986), 710. See also M. Thorogood and M. Vessey, 'Trends in use of oral contraceptives in Britain', *British Journal of Family Planning*, 16 (1990), 41–53, 46, table 4. By 1987 over 80 per cent of all British GPs' prescriptions of the pill were for women under the age of 30. M. Thorogood and L. Villard-Mackintosh, 'Combined oral contraceptives', *British Medical Bulletin*, 49/1 (1993), 124–39, at 125; R. Russel-Briefel et al., 'Prevalence and trends in oral contraceptive use in pre-menopausal females, ages 12–54, United States, 1971–1980', *American Journal of Public Health*, 75 (1985), 1173–6.

109 Dunnell, *Family Formation*; Bone, *The Family Planning Services*, 42–4.

110 'Fertility and contraception in 12 developed countries', *Family Planning Perspectives*, 13/3 (Mar./Apr. 1981), 93–103, at 100. E. F. Jones et al., 'Unintended pregnancy, contraceptive practice and family planning services in developed countries', *Family Planning Perspectives*, 20/2 (1988), 53–67, at 55.

111 'Lower-dose pills', *Population Reports*, Series A, no. 7 (Nov. 1988), 1–31, at 10.

112 Pratt and Bachrach, 'What do women use when they stop using the pill?', 259.

113 W. H. W. Inman and M. P. Vessey, 'Investigation of deaths from pulmonary, coronary, and cerebral thrombosis and embolism in women of child-bearing age', *BMJ*, 2 (27 Apr. 1968), 193–9; M. P. Vessey and R. Doll, 'Investigation of relations between use of oral contraceptives and thromboembolic disease: a further report', *BMJ*, 2 (14 June 1969), 651–7; W. H. W. Inman et al., 'Thromboembolic disease and the steroidal content of oral contraceptives', *BMJ*, 2 (25 Apr. 1970), 203–9; M. P. Vessey et al., 'Postoperative thromboembolism and the use of oral contraceptives', *BMJ*, 3 (1970), 123–6.

114 Interview with Mrs J. A. S. by O'Brien, transcript, 7.
115 Interview with Mrs M. F. by O'Brien, Summer 1997, 1, 3.
116 Betty Vincent, interview on *Timewatch*.
117 Mrs T., cited in B. Seaman, *The Doctors' Case against the Pill*, 19.
118 Seaman, *The Doctors' Case against the Pill*, 46.
119 Interview with Mrs R. T. by O'Brien, transcript, 5.
120 See chapter 4 above.
121 The case of C. G., cited in M. Benn and R. Richardson, 'Uneasy freedom', *Women's Studies International Forum*, 7/4 (1984), 219–25, at 223.
122 Seaman, *The Doctors' Case against the Pill*, 106.
123 Ibid., 106–7.
124 Ibid., 107.
125 The case of V., cited in Benn and Richardson, 'Uneasy freedom', 221.
126 Ibid.
127 The case of A. H., cited in Benn and Richardson, 'Uneasy freedom', 223.
128 Ibid.; see also S. Pollock, 'Refusing to take women seriously', in R. Arditti et al., eds, *Test-Tube Women* (London, 1984), 148–51, at 149–50.
129 Interview with Barbara Seaman by L. Marks, 12 May 1996 notes.
130 The case of C. G., cited in Benn and Richardson, 'Uneasy freedom', 221.
131 The case of G. T., cited in Benn and Richardson, 'Uneasy freedom', 223.
132 Seaman, *The Doctors' Case against the Pill*, 77–81.
133 Interview with Mrs R. T. by O'Brien, transcript, 6.
134 Cartwright, *Parents and Family Planning Services*, 232–4.
135 Seaman, *The Doctors' Case against the Pill*, 218.
136 See chapter 6 above. See also F. B. McCrea and G. E. Markle, 'The estrogen replacement controversy in the USA and UK', *Social Studies of Science*, 14 (1984), 1–26.
137 Jones, Beninger and Westoff, 'Pill and IUD discontinuation' 293–300; J. D. Forrest, 'The delivery of family planning services in the United States', *Family Planning Perspectives*, 20/2 (1988), 88–95, at 94.
138 UN, *Levels and Trends of Contraceptive Use as Assessed in 1994* (New York, 1996), 56.
139 Pratt and Bachrach, 'What do women use when they stop using the pill?', 258.
140 See, for instance, Hunt, 'The first pill-taking generation', 13–15.
141 Eleanor B., cited in Seaman, *The Doctors' Case against the Pill*, 60.
142 UN, *Recent Levels and Trends of Contraceptive Use as Assessed in 1983* (New York, 1984), 38.
143 Woman married to an architect, cited in Seaman, *The Doctors' Case against the Pill*, 48.
144 K. Hunt and E. Annandale, 'Predicting contraceptive method usage among women in West Scotland', *Journal of Biosocial Science*, 22 (1990), 405–21, at 418.

9 Divisive Device

1 Text of *Humanae Vitae*, Encyclical of Pope Paul VI on the Regulation of Birth, 25 July 1968.

2 E. Stourton, *Absolute Truth* (London, 1999); P. Allitt, *Catholic Intellectuals and Conservative Politics in America 1950–1985* (New York, 1993), 10, 122–3.

3 Cited in L. McLaughlin, *The Pill, John Rock and the Catholic Church* (Boston, 1982), 153.

4 Ibid., 147.

5 Stourton, *Absolute Truth*, 44.

6 McLaughlin, *The Pill*, 148, 151.

7 R. B. Kaiser, *The Encyclical that Never Was* (London, 1987), 70.

8 Cited in J. Rock, 'We can end the battle over birth control', *Good Housekeeping*, July 1961, JR-FCL; see also J. Rock, *The Time Has Come* (New York, 1963), 87–8.

9 Allitt, *Catholic Intellectuals*, 166.

10 E. Watkins, *On the Pill* (Baltimore, 1998), 47.

11 Allitt, *Catholic Intellectuals*, 168; B. Asbell, *The Pill* (New York, 1995), 246–7.

12 A. F. Guttmacher, 'Church, state, and babies', *The Register Leader* (Summer 1965), AG-FCL, Box 3.

13 S. M. Spencer, 'The birth control revolution', *Saturday Evening Post*, 15 Jan. 1966, 68; Kaiser, *The Encyclical that Never Was*, 41, 49–50.

14 Interview with Anne Biezanek in Asbell, *The Pill*, 219. See also the Introduction above for more on Anne Biezanek.

15 McLaughlin, *The Pill*, 130.

16 Kaiser, *The Encyclical that Never Was*, 47; McLaughlin, *The Pill*, 168; Asbell, *The Pill*, 226.

17 'Birth control: the pill and the church', *Newsweek*, 6 July 1964, 51.

18 Kaiser, *The Encyclical that Never Was*, 166; McLaughlin, *The Pill*, 175; Stourton, *Absolute Truth*, 45.

19 McLaughlin, *The Pill*, 175.

20 Address to the International Congress of Hematology, 12 Sept. 1958, cited in McLaughlin, *The Pill*, 159.

21 McLaughlin, *The Pill*, 159. The rhythm method relied on taking the daily body temperature to determine a woman's fertility. Intercourse was not to take place during the fertile period.

22 E. Ubell, 'Birth-control pill found effective', *New York Herald Tribune*, 28 May 1958.

23 Rock, *The Time Has Come*, 103.

24 'Notes on the Round Table Meeting of December 4 1936', Robert Dickinson papers, Francis Countway Library, cited in J. Reed, *The Birth Control Movement and American Society* (Princeton, 1984), 188; McLaughlin, *The Pill*, 124–5.

25 J. Rock, 'Medical and biological aspects of contraception', *Clinics*, 1 (Apr. 1943), 1601–2, cited in Reed, *The Birth Control Movement*, 353.

26 M. Sanger to M. Ingersoll, 18 Feb. 1954, MS-SS, cited in Reed, *The Birth Control Movement*, 352.

27 McLaughlin, *The Pill*, 124–5.

28 K. McCormick to M. Sanger, 19 July 1954, MS-SS, cited in Reed, *The Birth Control Movement*, 352.

29 M. Sanger to Mrs John D. Rockefeller Jr, 19 Feb. 1954, MS-SS, cited in Reed, *The*

Birth Control Movement, 352.

30 Cited in McLaughlin, *The Pill*, 156.
31 Rock, *The Time Has Come*, 103; Kaiser, *The Encyclical that Never Was*, 58.
32 'Birth control: the pill and the church', 51–2.
33 Rock, 'We can end the battle over birth control'.
34 Ibid.; see also J. Rock, 'It is time to end the birth control fight', *Saturday Evening Post*, 20 Apr. 1963, 10, 14.
35 Cited in McLaughlin, *The Pill*, 162.
36 Cited in ibid., 154–5.
37 McLaughlin, *The Pill*, 155.
38 J. Rock to K. McCormick, 4 Oct. 1961, JR-FCL.
39 McLaughlin, *The Pill*, 162.
40 Ibid., 164, 167; see also Allitt, *Catholic Intellectuals*, 166–7
41 McLaughlin, *The Pill*, 168; Allitt, *Catholic Intellectuals,* 166.
42 Kaiser, *The Encyclical that Never Was*, 43, 81.
43 Ibid., 47.
44 Stourton, *Absolute Truth*, 46.
45 Kaiser, *The Encyclical that Never Was*, 67–9.
46 Ibid., 103.
47 Stourton, *Absolute Truth*, 46.
48 Ibid.
49 Ibid.
50 Excerpts cited in ibid, 47.
51 Cited in Asbell, *The Pill*, 276.
52 Kaiser, *The Encyclical that Never Was*, 129–31.
53 Stourton, *Absolute Truth*, 48.
54 Ibid.
55 Allitt, *Catholic Intellectuals*, 172; McLaughlin, *The Pill*, 186–7.
56 Stourton, *Absolute Truth*, 50.
57 Allitt, *Catholic Intellectuals*, 169.
58 'Final report of the Pontifical Commission on Population, Family and Birth', *Tablet* (22 Apr. 1967), reprinted in Kaiser, *The Encyclical that Never Was*, 13.
59 McLaughlin, *The Pill*, 188.
60 Stourton, *Absolute Truth*, 52.
61 *Humanae Vitae*.
62 Ibid.
63 Kaiser, *The Encyclical that Never Was*, 83.
64 McLaughlin, *The Pill*, 189.
65 Stourton, *Absolute Truth*, 49.
66 Asbell, *The Pill*, 278–80; Stourton, *Absolute Truth*, 49.
67 Stourton, *Absolute Truth*, 5, 21, 31, 52; see also McLaughlin, *The Pill*, 189; Kaiser, *The Encyclical that Never Was*, 267.
68 J. Rock, cited in P. Vaughan, *The Pill on Trial* (London, 1972), 206–7.
69 Editorial, 'The birth control encyclical', *Commonweal* (9 Aug. 1968), 515–16, cited in Allitt, *Catholic Intellectuals*, 174.
70 Kaiser, *The Encyclical that Never Was*, 245–6; see also Asbell, *The Pill*, 289–90.
71 'The theologians retort', *Commonweal* (23 Aug. 1968), 553, cited in Allitt, *Catholic Intellectuals*, 175, and Kaiser, *The Encyclical that Never Was*, 244. See also McLaughlin, *The Pill*, 189–91.

72 Asbell, *The Pill*, 297.

73 Rock, cited in Vaughan, *The Pill on Trial*, 206–7.

74 Allitt, *Catholic Intellectuals,* 175.

75 Ibid.

76 See chapter 10 below.

77 UN, *Recent Levels and Trends of Contraceptive Use as Assessed in 1983* (New York, 1984), 60.

78 Watkins, *On the Pill*, 63.

79 Asbell, *The Pill*, 247–8.

80 McLaughlin, *The Pill*, 191.

81 Asbell, *The Pill*, 297.

82 Cited in Vaughan, *The Pill on Trial*, 205.

83 Allitt, *Catholic Intellectuals,* 175.

84 Kaiser, *The Encyclical that Never Was*, 42.

85 'Birth control: the pill and the church'.

86 Cited in J. Rock, 'Keynote address to Symposium on Progestogen-Estrogen Compounds', *Applied Therapeutics*, 6/5 (May 1964), 406–9, at 407.

87 Kaiser, *The Encyclical that Never Was*, 42.

88 Ibid.

89 'Birth control: the pill and the church'; John Rock, transcript, in A David Brinkley Journal Special, 'Birth control how?', JR-FCL; John Rock, 'Sex, science and survival', Seventh Oliver Bird Lecture, 8 Apr. 1964, delivered to London School of Hygiene, JR-FCL; see also Allitt, *Catholic Intellectuals*, 171–2.

90 Kaiser, *The Encyclical that Never Was*, 60.

91 *Humanae Vitae*.

92 Stourton, *Absolute Truth*, 58.

93 *Post*, 3 Apr. 1997. In 1965, John Paul II, then known as Cardinal Karol Wojtyla, had in fact been appointed as an expert to the Pontifical Commission. One of the reasons he had been selected for the commission was because he had published a book on the philosophy of relationships called *Love and Responsibility*. The book was remarkable because it combined the modern approach to sex, whereby sex could be seen as pleasurable, with the traditional teachings of the church. Nonetheless, he had never been present at the commission's discussions because he was too busy with his campaign against communism in Poland. See Stourton, *Absolute Truth*, 50–1.

10 Panacea or Poisoned Chalice?

1 S. M. Spencer, 'The birth control revolution', *Saturday Evening Post*, 15 Jan. 1966, 21–5, 66–70, at 22.

2 Pearl S. Buck, 'The pill and the teenage girl', *Reader's Digest* (Apr. 1968), 111; E. Watkins, *On the Pill* (Baltimore, 1998), 66.

3 'OCs – update on usage, safety, and side effects', *Population Reports*, Series A, no. 5 (Jan. 1979), A-136.

4 UN, *Levels and Trends of Contraceptive Use as Assessed in 1994* (New York, 1996), 56.

5 Ibid., table 11; UN, *Recent Levels and Trends of Contraceptive Use as Assessed in 1983* (New York, 1984), table 9.

6 R. Courey, 'Participants in the development, marketing and safety evaluation of the oral contraceptive, 1950–1965', Ph.D thesis, University of California, Berkeley, 1994, 180.

7 A. Guttmacher, 'The pill around the world', 5, prepared for *IPPF Medical Bulletin*, Sept. 1966, AG-FCL, Box 18.

8 'Oral contraceptives – 50 million users', *Population Reports*, Series A, no. 1 (Apr. 1974), A-17; Courey, 'Participants', 180–2.

9 Alliances between pharmaceutical companies and international agencies can be seen from the correspondence concerning the provision of free pills by Syntex and Searle to the Population Council; see 'Use of oral contraceptives in Population Council programs', Minutes of meeting, 22 Aug. 1966, and notes by B. Berelson, 11 Aug. 1966, Population Council Papers, Box 124, fo. 2263, record group IV; and J. W. Richter to H. Levin, 23 Mar. 1966, Population Council papers, Box 125, fo. 2302, record group IV, Rockefeller Archive.

10 The USA continued to be the world leader in providing funds for global family planning programmes, providing almost 40 per cent of the $1.2 billion in population aid for developing countries in 1994. Such funding, however, was later cut by about a third with the Republican takeover of Congress in the mid-1990s. 'Editorial: paying for family planning', *Lancet*, 352 (12 Sept. 1998), 831.

11 'Oral contraceptives – 50 million users', A-17.

12 'OCs – update on usage, safety, and side effects', A-136–41.

13 Ibid.

14 'Lower-dose pills', *Population Reports*, Series A, no. 7 (Nov. 1988), 1–31, at 10.

15 Geoffrey Venning, an official from Searle, retrospectively reflected that one of the reasons that India and other developing countries saw the imposition of the pill and other forms of contraception as a Western plot was because the West had failed to recognize their own problems. G. Venning, 'Family planning and population policies in developed and less developed countries', chapter for *Clinics in Endocrinology and Metabolism*, 2/3 (1973), 13, MS chapter 18. G. D. Searle papers, High Wycombe.

16 Courey, 'Participants', 179, 184, 188–9, 192–8, 202–3, 216–25. Venning blames these intricate medical regulations on 'British and American medical schools which have played a major part in exporting a philosophy and medical educational policy which is almost totally inappropriate for Indian needs. The example of contraceptive policies is but part of a wider picture of upside down policies.' What he criticizes is the ways in which the West has confined contraceptives, such as the pill, to distribution through medical clinics and not making them available on demand through commercial and other channels. Venning, 'Family Planning and Population policies', p. 14.

17 Watkins, *On the Pill*, 56; D. Roberts, 'Black women and the pill', *Family Planning Perspectives*, 32/2 (Mar./Apr. 2000), 92–3.

18 Ibid.

19 See chapter 6 above.

20 B. Zondek to G. Pincus, 27 June 1953, GP-LC, Box 15; Y. Koya to M. Sanger, 8 July 1954, K. McCormick to M. Sanger 12 Mar. 1955, K. McCormick's notes on conversation with Dr Pincus, 23 Apr. 1959, MS-SS; M. Matsuba to G. Pincus, 22 July 1954, Y. Koya to M. Sanger, 24 Oct. 1954, GP-LC, Box 17; M. Ishikawa to M. Sanger, 14 Jan. 1955, GP-LC, Box 18; M. Ishikawa to G. Pincus, 18 Feb. 1955, MS-SS; G. Pincus to Y. Koya, 18 Oct. 1957, I. Winter to M. Ishikawa, 21 Oct. 1957, M. Ishikawa et al., 'Report of experimental studies of SC 4642', M. Ishikawa,

'Clinical study of antifertility property of orally administered progesterone', GP-LC Box 26; McCormick, 'Notes on a conversation with Dr Pincus', 23 Apr. 1959, CG-FCL, Box 195, fo. 3080; G. Pincus to J. Ijiri and G. Tokuda, 18 Nov. 1959, GP-LC, Box 38; Y. Ued and K. Hayashi, 'Present state of oral contraception in Japan', *Journal of the Japanese Obstetrical and Gynecological Society*, 9/1 (Jan. 1962), 26–39; Family Planning Federation of Japan, 'Japan's experience in family planning – past and present', 1967, Ford Foundation Archive, Population Box 12532, in 'Various population papers 1963–67'.

21 M. Sanger to G. Pincus, 25 Feb. 1955, MS-SS; A. Guttmacher, 'The pill around the world', 5.

22 *Financial Times*, 26 Feb. 1997.

23 H. Maruyama, et al., 'Why Japan ought to legalize the pill', *Nature*, 379 (15 Feb. 1998), 579–80; 'Permission denied', *Far Eastern Economic Review* (14 Apr. 1994), 38.

24 M. Jitsukawa and C. Djerassi, 'Birth control in Japan: realities and prognosis'. I am grateful to Carl Djerassi for giving me a copy of this paper in manuscript form. See also *Japan Economic Newswire*, 8 Mar. 2000; *Worcester Sunday Times*, 5 Sept. 1999.

25 McCormick, 'Notes on a conversation with Dr Pincus', 23 Apr. 1959; Courey, 'Participants', 191.

26 'Oral Contraceptives – 50 million users', A-22.

27 Ibid.

28 'OCs – update on usage, safety, and side effects', A-141.

29 Chapter 4 above, and see J. C. Cobb to G. Pincus, 12 Aug. 1961, GP-LC, Box 47.

30 Cited in P. P. Gossel, 'Packaging the pill', in R. Bud, ed., *Manifesting Medicine* (Amsterdam, 1999), 105–122, 106.

31 Cited in ibid., 107–8.

32 Ibid.

33 Ibid.

34 In later years other prescriptive drugs were to follow suit; cited in ibid., 117–18.

35 Cited in ibid., 114.

36 Cited in ibid., 114.

37 Ibid.

38 D. Hubacher and L. Potter, 'Adherence to oral contraceptive regimens in four countries', *International Family Planning Perspectives*, 19/2 (June 1993), 49–53, at 50.

39 'Lower-dose pills', 4.

40 Gossel, 'Packaging the pill', 115.

41 In 1991 approximately two-thirds of women were suffering from anaemia during pregnancy worldwide; figure cited in B. Hartmann, *Reproductive Rights and Wrongs* (New York, 1995), 50.

42 'Oral contraceptives – 50 million users', A-23–4.

43 Ibid., A-2.

44 For more on this, see chapter 6 above.

45 M. Williams-Deane and L. S. Potter, 'Current oral contraceptive use instructions', *Family Planning Perspectives*, 24/3 (May/June 1992), 111–15, at 111.

46 Ibid.

47 Ibid., 112–14.

48 Ibid.

49 Hubacher and Potter, 'Adherence to oral contraceptive regimens', 49–53.

50 'Oral contraceptives – 50 million users', A-23–4.

51 The importance of racial characteristics in determining the effects of the pill on women's bodies was noted early on. One of the reasons that Pincus and G. D. Searle had been so enthusiastic to initiate trials in Japan had been because the FDA would not accept results of use purely on American women and because early studies had shown 'that women of different racial groups react differently and require different amounts of medication'. McCormick, 'Notes on a conversation with Dr Pincus', 23 Apr. 1959, CG-FCL, Box 195, fo. 3080.

52 'OCs – update on usage, safety, and side effects', A-134–6, A-164.

53 Ibid.

54 Ibid., A-135–6.

55 Cited in A. P. Hardon, 'Needs of women versus the interests of family planning personnel, policy-makers and researchers', *Social Science and Medicine*, 35 (1992), 753–66, at 761.

56 'Lower-dose pills', *Population Reports*, Series A, no. 7 (Nov. 1988), figs 1, 4, 6, pp. 4 and 9.

57 E. F. Jones et al., 'Unintended pregnancy, contraceptive practice and family planning services in developed countries', *Family Planning Perspectives*, 20/2 (Mar./Apr. 1988), 53–67, at 60, 65.

58 McCormick, McCormick's notes on conversation with Dr Pincus, 22 Feb. 1958, 16 Apr. 1958 and 29 May 1958, MS-SS.

59 'Oral contraceptives – 50 million users', A-1.

60 The number of liability claims made against contraceptive manufacturers increased between 1974 and 1984; for more information on this see L. B. Tyrer and J. E. Salas, 'Contraceptive problems unique to the United States', *Clinical Obstetrics and Gynaecology*, 32/2 (June 1989), 307–15, at 308.

61 Jones et al., 'Unintended pregnancy', 60.

62 'Editorial: paying for family planning', 831.

63 Jones et al., 'Unintended pregnancy', 60.

64 For an interesting history of family planning and government policy in the USA, see D. Critchlow, *Intended Consequences* (Oxford, 1999). Critchlow argues that one of the reasons that contraception has not been made universally free in the USA is rooted in the 1960s, when the government was afraid to fund family planning openly and thus established a piecemeal system which was to continue into the following years.

65 'Backbench fury at proposal to charge women for the pill', *Daily Telegraph*, 1 Jan. 1998.

66 Office of Health Economics, *Family Planning in Britain* (London, 1972), 19.

67 This was partly attributable to the general restructuring of family planning services overall, which were brought under the general framework of the National Health Service for the first time. Prior to this, family planning had been the responsibility of local authorities in conjunction with local family planning associations. Interestingly, medical practitioners could not give out condoms free under the new scheme. This policy had resulted from opposition on the part of medical practitioners themselves, who saw such provision as beyond their medical duties. By contrast, condoms could be obtained free from family planning clinics. This policy remains in place to this day.

68 *The Times*, 21 Dec. 1972, 30 Dec. 1972, 2 May 1973.

69 *The Times*, 21 Dec. 1972, 2 May 1973.

70 *Financial Times*, 10 May 1972; *The Times*, 7 Aug. 1974; *Evening News and Star (Cumberland)*, 28 Mar. 1974.

71 *The Times*, 13 Dec. 1972, 20 Dec. 1972.

72 *The Times*, 21 Dec. 1972, 2 May 1973. In later years the costs of oral contraceptives featured high on the political agenda. In 1995, for instance, the British government withdrew certain brands of the pill which were thought to be associated with venous thrombosis. These pills were some of the most expensive on the market, and many thought the decision to withdraw them was not so much to do with safety issues as to do with the expense to the National Health Service. Just three years before, the Secretary of State for Health, Virginia Bottomley, had proposed to restrict the range of oral contraceptives on the market to limit such costs, but she had failed to achieve the plan. *Independent on Sunday*, 22 Oct. 1995, 1. By the 1990s the free provision of oral contraceptives was seen as particularly important for guarding against teenage pregnancy. In 1997 it was estimated that the provision of oral contraceptives by general practitioners saved the government at least £466 per unplanned pregnancy avoided, and that the overall costs of providing contraception were far smaller than the health and social expenses involved in unplanned pregnancies. NHS Centre for Reviews and Dissemination, 'Preventing and reducing the adverse effects of unintended teenage pregnancies', *Effective Health Care*, 3/1 (Feb. 1997), 1–12, at 7.

73 'Backbench fury at proposal to charge women for the pill', *Daily Telegraph*.

74 D. J. Van de Kaa, 'Population prospects and population policy in the Netherlands', *Netherlands Journal of Sociology*, 17 (1981), 73–91, at 78–9.

75 Ibid.; E. Ketting and A. P. Visser, 'Contraception in the Netherlands', *Patient Education and Counselling*, 23 (1994), 161–71, at 163–5; E. Ketting, 'The "Dutch model" of family planning', *International Health Foundation Newsletter*, no. 3 (1992), 2–4; A. Torres and E. F. Jones, 'The delivery of family planning services in the Netherlands', *Family Planning Perspectives*, 20/2 (Mar./Apr. 1988), 75–9, at 78.

76 UN, *Levels and Trends of Contraceptive Use as Assessed in 1994*, 94–5.

77 Ibid.

78 In the USA, for example, the percentage of married women using a condom decreased from 22 per cent in 1965 to 11 per cent in 1976, largely due to the appearance of the pill and an increasing uptake of sterilization. By 1995, however, the percentage of married women using condoms had again risen to 17 per cent; A. Bankole, et al., 'Determinants of trends in condom use in the United States, 1988–95', *Family Planning Perspectives*, 31/6 (Nov./Dec. 1999), 264–71.

79 Interestingly the condom has become popular among women across the social classes in recent years; L. Peterson, 'Contraceptive use in the United States: 1982–90'. *Advance Data*, no. 260 (14 Feb. 1995), 1–16; L. J. Piccino and W. D. Mosher, 'Trends in Contraceptive Use in the United States: 1982–1995', *Family Planning Perspectives*, 30/1 (Jan./Feb. 1998), 4–10, at 4, 7.

80 See chapter 8 above.

81 M. Potts, 'Birth Control Methods in the United States', *Family Planning Perspectives*, 20/6 (Nov./Dec. 1988), 268–97; W. F. Pratt and C. A. Bachrach, 'What do women use when they stop using the pill?', *Family Planning Perspectives*, 19/6 (Nov./Dec. 1987), 257–66.

82 Ibid.; UN, *Levels and Trends of Contraceptive Use as Assessed in 1994*, 57.

83 See figure 8.2, p. 213 above.

84 Some of the most dramatic decline in pill use in Britain occurred in the aftermath

of adverse publicity. In 1967, for instance, when the pill became linked with thrombosis, the number of pill users fell by an estimated 16 per cent. Similarly, in 1977 when reports linked the medication with arterial disease, its number of takers dropped by 10 per cent. The number of takers also dropped by 14 per cent in 1983 when scares surfaced over the pill's possible associations with cancer. While the number of users was to climb again once the effect of the publicity had worn off, people's assumptions about the safety of the drug had nonetheless been shaken; see K. Wellings, 'Help or hype', *British Journal of Family Planning*, 11 (1985), 92–8.

85 Department of Health, 'NHS contraceptive services, England, 1998–99', *Bulletin* (Nov. 1999).

86 K. Wellings, 'Trends in contraceptive method usage since 1970', *British Journal of Family Planning*, 12 (1986), 57–64.

87 K. Kiernan, H. Land, and J. Lewis, *Lone Motherhood in Twentieth-Century Britain* (Oxford, 1998); S. Singh and J. E. Darroch, 'Trends in sexual activity among adolescent American women: 1982–1995', *Family Planning Perspectives*, 31/5 (Sept./Oct. 1999), 212–19.

88 Piccino and Mosher, 'Trends in contraceptive use', 9.

89 Bankole, et al., 'Determinants of trends in condom use', 264–71; J. E. Darroch, 'The pill and men's involvement in contraception', *Family Planning Perspectives*, 32/2 (Mar./Apr. 2000), 90–1.

90 UN, *Levels and Trends of Contraceptive Use as Assessed in 1994*, 38, 58.

91 'Lower-dose pills', 20.

92 UN, *Levels and Trends of Contraceptive Use as Assessed in 1994*, 61, table 17.

Bibliography

The materials listed below are restricted to those that have been mentioned in the text together with a selection of sources providing a general background to the history of the pill.

Archival collections

People

Mary Calderone, Schlesinger Library, Cambridge, Mass.
Clarence James Gamble, Francis Countway Library, Boston.
Alan Guttmacher, Francis Countway Library, Boston.
J. H., Hetherington, Archives and Manuscripts, Wellcome Library for the History and Understanding of Medicine, London.
Alan S. Parkes, Archives and Manuscripts, Wellcome Library for the History and Understanding of Medicine, London.
Gregory Pincus, Library of Congress, Washington DC.
John Rock, Francis Countway Library, Boston.
John Rockefeller III, Rockefeller Archive, Tarrytown, N.Y.
Margaret Sanger, Library of Congress, Washington DC.
Margaret Sanger, Sophia Smith Collection, Smith College, Northampton, Mass.
Alan Stone, Francis Countway Library, Boston.

Organizations

Abortion Law Reform Association, Archives and Manuscripts, Wellcome Library for the History and Understanding of Medicine, London.
Birth Control Campaign, Archives and Manuscripts, Wellcome Library for the History and Understanding of Medicine, London.
Council for the Investigation of Fertility Control, Family Planning Association papers, Archives and Manuscripts, Wellcome Library for the History and Understanding of Medicine, London.
Food and Drug Administration papers, Washington DC.

Ford Foundation, Ford Foundation Archive, New York.

Medical Letter, Rockefeller Archive Center, Tarrytown, N.Y.

Medical Research Council, Public Records Office, Kew, Surrey.

Ministry of Health, Public Records Office, Kew, Surrey.

Planned Parenthood Federation of America papers, Sophia Smith Collection, Smith College, Northampton, Mass.

Planned Parenthood League of Massachusetts papers, Sophia Smith Collection, Smith College, Northampton, Mass.

Population Council, Rockefeller Archive, Tarrytown, N.Y.

Population Council, Ford Foundation Archive, New York.

Royal College of Obstetricians and Gynaecologists, London.

G. D. Searle, company headquarters in High Wycombe, UK.

Smithsonian Collection, National Museum of American History, Washington DC.

Worcester Foundation for Experimental Biology, Worcester Foundation papers, Shrewsbury, Mass.

Personal papers, with the original people

Ridgeley C. Bennett, Washington DC.

Philip Corfman, Washington DC.

William Inman, Southampton.

Stephen Lock, London.

Klim McPherson, London.

Barbara Seaman, New York.

Susan Szasz, New York.

Geoffrey Venning, High Wycombe.

Martin Vessey, Oxford.

Victor Wynn, London.

Oral interviews

Interviewed by Lara V. Marks (transcripts to be deposited at the National Sound Archive)

Ridgeley C. Bennett, 30 Apr. 1996, Washington DC, notes.

Valerie Beral, 17 and 26 Dec. 1998, London, notes and tape.

Eliahu Caspi, 23 Mar. 1995, Worcester, Mass., notes.

Philip Corfman, May 1996, Washington DC., notes.

Emy Deva, 7 Nov. 1996, High Wycombe, transcript.

Carl Djerassi, 23 May 1994, London, notes and tape.

Celso Ramon Garcia, 16 Apr. 1995, Philadelphia, transcript.

Alejandro Hernandez, 8 Apr. 1997, Mexico City, tape (Spanish and English) notes, translator Felipe Lopez.

Roy Hertz, 21 Apr. 1995, Washington DC, notes.

Dot Hunt, 7 Apr. 1995, Worcester, Mass., transcript.

Jean Infield, 29 Jan. 1996, London, transcript.

William Inman, 13 Oct. 1994, Southampton, transcript.

Clifford Kay, 3 Dec. 1996, Manchester, transcript.

Francis Kelsey, 20 Feb. 1997, Washington DC, notes.
Judith McCann, 6 Apr. 1995, Worcester, Mass., notes.
John McCracken, 7 Apr. 1995, Worcester, Mass., notes.
Anne Merrill and Mary Ellen Fitts Johnson, 8 Apr. 1995, Worcester, Mass., transcript.
Luis Miramontes, 10 Apr. 1997, Mexico City, notes.
Joan Nabarro, 9 Dec. 1996, London, notes.
Denise Pullen, 16 Dec. 1996, Eastbourne, transcript.
Eli and Louisa Romanoff, 7 Apr. 1995, Worcester, Mass., tape, notes.
Adaline Satterthwaite, 27 Apr. 1995, Philadelphia, transcript.
Barbara Seaman, 12 May 1996, New York, notes.
Segal Sheldon,, 30 Apr. 1996, Washington DC, notes.
Roger Short, 13 Nov. 1995, Oxford, notes.
Bruce Stradel, 30 Apr. 1996, Washington DC, transcript.
Ellen Tyler May, 13 May 1996, Minnesota, notes from telephone interview.
Geoffrey Venning, 16 Oct. 1996 and 7 Nov. 1996, London, notes.
Aviva Wiseman, 3 Mar. 1997, Slough, notes.
Victor Wynn, 6 Apr. 1994, London, transcript.

Interviewed by Ros O'Brien on behalf of Lara V. Marks (transcripts to be deposited at the National Sound Archive)

Mrs M.B., 15 Mar. 1997, transcript.
Mrs A.C., Autumn 1997, transcript, includes letter from Mrs A.C. to Lara V. Marks, n.d.
Mrs B.F., Autumn 1997, transcript.
Mrs J.F., 25 Mar. 1997, transcript.
Mrs M.F., Summer 1997, transcript.
Mrs C.H., Winter 1997, transcript.
Mrs D.R., Autumn 1997, transcript.
Mrs J.S., 25 Mar. 1997, transcript.
Mrs J.A.S., Autumn 1997, transcript.
Mrs S.S., Winter 1997, transcript.
Mrs R.T., Winter 1997, transcript.
Mrs R.W., Winter 1997, transcript.

Interviewed by Wendy Neil on behalf of Lara V. Marks

Mrs P.C., 13 Nov. 1997, transcript.

Interviewed by Sylvia Frenk on behalf of Lara V. Marks

Luis Miramontes, Mar. 1995, tape (Spanish) transcript, translated by Pilar Sanchez.

Interviews for the Oral History Project (deposited at Schlesinger Library, Cambridge, Mass.)

Mary Calderone, interviewed by James Reed, 7 Aug. 1974, transcript.
Elizabeth Arnold Cohen, interviewed by James Reed, Nov. 1974, transcript.
Mrs Alan Guttmacher, interviewed by James Reed, 15 Nov. 1974, transcript.
Frances Ferguson Hand, interviewed by James Reed, June 1974, transcript.

Emily Mudd, interviewed by James Reed, n.d., transcript.
Stuart Mudd, interviewed by James Reed, 21 May 1974, transcript.
Edris Rice-Wray, interviewed by James Reed, 14 Mar. 1974, transcript.
Grant Sanger, interviewed by Ellen Chesler, Aug. 1976, transcript.
Adaline Satterthwaite, interviewed by James Reed, 19 June 1974, transcript.
Sarah and Christopher Tietze, interviewed by James Reed, 19 Dec. 1975, transcript.

Interviews for *Timewatch* TV programme 'The pill: prescription for revolution', deposited at the National Sound Archive

Heather Bailey, tape C612/05/C612/06, transcript.
Maureen Delenian, tape, C612/02/C612/03, transcript.
Helen Gurley Brown, tape C612, transcript.
Denise Pullen, C612/07/08, transcript.
Betty Vincent, excerpts from the TV programme.
Jan Williams, tape C612/04, transcript.

Additional interviews

Edris Rice-Wray, n.d. and no interviewer's name, transcript. Copy with Lynn Carson, daughter of Edris Rice-Wray, Mexico.
Contributers to Committee on Safety of Drugs (renamed Committee on Safety of Medicines), Witness Seminar, 12 Mar. 1996, Wellcome Institute, transcript.
Contributers to The Pill, Witness Seminar, June 1995, Wellcome Institute, transcript.

Newspapers and periodicals

United Kingdom

Birmingham Post
British Medical Journal
Business Newsweek
Daily Express
Daily Mail
Daily Telegraph
Evening Chronicle
Evening News and Star (Cumberland)
Evening Standard
Financial Times
Guardian
Hospital Doctor
Independent on Sunday
Investors Chronicle
IPPF Medical Bulletin
Lancet
Manchester Guardian
Mid-Sussex Times
MIMS (Monthly Index of Medical Specialities)

Nature
Pharmaceutical Journal
Solihull, Warwick News
Spare Rib
Spectrum (newspaper of Family Planning and Human Conservation, published for Ortho Pharmaceutical Ltd).
Sun
Sunday Telegraph
Sunday Times
The Times
Windsor, Slough and Eton Express

United States

Harpers
Journal of the American Medical Association
Medical News
New York Times
Newsweek
PDR (Physicians Desk Reference)
Post
Sunday Dispatch
Time
Washington Post
Worcester Sunday Telegram
Worcester Sunday Times

Elsewhere

Japan Economic Newswire

Official papers and printed reports

United Kingdom

Department of Health, 'NHS contraceptive services, England, 1998–99', *Bulletin* (Nov. 1999).
Government Act 1948, 11 and 12 Geo. 6, c. 26 (1947–48).
NHS Act 9 and 10 Geo. 6, c. 81 (1945–46), sec. 22.
Parliamentary Debates: House of Commons, vol. 685, 2 Dec. 1963; vol. 711, 26 Apr. 1965; vol 721, 29 Nov. 1965; vol. 729, 17 June 1966; vol. 744, 4 Apr. 1967; vol. 763, 30 Apr. 1968; vol. 783, 12 May 1969; vol. 793, 15 Dec. 1969. House of Lords, 5 June 1967.
The Population Problem: Correspondence between the Prime Minister the Rt. Hon. Harold Wilson MP and the Rt. Hon. Sir David Renton MP (Huntington, 1967).

United States

Composite Report of the President's Committee to Study the United States Military Assistance Program, Vol. 1 (Government Printing Office, Washington DC, 17 Aug. 1959).

FDA Advisory Committee on Obstetrics and Gynecology, *Report on Oral Contraceptives*, (1 Aug. 1966).

FDA Advisory Committee on Obstetrics and Gynecology, *Second Report on Oral Contraceptives*, (1 Aug. 1969).

FDA Advisory Committee on Obstetrics and Gynecology, *Minutes*, 17 May 1968, 1 Apr. 1970, 12 Oct. 1973, 6 Jan. 1977, 11 Feb. 1982.

FDA Fertility and Maternal Health Drugs Advisory Committee Meetings, *Minutes*, 15 Jan. 1988, 28 Oct. 1993.

Population and the American Future: The Report of the Commission on Population Growth and the American Future (New York, 1972).

US Congress, House of Representatives, *Hearings of the Subcommittee on Government Operations, Drug Safety*, 1964, part 1

US Congress, House of Representatives, *Intergovernmental Relations Subcommittee of the Committee on Government Operations, FDA Regulation of Oral Contraceptives*, 15 July 1970.

US Congress, House of Representatives, Select Committee on Population, *Report: Fertility and Contraception in the United States*, Dec. 1978.

US Congress, Senate, *Competitive Problems in the Drug Industry: Hearings before the Subcommittee on Monopoly of the Select Committee on Small Business, US Senate 91st Congress, Second Session, on Present Status of Competition in the Pharmaceutical Industry*, parts 15–17, Jan. –Mar. 1970 (Nelson hearings).

US Congress, Senate, *Hearings before the Subcommittee on Foreign Expenditures of the Committee on Government Operations*, 89th Congress, 2nd Session, June 1966.

US Congress, Senate, *Hearings before the Subcommittee on Small Business*, 90th Congress, 2nd Session, 1968, part 8.

US Congress, Senate, *Interagency Coordination in Drug Research and Regulation, Hearings before the Subcommittee on Reorganization and International Organizations of the Committee on Government Operations*, 1962–64, parts 1–5;

US Congress, *Senate Subcommittee on Patents, Trademarks, and Copyrights of the Committee on the Judiciary, Wonder Drugs, Hearings on S. Res. 167*, 84th Congress, 2nd Session, 1956.

US Congress, Senate, *World Population and Food Crisis: Hearings before the Consultative Subcommittee on Economic and Social Affairs of the Committee on Foreign Relations*, 29 June 1965.

Unpublished papers

Bennett, R. C., 'Impact of FDA regulation of oral contraceptives on public health: reduction of thromboembolism, myocardial infarction, and stroke', Remarks to the Society of Alumni, Johns Hopkins University School of Hygiene and Public Health Annual Meeting and Recognition Banquet, 14 Nov. 1988, Bennett's personal papers.

Bennett, R. C., 'Remarks to the Fertility and Maternal Health Drugs Advisory Committee', 15 Jan. 1988, Bennett's personal papers.

Bennett, R. C., 'The safety and utility of oral contraceptives containing 50 micrograms of estrogen', prepared for FDA Fertility and Maternal Health Drugs Advisory Committee meetings, 28 Oct. 1993.

Bennett, R. C., 'It's effective, but is it safe?: the pill', n.d., Bennett's personal papers.

Calderone, M. S., 'Family planning and sexuality: retrospect 1953–74', Worcester Foundation archives.

Guttmacher, A., 'The pill around the world', prepared for *IPPF Medical Bulletin*, Sept. 1966, AG-FCL, Box 18.

Harris, H., 'Clinical trials of Enovid in Kentucky, 1958–1969', presented to American Association for the History of Medicine, Apr. 1998.

Hertz, R. and Bailar, J. C., 'An appraisal of some unresolved problems involved in the use of estrogen-progestogen combinations for contraception', National Institutes of Health staff paper, Apr. 1964.

Inman, W., 'Memoirs', Inman's personal papers.

Jitsukawa, M. and Djerassi, C., 'Birth control in Japan: realities and prognosis'. I am grateful to Carl Djerassi for giving me a copy of this paper in manuscript form.

Sartwell, P., Masi, A. S., Arthes, F. G., Greene, G. R. and Smith, H. E. 'Thromboembolism and oral contraceptives: an epidemiological case-control study', in FDA Advisory Committee on Obstetrics and Gynecology, *Minutes*, 1 Aug. 1969.

Venning, G., 'Family planning and population policies in developed and less developed countries', for *Clinics in Endocrinology and Metabolism*, 2/3 (1973), G. D. Searle's papers, High Wycombe, UK.

Wiseman, A., 'The pill', n.d., *c.* 1966, Wiseman's personal papers.

Unpublished theses

Berg, S. M., 'Gregory Goodwin Pincus: from reproductive biology to the birth control pill. Underlying motivations and professional goals', B.A. thesis, Harvard University, 1989.

Courey, R. M., 'Participants in the development, marketing and safety evaluation of the oral contraceptive, 1950–1965: mythic dimension of a scientific solution', Ph.D. thesis, University of California, Berkeley, 1994.

Fisher, K., 'An oral history of birth control practice *c.* 1925–50: a study of Oxford and South Wales', D.Phil. thesis, Oxford, 1997.

Kelt, I., 'The medical profession and the pill', B.Sc. dissertation, Wellcome Institute, June 1998.

Vayena, E., 'Cancer detectors: an international history of the pap test and cervical cancer screening, 1928–1970', Ph.D thesis, University of Minnesota, Nov. 1999.

Vessey, M. P., 'Some epidemiological investigations into the safety of oral contraceptives', M.D. thesis, London University, 1970.

Published sources

Abraham, J., *Science, Politics, and the Pharmaceutical Industry: Controversy and Bias in Drug Regulation* (New York, 1995).

Ad Hoc Advisory Committee, 'FDA report on Enovid', *JAMA*, 185 (1963), 776.

'Advantages of orals outweigh disadvantages', *Population Reports*, Series A, no. 2 (Mar. 1975).

Allitt, P., *Catholic Intellectuals and Conservative Politics in America 1950–1985* (New York, 1993).

'Another look at the pill and breast cancer', *Lancet*, 2 (2 Nov. 1985), 985–7.

Applezweig, N., 'The big steroid treasure hunt', *Chemical Week*, 84 (21 Jan. 1959), 37–51.

Applezweig, N., *Steroid Drugs* (New York, 1962).

Asbell, B., *The Pill: A Biography of the Drug that Changed the World* (New York, 1995).

Astwood, E. B., 'Progesterone inhibition of ovulation in the rat', *American Journal of Physiology*, 127 (1939), 127.

Bachrach, C. A., 'Contraceptive practice among young American women, 1973–1982', *Family Planning Perspectives*, 16/6 (1984), 253–9.

'Backbench fury at proposal to charge women for the pill', *Daily Telegraph*, 1 Jan. 1998.

Bailey, B., 'Prescribing the pill: politics, culture, and the sexual revolution in America's heartland', *Journal of Social History* (Summer 1997), 827–56.

Baker, C. Looper and Kline, C. Baker, eds, *The Conversation Begins: Mothers and Daughters Talk about Living Feminism* (New York, 1996).

Bankole, A., Darroch J. E. and Singh, S., 'Determinants of trends in condom use in the United States, 1988–95', *Family Planning Perspectives*, 31/6 (Nov./Dec. 1999), 264–71.

Barrett, J., 'Product liability and the pill', *Cleveland State Law Review*, 19 (1970), 468–78, repr. in J. Katz, *Experimentation with Human Beings: The Authority of the Investigator, Subject, Professionals and State in the Human Investigation Process* (New York, 1972), 789–91.

Baum, J. F. et al., 'Possible association between benign hepatomas and oral contraceptives', *Lancet*, 2 (1973), 926–8.

Benn, M. and Richardson, R., 'Uneasy freedom: Women's experiences of contraception', *Women's Studies International Forum*, 7/4 (1984), 219–25.

Beral, V., 'Parity and susceptibility to cancer', in *Fetal Antigens and Cancer*, Ciba Foundation Symposium 96 (London, 1983), 182–203.

Beral, V., 'Childbearing, oral contraceptives and breast cancer', *Lancet*, 341 (1993), 110–12.

Beral, V., Fraser P., and Chilvers, C., 'Does pregnancy protect against ovarian cancer?', *Lancet* (20 May 1978), 1083–6.

Beral V. et al., 'Mortality associated with oral contraceptive use: 25-year follow-up of cohort of 46,000 women from Royal College of General Practitioners' oral contraception study', *BMJ*, 318 (9 Jan. 1999), 96–100.

Bertina, R. M. et al., 'Mutation in blood coagulation factor V associated with resistance to activated protein C', *Nature* 369/6475 (5 May 1994), 64–7.

Bhrolcháin, M. N., 'The contraceptive confidence idea: an empirical investigation', *Population Studies*, 42 (1988), 205–25.

Bielschowsky F. and Horning, E. S., 'Aspects of endocrine carcinogenesis', *British Medical Bulletin*, 14/2 (1958), 106–15.

Biezanek, A., *All Things New* (New York, 1965).

Birch, A. J., 'Steroid hormones and the Luftwaffe. A venture into fundamental strategic research and some of its consequences: The Birch reduction becomes a birth reduction', *Steroids*, 57 (Aug. 1992), 363–77.

'Birth control pills boom', *Business Week*, 23 Feb. 1963, 62–3.

'Birth control: The pill and the church', *Newsweek*, 6 July 1964, 51–4.

Bland, L., *Banishing the Beast: English Feminism and Sexual Morality 1885–1914* (London, 1995).

Blom, I., 'Voluntary motherhood 1900–1930: Theories and politics of a Norwegian feminist in an international perspective', in G. Bock and P. Thane, eds, *Maternity and Gender Policies* (London, 1991).

Bock, G., 'Antinatalism, maternity and paternity in National Socialist racism', in G. Bock and P. Thane, eds, *Maternity and Gender Policies* (London, 1991), 233–55.

Bock, G. and Thane, P., eds, *Maternity and Gender Policies: Women and the Rise of European Welfare States, 1880s–1950s* (London, 1991).

Bone, M., *Family Planning Services in England and Wales* (London, 1973).

'The book that brought consumer advocacy to the medical system', *Health Facts: Center for Medical Consumers*, 20/196 (Sept. 1995), 3–4.

Borell, M., 'Brown-Sequard's organotherapy and its appearance in America at the end of the nineteenth century', *Bulletin of the History of Medicine*, 50/3 (Fall 1976), 309–20.

Borell, M., 'Organotherapy, British physiology, and the discovery of internal secretions', *Journal of the History of Biology*, 9/2 (Fall 1976), 235–68.

Boston Collaborative Drug Surveillance Programme, 'Oral contraceptives and venous thromboembolic disease, surgically confirmed gallbladder disease, and breast tumours', *Lancet* (23 June 1973), 1399–404.

Boston Women's Health Collective, *Our Bodies, Ourselves* (Boston, 1984).

Boyle, T. C., *Riven Rock* (Viking, 1998).

'Breast cancer and the pill – a muted reassurance', *BMJ*, 282/6282 (27 June 1981), 2075–6.

Brinton L. A. et al., 'Risk factors for benign breast disease', *American Journal of Epidemiology*, 113/3 (Mar. 1981), 203–14.

Brinton L. A. et al., 'Oral contraceptives and breast cancer', *International Journal of Epidemiology*, 11/4 (1982), 316–22.

Brookes, B., *Abortion in England, 1900–1967* (London, 1988).

Buck, P. S. 'The pill and the teenage girl', *Reader's Digest* (Apr. 1968), 111.

Buehring, G. C., 'Oral contraceptives and breast cancer: What has 20 years of research shown?', *Biomedicine and Pharmacotherapy*, 42 (1988), 525–30.

Bullough, V. N., *Science in the Bedroom: A History of Sex Research* (New York, 1994).

Burt Gerstman, B. et al., 'Trends in the content and use of oral contraceptives in the United States, 1964–88', *American Public Health Journal*, 81/1 (Jan. 1991), 89–96.

Caldwell, J. and Caldwell, P., *Limiting Population Growth and the Ford Foundation Contribution* (London, 1986).

Cantor, D., 'Cortisone and the politics of empire: Imperialism and British medicine, 1918–1955', *Bulletin of the History of Medicine*, 67/3 (1993), 463–93.

Cartwright, A., *Parents and Family Planning Services* (London, 1970).

Cartwright, A., *How Many Children?* (London, 1976).

Cartwright, A., 'Family size, contraceptive practice and fertility intentions in England and Wales, 1967–1975, *Family Planning Perspectives*, 11/2 (1979), 128–37.

Cartwright, A., 'Trends in family intentions and the use of contraception among recent mothers, 1967–84', Population Trends, 49 (1987), 31–4, 33.

CASH, 'Long-term oral contraceptive use and risk of breast cancer', *JAMA*, 249 (1983), 1591–5.

CASH, 'Oral contraceptive use and the risk of ovarian cancer', *JAMA*, 249 (1983), 1596–9.

CASH, 'Oral contraceptive use and the risk of breast cancer', *New England Journal of Medicine*, 315/7 (1986), 405–11.

CASH, 'Breast cancer and hormonal contraceptives: Further results', *Contraception,* 53/3s (1996), 1s–106s.

CASH, 'Breast cancer and hormonal contraceptives', *Lancet,* 347 (22 June 1996), 1713–27.

Cassagrande, J. T. et al., '"Incessant ovulation" and ovarian cancer', *Lancet* (28 July 1979), 170–3.

Chang, M. C. and Pincus, G., 'Does phosphorylated hesperidin affect fertility?', *Science,* 117 (13 Mar. 1953), 274–6.

ChenSee, S., *Women in Science* (Canadian Science Writers' Association, 1999).

Chesler, E., *Woman of Valor: Margaret Sanger and the Birth Control Movement in America* (New York, 1992).

Chivers C. E. D. and Deacon, J. M., 'Oral contraceptives and breast cancer', *British Journal of Cancer* 61/1 (1990), 1–4.

Clarke, A., 'Controversy and the development of reproductive sciences', *Social Problems,* 37 (1990), 18–37.

Colton, F. B., 'Steroids and "the Pill": Early steroid research at Searle', *Steroids,* 57 (Dec. 1992), 624–30.

Committee on Safety of Medicines, *Combined Oral Contraceptives and Thromboembolism* (London, 1995).

Cook, R., *Human Fertility: The Modern Dilemma* (New York, 1951).

Cookson, C., 'The nature of things: new conclusions from old studies', *Financial Times,* 26–27 Nov. 1994, 3.

Coughlan, R., 'Control challenge: Science is near success in a search for way to curb runaway population', *Life,* 21 Nov. 1959, 159–76.

Cova, A., 'French feminism and maternity: theories and policies 1890–1918', in G. Bock and P. Thane, eds, *Maternity and Gender Policies* (London, 1991).

Crapo, L., *Hormones: The Messengers of Life* (Stanford, 1985).

Critchlow, D., *Intended Consequences: Birth Control, Abortion, and the Federal Government in Modern America* (Oxford, 1999).

Crossman, R., *The Diaries of a Cabinet Minister, vol. 3: Secretary of State for Social Services, 1968–70* (London, 1977).

Curtis Wood, H., 'Unplanned children: Whose burden? Whose care?', *Medical Opinion and Review* (Mar. 1966), 28–35.

Cutler, B. S., 'Endometrial carcinoma after stilboestrol therapy in gonadal dysgenesis', *New England Journal of Medicine,* 287 (1972), 628.

Dahlback, B., 'Factor V and protein S as cofactors to activated protein C', *Haemotologica,* 82/1 (Jan.–Feb. 1997), 91–5.

Dale, H. E., 'The chemistry of sex hormones', *Pharmaceutical Journal* (29 Apr. 1939), 432–41.

Darroch, J. E., 'The pill and men's involvement in contraception', *Family Planning Perspectives,* 32/2 (Mar./Apr. 2000), 90–1.

Davey, J., 'How safe are the birth control pills?', *Redbook,* Feb. 1963.

Davin, A., 'Imperialism and motherhood', *History Workshop Journal,* 5 (1978), 9–66.

De Lee, J., 'The prophylactic forceps operation', *American Journal of Obstetrics and Gynecology,* 1 (1920–1), 34–44, 77–84.

Deverell, C., 'The International Planned Parenthood Federation – its role in developing countries', *Demography,* 5/2, (1968), special issue, 574–7.

Devesa S. S. et al., 'Cancer incidence and mortality trends among whites in the United States, 1947–84', *Journal of National Cancer Institute,* 79 (1987), 701–70.

Diczfalusy, E., 'Gregory Pincus and steroidal contraception: a new departure in the history of mankind', *Journal of Steroid Biochemistry*, 11 (1979), 3–11.

Direcks, A. and Hoen, E., 'DES: The crime continues', in K. Donnell, ed., *Adverse Effects: Women and the Pharmaceutical Industry* (Toronto, 1986).

Djerassi, C., *The Politics of Contraception* (London, 1979).

Djerassi, C., *The Pill, Pygmy Chimps, and Degas' Horse* (New York, 1992).

Djerassi, C., 'Steroid research at Syntex: "The pill" and cortisone', *Steroids*, 57 (Dec. 1992), 631–41.

Djerassi, C., *From the Lab into the World* (Washington DC, 1994).

Djerassi, C., 'The mother of the pill', *Recent Progress in Hormone Research*, 50 (1995), 1–18.

Draper, E., *Birth Control in the Modern World* (Harmondsworth, 2nd edn, 1972).

Drill, V. A., 'History of the first oral contraceptive', *Journal of Toxicology and Environmental Health*, 3 (1977), 133–8.

Dunnell, K., *Family Formation* (London, 1976).

Dutt, R. H. and Casida, L. E., 'Alteration of estrual in sheep by use of progesterone and its effects upon subsequent ovulation and fertility', *Endocrinology*, 43 (1943), 208–217.

Dutton, D. B., *Worse than the Disease: Pitfalls of Medical Progress* (Cambridge, 1988).

Economist Intelligence Unit, 'Special Report no. 1: Contraceptives', *Retail Business Market Surveys*, no. 138 (Aug. 1969), 12–27.

Edgren, R. A., 'Early oral contraceptive history: Norethynodrel is not a prohormone', letter to the editor, *Steroids*, 59 (Jan. 1994), 58–9.

Editorial, 'Oral contraceptives: The good news', *JAMA*, 249/12 (25 Mar. 1983), 1624–5.

'Editorial: Paying for family planning', *Lancet*, 352 (12 Sept. 1998), 831.

Edmonsen, H. A., Henderson, B. and Benton, B., 'Liver-cell adenomas associated with the use of oral contraceptives', *New England Journal of Medicine*, 294 (1976), 470–2.

Ehrenstrom, P., 'Eugenics and the law in Switzerland', *Galton Institute Newsletter* (Sept. 1997), 4–5.

Elkas J. and Farias-Eisner, R., 'Cancer of the uterine cervix', *Current Opinion, Obstetrics and Gynecology*, 10 (1998), 47–50.

Encyclopedia of Chemical Technology, 3rd edn (New York, 1978–84), vol. 6.

Encyclopedia of Chemical Technology, 4th edn (New York, 1991–8), vol. 7.

Engelmann, G. J., *Labour among Primitive Peoples* (St Louis, Ind., 1882).

Ernster, V. L., 'The epidemiology of benign breast disease', *Epidemiological Reviews*, 3 (1981), 184–202.

'Experimental interruption of pregnancy', *BMJ* (10 Sept. 1938), 580.

Farmer, R. D. T. and Preston, T. D., 'The risk of venous thromboembolism associated with low oestrogen oral contraceptives', *Journal of Obstetrics and Gynaecology*, 15 (1995), 195–200.

Fasal, E. and Paffenberger, R. S., 'Oral contraceptives as related to cancer and benign lesions of the breast', *JNCI*, 55/4 (Oct. 1975), 767–73.

'Fertility and contraception in 12 developed countries', *Family Planning Perspectives*, 13/3 (Mar./Apr. 1981), 93–103.

'Fertility and infertility', transcript of a panel meeting, *Bulletin of New York Academy of Medicine*, 37/10 (Oct. 1961), 689–712.

Forrest, J. D., 'The delivery of family planning services in the United States', *Family Planning Perspectives*, 20/2 (1988), 88–95.

Fortes J. and Adler Lomnitz, L., *Becoming a Scientist in Mexico: The Challenge of Creating a Scientific Community in an Underdeveloped Country*, trans. A. P. Hynds,

(Philadelphia, 1994).

Fortney, J. A., Harper J. M. and Potts, M., 'Oral contraceptives and life expectancy', *Studies in Family Planning*, 17/3 (May/June 1986), 117–25.

FPA, 'Joint statement on oral contraception and breast cancer', 20 Nov. 1987.

Fryer, P., *The Birth Controllers* (London, 1967).

Galewitz, P., '"The Pill" might prevent acne too', 30 Jan. 2000, Associated Press, Yahoo, http://biz.com.apf/000130/the_pill_3.html.

Gardner, W. U., 'Tumors in experimental animals receiving steroid hormones', *Surgery*, 16 (1944), 8–32.

Gardner, W. U., 'Studies on steroid hormones in experimental carcinogenesis', *Recent Progress in Hormone Research*, 1 ((1946), 217–60.

Garnall, D., 'Controversy rages over new contraceptive data', *BMJ*, 311, (28 Oct. 1995), 1117–18.

General Household Survey (London, 1983).

General Register Office, *Registrar General's Statistical Review of England and Wales*, part 1 (London, 1969).

Ghosh, S. and Gupta, A., 'The effectiveness as an oral contraceptive of synthetic metax/ylohydroquinone, the active principle of the field pea (Pisum Sativum Linn): A preliminary report', *International Medical Abstracts and Reviews* (16 Nov. 1954), 89–90.

Gillmer, M. D. G., 'Metabolic effects of combined oral contraceptives', in M. Filshie and J. Guillebaud, eds, *Contraception: Science and Practice* (London, 1989).

Glantz, L. H., 'The influence of the Nuremberg Code on U.S. statutes and regulations', in G. J. Annas and M. A. Grodin, eds, *The Nazi Doctors and the Nuremberg Code: Human Rights in Human Experimentation* (Oxford, 1992).

Goldzeiher, J. W., 'Estrogens in oral contraceptives: historical perspectives', *Johns Hopkins Medical Journal*, 150 (1982).

Goldzieher, J. W., 'The history of steroidal contraceptive development: The estrogens', *Perspectives in Biology and Medicine*, 36/3 (Spring 1993), 363–8.

Goldzieher, J. W., 'Are low-dose oral contraceptives safer and better?', *AJOG*, 171/3 (Sept. 1994), 587–90.

Goldzieher, J. W., Moses, L. E. and Ellis, L. T., *JAMA*, 180 (1962), 352.

Goodman L. S. and Gilman, A., *The Pharmacological Basis of Therapeutics*, 2nd edn (New York, 1960).

Gordon, L., *Woman's Body, Woman's Right: A Social History of Birth Control in America* (New York, 1976).

Gossel, P. P. 'Packaging the pill', in R. Bud, ed., *Manifesting Medicine: Bodies and Machines* (Amsterdam, 1999), 105–22.

Gould, S. J., *The Mismeasure of Man* (London, 1992).

Grant, L., *Sexing the Millennium* (London, 1993).

Grant, N. J., *The Selling of Contraception: The Dalkon Shield Case, Sexuality, and Women's Autonomy* (Columbus, Ohio, 1992).

Graves, R., *Greek Myths* (Wakefield, R.I., 1988).

Gray, M., *Margaret Sanger. A Biography of the Champion of Birth Control* (New York, 1979).

Greenblatt, E. R., et al., 'Breast cancer in mothers given diethylstilboestrol in pregnancy', *New England Journal of Medicine*, 311 (1984), 1393–7.

Greep, R. O., ed., *Human Fertility and Population Problems* (New York, 1963).

Greer, G., *The Change: Women, Ageing and the Menopause* (London, 1993).

Grigg, D., *The World Food Problem* (Oxford, 1993).

Grimes, D., 'The safety of oral contraceptives: Epidemiological insights from the first 30 years', *AJOG*, 166/6 (June 1992), part 2, 1950–4.

Guillebaud, J., *The Pill* (Oxford, new edn 1991).

Guillebaud, J., 'Advising women on which pill to take', *BMJ*, 311 (28 Oct. 1995), 1111–12.

Gurewich, V. et al., 'Risk of idiopathic cardiovascular death and non-fatal venous thromboembolism in women using oral contraceptives with different progestagen components', *Lancet*, 346 (1995), 1589–93.

Halberstam, D., *The Fifties* (New York, 1993).

Hall, L., 'Women, feminism and eugenics', in R. Peel, ed., *Essays in the History of Eugenics* (London, 1998), 36–51.

Hall, L., '"A suitable job for a woman?": Women doctors and birth control before 1950', in L. Conrad and A. Hardy, eds, *Women and Modern Medicine* (Amsterdam, 2000).

Hall, L., 'Malthusian mutations: The changing politics and moral meanings of birth control in Britain', in B. Dolan, ed., *Malthus, Medicine and Morality: 'Malthusianism' after 1798* (Amsterdam, 2000), 141–63.

Hancock and Co. Ltd, *The Ravages of Time Defied: A Handbook of English, Foreign and Continental Animal Gland Prescriptions* (London, 1934).

Hardon, A. P., 'Needs of women versus the interests of family planning personnel, policy-makers and researchers: Conflicting views on safety and acceptability of contraceptives', *Social Science and Medicine*, 35 (1992), 753–66.

Harkavy, O., *Curbing Population Growth: An Insider's Perspective on the Population Movement* (New York, 1995).

Harris, R., *The Real Voice* (New York, 1964).

Hartmann, B., *Reproductive Rights and Wrongs: The Global Politics of Population Control* (Boston, 1995).

Harvey Young, J., *The Toadstool Millionaires: A Social History of Patent Medicines in America before Federal Regulation* (Princeton, 1961).

Hawkins, D. F., 'Thromboembolic risks in contraception', *Spectrum* (newspaper of Family Planning and Human Conservation, published for Ortho Pharmaceutical Ltd), no. 1, 1973.

Hennekens C. H. et al., 'A case-control study of oral contraceptive use and breast cancer', *JNCI*, 72/1 (Jan. 1984), 39–42.

Henshaw, P. S., 'Physiologic control of fertility', *Science*, 117 (29 May 1953), 572–82.

Henzl, M. R., letter to editor, *Lancet*, 347 (27 Jan. 1996), 257–8.

Hertz, R., 'Experimental and clinical aspects of the carcinogenic potential of steroid contraceptives', *International Journal of Fertility*, 13 (Oct./Dec. 1968), 273–86.

Hertz, R. and Bailar, J. C., 'Estrogen-progestogen combinations for contraception', *JAMA*, 198 (Nov. 1966), 136–42.

Hertz, R., Waite, J. H., and Thomas, L. B., 'Progestational effectiveness of 19-nor-ethinyl-testosterone by oral route in women', *Proceedings of Experimental Biology and Medicine*, 91 (1956), 418–20.

Hertz, R. et al., 'Observations on the effect of progesterone on carcinoma of the cervix', *JNCI*, 11 (Apr. 1951), 867–75.

Hodges, A., *Alan Turing: The Enigma of Intelligence* (London, 1983).

Hope, S., '12 per cent of women stopped taking their pill immediately they heard CMS's warning', letter, *BMJ*, 312 (1996), 576.

Horvath, E., Kovacs, K. and Ross, R. C., 'Ultrastructural findings in a well differentiated hepatoma', *Digestion*, 7 (1972), 74.

'How safe are the birth control pills?', *Vogue*, 8 Jan. 1961, 90–1, 128.

Hubacher, D. and Potter, L., 'Adherence to oral contraceptive regimens in four countries', *International Family Planning Perspectives*, 19/2 (June 1993), 49–53.

Huggins, G. R. and Giuntoli, R. L., 'Oral contraceptives and neoplasia', *Fertility and Sterility*, 32/1 (July 1979), 1–23.

Humphries, S., *A Secret World of Sex* (London, 1991).

Hunt, K., 'The first pill-taking generation: past and present use of contraception amongst a cohort of women born in the early 1950s', *British Journal of Family Planning*, 16 (1990), 3–15.

Hunt, K. and Annandale, E., 'Predicting contraceptive method usage among women in West Scotland', *Journal of Biosocial Science*, 22/4 (1990), 405–21.

Huxley, A., *Brave New World* (London, 1994).

Inman, W. H. W., 'Role of drug-reaction monitoring in the investigation of thrombosis and "the pill"', *British Medical Bulletin*, 26/3 (1970), 248–56.

Inman, W. H. W. and Vessey, M. P., 'Investigation of deaths from pulmonary, coronary, and cerebral thrombosis and embolism in women of child-bearing age', *BMJ*, 2 (27 Apr. 1968), 193–211.

Inman, W. H. W., Vessey, M. P., Westerholm, B. and Engelund, A., 'Thromboembolic disease and the steroidal content of oral contraceptives', *BMJ*, 2 (25 Apr. 1970), 203–9.

'Is the pill too dependent on wild yams?', *New Scientist* (3 May 1973), 281.

Iverson, O. and Nilsen, S., 'Abortions increased by nearly 8 per cent in Norway', letter, *BMJ*, 313 (1996), 363–4.

Jackson, C. O., *Food and Drug Legislation in the New Deal* (Princeton, 1970).

Jackson, H., 'Antifertility substances', *Pharmacological Reviews*, 2 (1959), 135–72.

Jick, S. S. et al., 'Oral contraceptives and breast cancer', *British Journal of Cancer*, 59 (1989), 618.

Johnson, R. C., 'Feminism, philanthropy and science in the development of the oral contraceptive pill', *Pharmacy in History*, 19/2 (1977), 63–77.

Johnson, S. P., *World Population and the United Nations: Challenge and Response* (Cambridge, 1987).

Jones, E. F., Beninger J. R., and Westoff, C. F., 'Pill and IUD discontinuation in the United States, 1970–1975: The influence of the media', *Family Planning Perspectives*, 12/6 (1980), 293–300.

Jones E. F. et al., 'Unintended pregnancy, contraceptive practice and family planning services in developed countries', *Family Planning Perspectives*, 20/2 (Mar./Apr. 1988), 53–67.

Jordanova, L., *Sexual Visions: Images of Gender in Science and Medicine between the Eighteenth and Twentieth Centuries* (London, 1989).

Junod, S. W. and Marks, L. V., 'Women on trial: approval of the first oral contraceptive in the United States and Great Britain', forthcoming.

Kaiser, R. B. *The Encyclical that Never Was: The Story of the Pontifical Commission on Population, Family and Birth* (London, 1987).

Kalache, A. et al., 'Oral contraceptives and breast cancer', *British Journal of Hospital Medicine* (Oct. 1983), 278–84.

Katz, H., 'British jump gun on pill data', *Montreal Gazette*, 21 Oct. 1995.

Kay, C. R., 'Oral contraceptives and cancer', letter to the editor, *Lancet* (29 Oct. 1983), 1018.

Kay, C. R., 'Latest views on Pill prescribing', *Journal of the Royal College of General*

Practitioners (Nov. 1984), 611–14.

Kennedy, D. M., *Birth Control in America: The Career of Margaret Sanger* (New Haven, 1970).

Ketting, E., 'The "Dutch model" of family planning', *International Health Foundation Newsletter*, no. 3 (1992), 2–4.

Ketting, E., 'CMS's advice will harm women's health world-wide', letter, *BMJ*, 312 (1996), 576.

Ketting, E., and Visser, A. P. 'Contraception in the Netherlands: The low abortion rate explained', *Patient Education and Counselling*, 23 (1994), 161–71.

Kevles, D., *In the Name of Eugenics: Genetics and the Uses of Human Heredity* (Los Angeles, 1985).

Kiernan, K., Land, H. and Lewis, J., *Lone Motherhood in Twentieth-Century Britain* (Oxford, 1998).

Kleinman, R. L., *Directory of Hormonal Contraceptives* (Carnforth, Lancs., 1992).

Klopper, A., 'Advertisement and classification of oral contraceptives', *BMJ* (16 Oct. 1965), 932–3.

Kostering, S., 'Etwas Besseres als das Kondom', in G. Staupe and L. Vieth, eds, *Die Pille: Von der Lust und von der Liebe* (Berlin, 1996).

Kuhl, S., *The Nazi Connection: Eugenics, American Racism and German National Socialism* (Oxford, 1994).

Lader, L., *The Margaret Sanger Story and the Fight for Birth Control* (New York, 1955).

Langford, C. M., *Birth Control Practice and Marital Fertility in Great Britain* (Oxford, 1976).

Laqueur, T., *Making Sex: Body and Gender from the Greeks to Freud* (Cambridge, Mass., 1990).

Laurence, J., 'More bad news for the Pill', *New Society*, 22/29 (Dec. 1983), 50.

Leathard, A., *The Fight for Family Planning* (London, 1980).

Leavitt, J., 'Joseph DeLee and the practice of preventive obstetrics', *American Journal of Public Health*, 78/10 (1988), 1353–9.

Lederer, S. E., *Subjected to Science: Human Experimentation in America before the Second World War* (Baltimore, 1995).

Lee, L. T., 'Law and family planning', *Studies in Family Planning* (Population Council), 2, no.2 (Apr. 1971), 81–98.

Lehmann, P. A., Bolivar A. and Quinteron, R., 'Russell E. Marker: pioneer of the Mexican steroid industry', *Journal of Chemical Education*, 50/3 (Mar. 1973), 195–9.

Leis, H. P., 'Endocrine prophylaxis of breast cancer with cyclic estrogen and progesterone', *International Surgery*, 45/5 (May 1966), 496–503.

Lewis, M. A., 'The epidemiology of oral contraceptive use: A critical review of the studies on oral contraceptives and the health of young women', *AJOG*, 179/4 (Oct. 1998), 1086–97.

Lilienfeld, A., 'Epidemiology of infectious and non-infectious disease: some comparisons', *American Journal of Epidemiology*, 97 (1973), 135–47.

Lincoln, R., 'The pill, breast and cervical cancer, and the role of progestogens in arterial disease', *Family Planning Perspectives*, 16/2 (Mar./Apr. 1984), 55–63.

Lipnick, R. J., 'Oral contraceptives and breast cancer: A prospective cohort study', *JAMA*, 255/1 (3 Jan. 1986), 58–61.

Lippincott, J. P. and Co., *New and Nonofficial Remedies* (Philadelphia, 1951).

Loudon, I., *Deaths in Childbirth: An International Study of Maternal Care and Maternal Mortality 1800–1950* (Oxford, 1992).

Loudon, I., 'Some international features of maternal mortality, 1880–1950', in V. Fildes, L. V. Marks and H. Marland, eds, *Women and Children First: International Maternal and Infant Welfare, 1870–1945* (London, 1992).

'Lower-dose pills', *Population Reports*, Series A, no. 7 (Nov. 1988), 1–31.

Luker, K., *Taking Chances: Abortion and the Decision Not to Contracept* (Berkeley, 1975).

McCann, C. R., *Birth Control Politics in the United States* (Ithaca, 1994).

McCrea, F. B., and Markle, G. E., 'The estrogen replacement controversy in the USA and UK: Different answers to the same question?', *Social Studies of Science*, 14 (1984), 1–26.

McFadyen, R., 'Thalidomide in America: A brush with tragedy', *Clio Medica*, 11/2 (1976), 79–93.

McLaren, A., *A History of Contraception: From Antiquity to the Present Day* (Oxford, 1994).

McLaughlin, L., *The Pill, John Rock, and the Catholic Church: The Biography of a Revolution* (Boston, 1982).

MacMahon, B., Cole P. and Brown, J., 'Etiology of human breast cancer: a review', *JNCI*, 50 (1973), 21–42.

McNeill, P. M., *The Ethics and Politics of Human Experimentation* (Cambridge, 1993).

Macnicol, J., 'Eugenics and the campaign for voluntary sterilization in Britain between the wars', *Social History of Medicine*, 2/2 (Aug. 1989), 147–70.

McPherson, K., 'Modelling latent effects in any association between oral contraceptives and breast cancer', in H. Morgenstern et al., eds, *Models of Non-Communicable Diseases: Health Status and Health Service Requirements* (Heidelberg, 1992), 74–5.

McPherson, K. and Owen J., letters to the editor, *British Medical Journal* (20 Sept. 1986), 710.

McPherson K. et al., 'Oral contraceptives and breast cancer', *Lancet*, 2 (1983), 1414–15.

McPherson K. et al., 'Early oral contraceptive use and breast cancer: Results of another case-control study', *British Journal of Cancer*, 56 (1987), 653.

Maeder, T., *Adverse Reactions* (New York, 1994).

Maisel, A. Q., *The Hormone Quest* (New York, 1965).

Makepeace, A. W., Weinstein, C. L. and Friedman, M. H., 'The effect of progestin and progesterone on ovulation in the rabbit', *American Journal of Physiology*, 119 (1937), 512–16.

Mann C. C. and Plummer, M. L., *The Aspirin Wars: Money, Medicine, and One Hundred Years of Rampant Competition* (New York, 1991).

Mann, R. D., 'Breast cancer risk and the administration of human hormones: Part 1. Hormone replacement therapy', *Adverse Drug Reaction Toxicology Review*, 11/3 (1992), 149–72.

Marks, H. M., 'Cortisone, 1949: A year in the political life of a drug', *Bulletin of the History of Medicine* 6/3 (1992), 419–40.

Marks, H. M., *The Progress of Experiment: Science and Therapeutic Reform in the United States, 1900–1990* (Cambridge, 1997).

Marks, L. V., 'Historical perspectives: The oral contraceptive pill and its controversies', *British Journal of Sexual Medicine*, 22/ 5 (Sept./Oct. 1995), 25–7.

Marks, L. V., 'Controversial contraception: The international history of the oral contraceptive pill', *Wellcome Trust Review*, 5 (1996), 51–3.

Marks, L. V. '"A 'cage' of ovulating females": The history of the early oral contraceptive pill clinical trials, 1950–59', in H. Kamminga and S. de Chadarevian, eds, *Molecularising Biology and Medicine, 1930s – 1970s* (Amsterdam, 1998), 221–47.

Marks, L. V., 'Human guinea pigs? The history of the early oral contraceptive clinical trials', *History and Technology*, 15 (1999), 1–26.

Marks, L. V., 'The migration of scientific knowledge in the making of the contraceptive pill', *Proceedings of the American Historical Association*, (1999), ref: 10485.

Marks, L. V., '"Not Just a Statistic": The history of USA and UK policy over thrombotic disease and the oral contraceptive pill, 1960s–1970s', *Social Science and Medicine*, 49 (1999), 1139–55.

Marks, L. V., 'Parenting the pill: The early testing of the contraceptive pill', in A. R. Saetnan, N. Oudshoorn and M. Kirejczyk, eds, *Localizing and Globalizing Technologies* (Ohio, 2000).

Marks, L. V., '"Andromeda freed from her chains": medical attitudes towards women and the pill, 1950–1970', in L. Conrad and A. Hardy, eds, *Women and Modern Medicine*, (Amsterdam, 2001).

Marks, L. V., '"Public-spirited and enterprising volunteers": The council for the investigation of fertility control and the British clinical trials of the oral contraceptive pill, 1959–1973', in M. Gijswijt-Hofstra and T. Tansey, eds, *Remedies and Healing Cultures in Britain and the Netherlands in the Twentieth Century*, (Amsterdam, 2001).

Martin, E., *The Woman in the Body: A Cultural Analysis of Reproduction* (Milton Keynes, 1987).

Martin, G., 'Phosphorylated hesperdin', *Science*, 117 (3 Apr. 1953), 363.

Maruyama, H., Raphael J. H., and Djerassi, C., 'Why Japan ought to legalize the pill', *Nature*, 379 (15 Feb. 1998), 579–80.

Mays, E. T. et al., 'Hepatic changes in young women ingesting contraceptive steroids. Hepatic hemorrhage and primary hepatic tumors', *JAMA*, 235 (1976), 730–2.

Medical Research Council, 'Risk of thromboembolic disease in women taking oral contraceptives', *BMJ*, 2 (6 May 1967), 355–9.

Meirik, O. et al., 'Oral contraceptive use and breast cancer in young women: A joint national case-control study in Sweden and Norway', *Lancet* (20 Sept. 1986), 650–3.

Melamed M. R. et al.,'Prevalence rates of uterine cervical carcinoma in situ for women using the diaphragm or contraceptive oral steroids', *BMJ*, 3 (1969), 195–200.

Meldrum, M., '"Simple Methods" and "Determined Contraceptors": The statistical evaluation of fertility control, 1957–1968', *Bulletin for the History of Medicine*, 70 (1996), 266–95.

'Microbes may replace yams for making the pill', *New Scientist* (5 Sept. 1974), 589.

Miller, D. R. et al., 'Breast cancer risk in relation to early oral contraceptive use', *Obstetrics and Gynecology*, 68/6 (Dec. 1986), 863–8.

Millman N. and Rosen, F., 'Failure of phosphorylated hesperidin to influence fertility in rodents', *Science*, 118 (21 Aug. 1953), 212–13.

Mintz, M., 'The pill, press and public at the experts' mercy', *Columbia Journalism Review* (Winter 1968–9), 4–10.

Moore, F. D., 'Ethical boundaries in initial clinical trials', in P. A. Freund, ed., *Experimentation with Human Subjects* (New York, 1970).

Morgenstern, H. et al., eds, *Models of Non-Communicable Diseases: Health Status and Health Service Requirements* (Heidelberg, 1992).

Moscucci, O., *The Science of Woman: Gynaecology and Gender in England, 1800–1929* (Cambridge, 1990).

Mosher, W., 'Fertility and family planning in the 1970s: The national survey of family growth', *Family Planning Perspectives*, 14/6 (1982), 314–20.

Mumford, S. D., 'The Vatican and world population policy: An interview with Milton

P. Siegel' on http://www.kzpg.com/Lib/Pages/Books/NSSM-200/29-APP3.html

Murphy, M., 'The contraceptive pill and women's employment as factors in fertility change in Britain 1963–1980: A challenge to the conventional view', *Population Studies*, 47 (1993), 221–43.

Murphy, M., 'Sterilisation as a method of contraception: Recent trends in Great Britain and their implications', *Journal of Biosocial Science*, 27 (1995), 31–46.

Murray C. J. L. and Lopez, A. D., eds, *Global Health Statistics*, Global Burden of Disease and Injury Series, vol. 2, Harvard School of Public Health on behalf of WHO and the World Bank (Boston, 1996).

Murty, J. and Firth, S., 'Contraceptive effectiveness may be being sacrificed for safety', letter, *BMJ*, 313 (1996), 363.

Nash, M., 'Pronatalism and motherhood in Franco's Spain', in G. Bock and P. Thane, eds, *Maternity and Gender Policies*, (London, 1991), 160–77.

National Science Foundation, *Technology in Retrospect and Critical Events in Science*, vol.1 (15 Dec. 1968) and vol. 2 (30 Jan. 1969).

Newhouse, M. L. et al., 'A case-control study of carcinoma of the ovary', *British Journal of Preventive Social Medicine*, 31 (1977), 148–53.

NHS Centre for Reviews and Dissemination, 'Preventing and reducing the adverse effects of unintended teenage pregnancies', *Effective Health Care*, 3/1 (Feb. 1997), 1–12.

'OCs – update on usage, safety, and side effects', *Population Reports*, Series A, no. 5 (Jan. 1979).

Offen, K., 'Body politics: women, work and the politics of motherhood in France, 1920–1950', in G. Bock and P. Thane, eds, *Maternity and Gender Policies* (London, 1991).

Office of Health Economics, *Family Planning in Britain* (London, 1972).

Ohlander, A. S., 'The invisible child? The struggle for a Social Democratic family policy in Sweden, 1900–1960s', in G. Bock and P. Thane, eds, *Maternity and Gender Policies* (London, 1991).

'Oral contraceptives', *Population Reports*, Series A, No. 2 (Mar. 1975).

'Oral contraceptives – 50 million users', *Population Reports*, Series A, no. 1 (Apr. 1974).

'Oral contraceptives in the 1980s', *Population Reports*, Series A, 10/3 (May–June 1982).

Ory, H. W., *Making Choices: Evaluating the Health Risks and Benefits of Birth Control Methods* (New York, 1983).

Oudshoorn, N., *Beyond the Natural Body: An Archaeology of Sex Hormones* (London, 1994).

Ovid, *Metamorphoses Book IV*, trans. R. Graves (Cambridge, Mass., 1985).

Paffenberger, R. S. et al., 'Cancer risk as related to use of oral contraceptives during fertile years', *Cancer*, 39 (1977), 1887–91.

Parkes, A. S., 'The Biology of Fertility', in Greep, R. O., ed., *Human Fertility and Population Problems* (New York, 1963).

Parkes, A. S., Dodds, E. S. and Noble, R. L., 'Interruption of early pregnancy by means of orally active oestrogens', *BMJ* (10 Sept. 1938), 557–8.

Parkin, D. M., Laara, E. and Muir, C. S., 'Estimates of worldwide frequency of sixteen major cancers in 1980', *International Journal of Cancer*, 41 (1988), 184–97.

Paul, C., Skegg, D. C., and Spears, G. F. C., 'Oral contraception and breast cancer in New Zealand', in R. D. Mann, ed., *Oral Contraceptives and Breast Cancer* (Carnforth, Lancs, 1990), 85–94.

Paul C. et al., 'The pill and breast cancer: why the uncertainty?', letter to editor, *BMJ*,

293/29 Nov. 1986, 1433.

Payer, L., *Medicine and Culture: Notions of Health and Sickness* (London, 1989).

Pedro, A. and Lehmann, P. A., 'Early history of steroid chemistry in Mexico: The story of three remarkable men', *Steroids*, 57 (Aug. 1992), 403–8.

Pedro, A. et. al., 'Russell E. Marker: Pioneer of the Mexican steroid industry', *Journal of Chemical Education*, 50/3, (3 Mar. 1973), 198.

Peel, J. and Potts, M., *Textbook of Contraceptive Practice* (Cambridge, 1969).

Perley, S., Fluss, S. S., Bankowski, Z. and Simon, F., 'The Nuremberg Code: An international overview', in G. J. Annas and M. A. Grodin, eds, *The Nazi Doctors and the Nuremberg Code: Human Rights in Human Experimentation* (Oxford, 1992).

'Permission denied', *Far Eastern Economic Review* (14 Apr. 1994), 38.

Perone, N., 'The history of steroidal contraceptive development: The progestins', *Perspectives in Biology and Medicine*, 36/3 (Spring 1993), 347–68.

Peterson, L., 'Contraceptive use in the United States: 1982–90'. *Advance Data* (Centers for Disease Control and Prevention), no. 260 (14 Feb. 1995), 1–16.

Peto, J., 'Oral contraceptives and breast cancer: Is the CASH study really negative?', *Lancet*, 1 (1989), 552.

Pfeffer, N., 'Lessons from history: The salutary tale of stilboestrol', in P. Alderson, ed., *Consent to Health Treatment and Research: Differing Perspectives*, Report of the Social Science Research Unit Consent Conference Series, no. 1 (Dec. 1992).

Pfeffer, N., *The Stork and the Syringe* (Cambridge, 1993).

Piccino L. J., and Mosher, W. D., 'Trends in contraceptive use in the United States: 1982–1995', *Family Planning Perspectives*, 30/1 (Jan./Feb. 1998), 4–10.

Pike, M. C. et al., 'Oral contraceptive use and early abortion as risk factors for breast cancer in young women', *British Journal of Cancer*, 43 (1981), 72–6.

Pike, M. C. et al., 'Breast cancer in young women and use of oral contraceptives; Possible modifying effect of formulation and age at use', *Lancet*, 2 (1983), 926–30.

'Pill pariah', *In These Times* (7 Aug. 1995), 10–11.

'Pill scares and public responsibility', *Lancet*, 347 (22 June 1996), 1707.

Pincus, G., 'Factors controlling the growth of rabbit blastocysts', *American Journal of Physiology*, 133 (1941), 412–13.

Pincus, G., 'The physiology of ovarian hormones', *The Hormones*, 2 (1950).

Pincus, G., 'Fertilization in mammals', *Scientific American*, 184/3 (1951).

Pincus, G. 'Progestational agents and the control of fertility,' *Vitamins and Hormones*, 169 (1959), 81.

Pincus, G., *The Control of Fertility* (New York, 1965).

Pincus, G., 'Control of contraception by hormonal steroids', *Science*, 153 (19 July 1966), 493–500.

Pincus, G. and Garcia, C. R., 'Studies in vaginal, cervical and uterine histology', *Metabolism*, 3 (1965), 344–7.

Pincus, G. and Kirsch, R. E., 'The sterility in rabbits produced by injections of oestrone and related compounds', *Journal of Experimental Physiology*, 115 (1936), 219–28.

Pincus G. and Werthenssen, N. T., 'The comparative behaviour of mammalian eggs *in vivo* and *in vitro*. III. Factors controlling the growth of the rabbit blastocyst', *Journal of Experimental Zoology*, 78 (1938), 1–18.

Pincus G. and Werthenssen, N. T., 'An analysis of the mechanism of oestrogenic activity', *Proceedings of the Royal Society*, 126 (1939), 506.

Pincus, G., Rock, R. and Garcia, C. R., 'Field trials with norethynodrel as an oral contraceptive', *Report of the Proceedings of the Sixth International Conference on Planned*

Parenthood, 14–21 Feb. 1959, New Dehli, India.

Pincus, G. et al., 'Fertility control with oral medication', *AJOG*, 75 (June 1958), 1333–46.

Piotrow, P., *World Population Crisis: The United States Response* (New York, 1973).

Piper J. M. and Kennedy, D. L., 'Oral contraceptives in the United States: Trends in content and potency', *International Journal of Epidemiology*, 16/2 (1987), 215–21.

Pollock, S., 'Refusing to take women seriously: Side effects and the politics of contraception', in R. Arditti et al., eds, *Test-Tube Women: What Future for Motherhood?* (London, 1984), 148–51.

Pope Paul VI, *Humanae Vitae*, Encyclical of Pope Paul VI on the Regulation of Birth, 25 July 1968, CM 66 (Sept. 1968).

Potts, M., 'Birth Control Methods in the United States', *Family Planning Perspectives*, 20/6 (Nov./Dec. 1988), 268–97.

Pratt W. F. and Bachrach, C. A., 'What do women use when they stop using the pill?', *Family Planning Perspectives*, 19/6 (1987), 257–66.

Prentice, R. L. and Thomas, D. B., 'On the epidemiology of oral contraceptives and disease', *Advances in Cancer Research*, 19 (1987), 342–59.

President's Advisory Committee, *The Human Radiation Experiments: Final Report of the President's Advisory Committee* (New York, 1996).

Proctor, R., *Racial Hygiene: Medicine under the Nazis* (Cambridge, Mass., 1989).

Ramcharan, S., ed., *The Walnut Creek Contraceptive Drug Study: A Prospective Study of the Side-Effects of Oral Contraceptives*, Vol. 1 (Washington DC, 1974).

Ramirez de Arellano, A. B. and Seipp, C., *Colonialism, Catholicism and Contraception: A History of Birth Control in Puerto Rico* (London, 1983).

Ravenholt, R. T., 'The A.I.D. population and family planning program – goals, scope and progress', *Demography*, 5/2 (1968).

Ray, J., and Gosling, F. G., 'American physicians and birth control, 1936–47', *Journal of Social History*, 18 (1985), 399–411.

Reed, J., *The Birth Control Movement and American Society: From Private Vice to Public Virtue* (Princeton, 1984).

Report of the Committee of Enquiry into the Relationship of the Pharmaceutical Industry with the National Health Service, 1965–7, Cmnd. 3410 (London, 1967).

Rice-Wray, E., Becerra, C., Esquivel J. and Maqueo, M., 'Clinical trials of a combination of lynestrenol and menstranol (lyndiol) as an oral contraceptive agent', *Canadian Medical Association Journal*, 9 (12 Nov. 1966), 1024–30.

Richart, R. M., 'Cervical cancer in developing countries', in *Special Challenges in Third World Women's Health*, presentations at the 1989 annual meeting of the American Public Health Association, published at http://www.iwhc.org/sc_cc.html.

Ridker, P. M., Miletich, J. P., Hennekens, C. H., and Buring, J. E., 'Ethnic distribution of factor V Leiden in 4047 men and women: Implications for venous thromboembolism screening.' *Journal of the American Medical Association*, 277/16 (23–30 Apr. 1997), 1305–7.

Roberts, D., 'Black women and the pill', *Family Planning Perspectives*, 32/2 (Mar./Apr. 2000), 92–3.

Rock, J., 'Medical and biological aspects of contraception', *Clinics*, 1 (Apr. 1943), 1601–2.

Rock, J., 'We can end the battle over birth control', *Good Housekeeping*, July 1961.

Rock, J., 'It is time to end the birth control fight', *Saturday Evening Post*, 20 Apr. 1963, 10, 14.

Rock, J., *The Time Has Come: A Catholic Doctor's Proposals to End the Battle over Birth Control* (New York, 1963).

Rock, J., 'Keynote address to Symposium on Progestogen-Estrogen Compounds', *Applied Therapeutics*, 6/5 (May 1964), 406–9.

Rock, J., 'Science and charity to the rescue of humanity', *Pacific Medicine and Surgery (Ortho-Symposium)*, 73 (Feb. 1965), 1-A-25-27.

Rosenberg, L. et al., 'Breast cancer and oral contraceptive use', *American Journal of Epidemiology*, 119 (1984), 167.

Rosenkrantz, G., 'From Ruzicka's terpenes in Zurich to Mexican steroids via Cuba', *Steroids*, 57 (Aug. 1992), 409–18.

Royal College of General Practitioners, *Oral Contraceptives and Health: An Interim Report from the Oral Contraception Study of the Royal College of General Practitioners* (Oxford, 1974).

Rupke, R., ed., *Vivisection in Historical Perspective* (London, 1987).

Russel-Briefel, R., Ezzarati T. and Pelman, J., 'Prevalence and trends in oral contraceptive use in pre-menopausal females, ages 12–54, United States, 1971–1980', *American Journal of Public Health*, 75 (1985), 1173–6.

Salas, R. M., *International Population Assistance: The First Decade* (New York, 1979).

Sanger, M., *The New Motherhood* (London, 1922).

Sanger, M., *The Pivot of Civilization* (New York, 1922).

Sanyal, S. N., 'Functional uterine bleeding', *Journal of Medicine and International Medical Abstract Review*, 24/5 (1960), 5–11.

Sanyal, S. N., 'Ten years of research on an oral contraceptive from *Pisum Sativum Linn*', *Science and Culture*, 25 (June 1960), 661–5.

Sanyal, S. N. and Ghosh, S., 'Further clinical results with metaxylohydroquinone as an oral contraceptive', *International Medical Abstracts and Reviews*, 18/5 (Nov. 1955), 101–4.

Sartwell, P. E., Arthes, F. G. and Tonascia, J. A., 'Epidemiology of benign breast lesions; Lack of association with oral contraceptive use', *New England Journal of Medicine*, 288 (1973), 551.

Sax, K., 'The world's exploding population', *Perspectives in Biology and Medicine*, 7 (1963), 326–7.

Sayer, S. L. and Bausch, J. J. *Towards Safe, Convenient and Effective Contraceptives: A Policy Perspective*, Population Council (New York, 1978).

Schlesselman, J. J., et al., 'Breast cancer in relation to early use of oral contraceptives: No evidence of a latent effect', *JAMA*, 259/12 (25 Mar. 1988), 1828–33.

Schlesselman, J. J., 'Oral contraceptives and breast cancer', *AJOG*, 163/4, part 2 (Oct. 1990), 1379–87.

Schlesselman, J. J. et al., 'Breast cancer in relation to type of estrogen contained in oral contraceptives', *Contraception*, 36 (1987), 595.

Schrecker, E., *The Age of McCarthyism: A Brief History with Documents* (Boston, 1994).

Schwarz, R., 'FDA panel recommends limiting estrogen dose in contraceptives', *Medical World News* (14 Mar. 1988), 13.

Scrimshaw, S. M., 'Women and the pill: From panacea to catalyst', *Family Planning Perspectives*, 13/6 (Nov./Dec. 1981), 254–62.

Seaman, B., *The Doctors' Case against the Pill* (Alameda, Calif., 1995).

Seaman, B. and Seaman, G., *Women and the Crisis in Sex Hormones* (New York, 1977).

G. D. Searle and Co. *Proceedings of a Conference: Thromboembolic Phenomena in Women* (Chicago, 1962).

Second Reading of Colonial Development and Welfare Bill, *Parliamentary Debates*, House of Commons, 2 Feb. 1955.

Seigel, D. and Corfman, P., 'Epidemiological problems associated with studies of the safety of oral contraceptives', *JAMA*, 203/11 (11 Mar. 1963), 950–4.

Sen, A., 'Population: delusion and reality', *New York Review of Books*, 22 Sept. 1992, 1–7.

Sen, A., 'Population and reasoned agency: Food, fertility, and economic development', in K. Lindahl-Kiessling and H. Landberg, eds, *Population, Economic Development and the Environment* (Oxford, 1994), 52–5.

Shaw, R. W., 'Adverse long-term effects of oral contraceptives: A review', *British Journal of Obstetrics and Gynaecology*, 94 (Aug. 1987), 724–30.

Shen, L. and Dahlback, B., 'Factor V and protein S as synergistic cofactors to activated protein C in degradation of factor VIIIa', *Journal of Biological Chemistry*, 269/29 (22 July 1994), 18735–8.

Sherris, J. D., 'Cervical cancer prevention: A strategic opportunity to improve women's reproductive health', *Family Planning Perspectives*, 25 (Jan. 1999), supplement.

Sieve, B. F., 'A new antifertility factor (a preliminary report)', *Science* (10 Oct. 1952), 373–85.

Silverman J. and Jones, E. F., 'The delivery of family planning and health services in Great Britain', *Family Planning Perspectives*, 20/2 (Mar./Apr. 1988), 68–79.

Simmer, H. H., 'On the history of hormonal contraception I. Ludwig Haberlandt (1885–1932) and his concept of hormonal sterilization', *Contraception*, 1/1 (Jan. 1970), 3–27.

Simmer, H. H., 'On the history of hormonal contraception II. Otfried Otto Fellner (1873–n.d.) and estrogens as antifertility hormones', *Contraception*, 3/1 (Jan. 1971), 1–21.

Singh S. and Darroch, J. E., 'Trends in sexual activity among adolescent American women: 1982–1995', *Family Planning Perspectives*, 31/5 (Sept./Oct. 1999), 212–19.

Sjöström, H. and Nilsson, R., *Thalidomide and the Power of the Drug Companies* (Harmondsworth, 1972).

Skegg, D. C. G., 'Risks and benefits of oral contraceptives: Will breast cancer tip the balance?', in Institute of Medicine, *Oral Contraceptives and Breast Cancer* (Washington, 1991).

Skouby, S. O., 'Oral contraceptives and venous thrombosis: End of the debate?' *European Journal of Contraception and Reproductive Health Care*, 3/2 (June 1998), 59–64.

Sneader, W., *Drug Discovery: The Evolution of Modern Medicines* (Chichester, N.Y., 1985).

Sneader, W., *Drug Prototypes and their Exploitation*, (Chichester, N.Y., 1996).

Snider, S., 'The pill: 30 years of safety concerns', *FDA Consumer*, 24/10 (1990), 8–11.

Soloway, R. A., *Demography and Degeneration: Eugenics and the Declining Birthrate in Twentieth Century Britain* (Chapel Hill, N.C., new edn. 1995).

Spencer, S. M., 'The birth control revolution', *Saturday Evening Post*, 15 Jan. 1966, 21–5, 66–70.

Spitzer, W. O., 'The 1995 pill scare revisited: Anatomy of a non-epidemic', *Human Reproduction* 12/11 (Nov. 1997), 2347–57.

Spitzer, W. O. et al., 'Third generation oral contraceptives and risks of venous thromboembolic disorders: an international case-control study', *BMJ*, 312 (13 Jan. 1996), 83–8.

Stadel, B. V. et al., 'Oral contraceptives and breast cancer in young women', *Lancet* (2 Nov. 1985), 970–3.

Stanford, J. L., 'Oral contraceptives and neoplasia of the ovary', *Contraception*, 43/6 (1991), 543–56.

Stepan J. and Kellogg, E. H., *The World's Laws on Contraceptives*, Law and Population Monograph Series, no. 17 (Medford, Mass., 1974).

Stepan, N., *The Hour of Eugenics: Race, Gender and Nation in Latin America* (Ithaca, 1991).

Stockley, I. 'Drugs in use: Interactions with oral contraceptives', *Pharmaceutical Journal*, I (1976), 140–3.

Stolley, P. D., Schapiro, S., Sloane, D. and Schinnar, R., 'Cardiovascular effects of oral contraceptives', *Southern Medical Journal*, 71/7 (July 1978), 821–4.

Stone, A., 'The teaching of contraception in medical schools', *Human Fertility*, 7 (Aug. 1942), 108.

Stopes, M., *Enduring Passion* (London, 1928).

Stourton, E., *Absolute Truth: The Catholic Church in the World Today* (London, 1999).

Sturtevant, F. M., 'Breast cancer and oral contraceptives: Critique of the proposition that high potency progestogen products cover excess risk', *Biomedicine and Pharmacotherapy*, 38 (1984), 371–9.

Suissa, S. et al., 'First-time use of newer oral contraceptives and the risk of venous thromboembolism', *Contraception*, 56/3 (Sept. 1997) 114–6.

Surface, B., 'Controversy over "the pill"', *Good Housekeeping*, Jan. 1970, 64–5, 123–7.

Susser, M., 'Epidemiology in the United States after World War II: Evolution of technique', *Epidemiologic Reviews* 7 (1985), 147–77.

Syntex Corporation, *A Corporation and a Molecule: The Story of Research at Syntex* (Palo Alto, 1966).

Szarewski, A., 'New evidence of risk of VTE and combined oral contraceptives', *Clinical Pulse* (2 Sept. 2000), 53, 57, 61.

Szpilfogel, S. A. and Zeelen, F. J., 'Steroid research at Organon in the golden 1950s and the following years', *Steroids*, 61 (1996), 483–91.

Szreter, S., 'The ideas of demographic transition and the study of fertility change: A critical intellectual history', *Population and Development Review*, 19/4 (Dec. 1993), 659–701.

Taylor, T. 'Opening statement of the prosecution December 9, 1946', in G. J. Annas and M. A. Grodin, eds, *The Nazi Doctors and the Nuremberg Code: Human Rights in Human Experimentation* (Oxford, 1992).

Temin, P., *Taking your Medicine: Drug Regulation in the United States* (Cambridge, Mass., 1980).

Thomas, D. B., 'Do hormones cause breast cancer?', *Cancer*, 53 (1 Feb. 1984), supplement, 595–601.

Thomas, J. D. and Williams, S., 'Women and abortion in 1930s Britain: A survey and its data', *Social History of Medicine*, 11/2 (1988), 283–310.

Thorogood, M. and Vessey, M. P., 'Trends in use of oral contraceptives in Britain', *British Journal of Family Planning*, 16 (1990), 41–53.

Thorogood, M. and Villard-Mackintosh, L., 'Combined oral contraceptives: Risks and benefits', *British Medical Bulletin*, 49/1 (1993), 124–39.

Tone, A., 'Contraceptive consumers: Gender and the political economy of birth control in the 1930s', *Journal of Social History*, 29/3 (1996), 485–506.

Torres, A. and Jones, E. F., 'The delivery of family planning services in the Netherlands', *Family Planning Perspectives*, 20/2 (Mar./Apr. 1988), 75–9.

Tullner, W. M., and Hertz, R., 'High progestational activity of 19-norprogesterone', *Endocrinology*, 52 (1953), 359–60.

Tullner, W. M. and Hertz, R., 'Progestational activity of 19-norprogesterone and

19-norethisterone in the rhesus monkey', *Proceedings of the Society of Experimental Biology and Medicine*, 94 (1957), 298–300.

Turney, J., *Frankenstein's Footsteps: Science, Genetics and Popular Culture* (New Haven, 1998).

Tyler, E. T., 'Eight years' experience with oral contraceptives and an analysis of use of low-dosage norethisterone', *BMJ* (3 Oct. 1964), 843–7.

Tyler, E. T., 'Oral contraceptives', *JAMA*, 175 (1961), 225.

Tyler May, E., *Homeward Bound: American Families in the Cold War Era* (New York, 1988).

Tyrer, L. B. and Salas, J. E., 'Contraceptive problems unique to the United States', *Clinical Obstetrics and Gynaecology*, 32/2 (June 1989), 307–15.

Ubell, E., 'Birth-control pill found effective', *New York Herald Tribune*, 28 May 1958.

UK National Case-Control Study Group, 'Oral contraceptive use and breast cancer risk in young women', *Lancet*, 1 (1989), 973–82.

UN, *Levels and Trends of Contraceptive Use as Assessed in 1994* (New York, 1996).

UN, *Recent Levels and Trends of Contraceptive Use as Assessed in 1983* (New York, 1984).

Usbourne, C., *The Politics of the Body in Weimar Germany* (London, 1992).

Van de Kaa, D. J., 'Population prospects and population policy in the Netherlands', *Netherlands Journal of Sociology*, 17 (1981), 73–91.

Vaughan, P., *The Pill on Trial* (Harmondsworth, 1972).

Vaughan, P., 'The pill turns twenty', *New York Times Magazine*, 13 June 1976.

Vessey, M. P., 'Female hormones and vascular disease – an epidemiological overview', *British Journal of Family Planning, Supplement*, 6/1 (Oct. 1980), 1–12.

Vessey, M. P., 'Oral contraceptives and breast cancer', *IPPF Medical Bulletin*, 21/6 (Dec. 1987), 1–2.

Vessey, M. P., 'Epidemiologic studies of oral contraception', *International Journal of Fertility, Supplement*, 34 (1989), 64–70.

Vessey, M. P. and Doll, R., 'Investigation of relations between use of oral contraceptives and thromboembolic disease: A further report', *BMJ*, 2 (14 June 1969), 651–7.

Vessey, M. P. and Doll, R., 'Evaluation of existing techniques: Is "the pill" safe enough to continue using?', *Proceedings of the Royal Society of London*, 195 (1976), 69–80.

Vessey, M. P. and Inman, W. H. W., 'Speculations about mortality trends from venous thromboembolic disease in England and Wales and their relation to the pattern of oral contraceptive usage', *Journal of Obstetrics and Gynaecology of the British Commonwealth*, 80 (June 1973), 562–6.

Vessey, M. P. and Mann, J. I., 'Female sex hormones and thrombosis: Epidemiological aspects', *British Medical Bulletin*, 34/2 (1978), 157–62.

Vessey, M. P., Doll R., and Sutton, P. M., 'Investigations of the possible relationship between oral contraceptives and benign and malignant breast disease', *Cancer*, 28 (1971), 1395.

Vessey, M. P., Doll, R. and Sutton, P. M., 'Oral contraceptives and breast neoplasia: A retrospective study', *BMJ*, 3 (1972), 719–34.

Vessey, M. P., Doll, R., Fairbairn A. S. and Glober, G., 'Postoperative Thromboembolism and the Use of Oral Contraceptives', *BMJ*, 3 (1970), 123–6.

Vessey, M. P., Villard-Mackintosh, L., McPherson, K. and Yeates, D., 'Mortality among contraceptive users: 20 year follow-up of women in a cohort study', *BMJ*, 299 (16 Dec. 1989), 1487–91.

Vessey, M. P. et al., 'A long term follow-up study of women using different methods of contraception: an interim report', *Journal of Biosocial Science*, 8 (1976), 373.

Vessey, M. P. et al., 'Oral contraceptive use and abortion before first term pregnancy in relation to breast cancer risk', *British Journal of Cancer*, 45 (1982), 327–31.

Vessey, M. P. et al., 'Oral contraceptives and breast cancer: Latest findings in a large cohort study', *British Journal of Cancer*, 59 (1989), 613–17.

Villar Borja, A., 'Productos Quimicos Vegetales Mexicanos, S.A. De C.V. (Proquivemex)', in X. Lozoya, *Estado Actual Del Conocimeiento en Plantas Medicanas* (Mexico City, 1976).

Vogt, W., *The Road to Survival* (New York, 1948).

Wall, M. E. et al., 'Steroidal Sapogenins. VII. Survey of plants for steroidal sapogenins and other constituents', *Journal of the American Pharmaceutical Association: Scientific Edition*, 43/1 (Jan. 1954), 1–7.

Watkins, E., *On the Pill: A Social History of Oral Contraceptives, 1950–1970* (Baltimore, 1998).

Wellings, K., 'Help or hype: an analysis of media coverage of the 1983 "pill scare"', *British Journal of Family Planning*, 11 (1985), 92–8.

Wellings, K., 'Trends in contraceptive method usage since 1970', *British Journal of Family Planning*, 12 (1986), 57–64.

Westoff, L. A. and. Westoff, C. F., *From Now to Zero: Fertility, Contraception and Abortion in America* (Boston, 1971).

'What do consultants think of the pill?', *World Medicine* (27 Feb. 1968), 82–3.

WHO, *Technology of Reproduction Series. World Health Organization* (1966), no. 326.

WHO (collaborative study of neoplasia and steroid contraceptives), 'Epithelial ovarian cancer and combined oral contraceptives', *International Journal of Epidemiology*, 18 (1989), 538–45.

WHO, 'WHO publishes research findings on oral contraceptives and risk of venous thromboembolism', press release, WHO/92, 15 Dec. 1995.

WHO (collaborative study of cardiovascular disease and steroid hormone contraception), 'Effect of different progestogens in low oestrogen oral contraceptives on venous thromboembolic disease', *Lancet*, 364 (1995): 1582–8.

WHO, 'The dimensions of reproductive ill-health. 1990–1995', Geneva, 1995.

WHO, 'Fifty facts from The World Health Report 1998: Global health situation and trends 1955–2025', Geneva, 1998.

Williams, D. and Williams, G., *Every Child a Wanted Child: Clarence James Gamble, M.D., and his Work in the Birth Control Movement*, ed. E. P. Flint (Boston, 1978).

Williams, D. et al., 'Effect of the British warning on contraceptive use in the General Medical Service in Ireland', *Irish Medical Journal*, 91/6 (Dec. 1999).

Williams-Deane, M. and Potter, L. S., 'Current oral contraceptive use instructions: An analysis of patient package inserts', *Family Planning Perspectives*, 24/3 (May/June 1992), 111–15.

Wilmsen, E., *Journeys with Flies* (Chicago, 1999).

Wingo, P. A. et al., 'Age specific differences in the relationship between oral contraceptive use and breast cancer', *Obstetrics and Gynaecology*, 78/2 (1991) 161–70.

Wiseman, A., 'Oral contraceptives in family planning', *Journal of the College of General Practice of Canada* (June 1966), 18–21.

Wiseman, A., 'Should you tell your daughter?', *Evening Standard*, 4 Nov. 1966.

Wiseman, A., 'Six years' experience of oral contraception in a family planning clinic', *Clinical Trials Journal*, 5 (Jan. 1968), 117–24.

'Women as guinea pigs, the continuing saga', *Critical List* (Summer 1977), 25–6.

Wood, C., *Birth Control Now and Tomorrow* (Gateshead, 1969).

Woolf, M., *Family Intentions* (London, 1971).

Wynn, V. and Doar, J. W. H., 'Some effects of oral contraceptives on carbohydrate metabolism', *Lancet*, 2 (1 Oct. 1966), 715–23.

Yuncker, B., 'Researcher predicts ban on the pill', *New York Post*, 22 Dec. 1969, 3.

Yuncker, B., 'A reporter finds a cause', *New York Post*, 24 Jan. 1970, 21.

Zaffaroni, A., 'From Paper Chromatography to Drug Discovery', *Steroids*, 57 (Dec. 1992), 642–8.

Zaremba, M., 'A victim of the record-years', *Dagens Nyheter*, trans. S. Croall (27 Sept. 1997).

Index